Proceedings of the
Third International Symposium of the Canadian Society for Immunology;
Toronto, October 3–5, 1968

Cellular and Humoral Mechanisms in Anaphylaxis and Allergy

Edited by:

HENRY Z. MOVAT, M.D., Ph.D., F.R.C.P. (C)
Division of Experimental Pathology
Department of Pathology
University of Toronto
Toronto, Ont., Canada

With 51 figures and 30 tables

19   69

BASEL (Switzerland)   S. KARGER   NEW YORK

The Symposium was organized with the financial support of:

the Medical Research Council of Canada
the Ontario Heart Foundation
the Canadian Arthritis and Rheumatism Society
the School of Graduate Studies and
the Division of Post-Graduate Medical Education University of Toronto

S. Karger AG, Arnold-Böcklin-Strasse 25, 4000 Basel 11 (Switzerland)

Table of Contents

Editorial Foreword

The International Symposia of the Canadian Society for Immunology were initiated in order to further Immunology in Canada.

The aim of the third symposium was to have presentations and discussions on the cellular and humoral mediators of anaphylaxis and allergy, encompassing the chemical mediators of acute inflammation. The first day dealt with the antibodies inducing anaphylaxis and allergy. Then four half-day sessions were devoted to the chemical mediators. These dealt first with mediators released from cells, particularly vasoactive amines, but also more recently recognized substances, derived from PMN-leukocytes and platelets. Humoral mediators generated in plasma, i.e. kinins and anaphylatoxin, were covered on the last day. Whenever timely and appropriate a general review preceded the session.

The success of the symposium was perhaps attributable first of all to the multidisciplinary nature of the subject that was chosen. Participants, invited discussants and members of the audience ranged from immunochemists to pharmacologists, pathologists, biochemists, parasitologists and clinicians. Immunology seems to have made enormous strides in recent years because it cuts across and encompasses so many disciplines of biology and medicine.

The technical success of our symposium was attributable to the invaluable contribution and help of many friends and colleagues. Former symposia, as well as the present one, were initiated by Dr. BERNHARD CINADER, president of the Canadian Society for Immunology. The preliminary program was laid down at a 'breakfast session' in Atlantic City, in which Drs. FRANK AUSTEN, ELMER BECKER, IRVIN BRODER, ERVIN ERDÖS, ABE OSLER and myself participated. I wish to thank these for their valuable suggestions. Thanks are due to my colleagues, Drs. NORTON TAICHMAN, YUKO TAKEUCHI and KEIJI UDAKA who helped in various phases of the organization. I wish to express my particular gratitude to my secretary, Miss MARICA MICHAEL, for performing inumerable organizational tasks, Miss RUTH SAISON for organizing the registration and our administrative assistant, Mr. RICHARD AUSTIN, for acting as treasurer and general manager of the symposium.

HENRY Z. MOVAT
Toronto, November, 1968

Participants

K. Frank Austen
Associate Professor of Medicine
Harvard Medical School
Physician-in-Chief
Robert B. Brigham Hospital
Boston, Mass. (USA)

Elmer L. Becker
(Chairman, Cellular events in anaphylaxis
and Slow reacting substance)
Chief, Division of Immunochemistry
Walter Reed Institute of Research
Walter Reed Army Medical Center
Washington, D.C. (USA)

A. M. J. N. Blair
Chief Pharmacologist
Fisons Pharmaceuticals Research Labs.
Bakewell Road, Loughborough
Leics. (England)

Kurt J. Bloch
Assistant Physician and
Assistant Professor of Medicine
Massachusetts General Hospital
Harvard Medical School
Boston, Mass. (USA)

Irvin Broder
Assistant Professor of Medicine,
Pathology and Pharmacology
University of Toronto
The Toronto Western Hospital
Toronto, Ont. (Canada)

Ervin G. Erdös
(Chairman, The kinin system)
Professor of Pharmacology
Department of Pharmacology
The University of Oklahoma
Medical Center
Oklahoma City, Okla. (USA)

H. Giertz
Professor of Pharmacology
Pharmakologisches Institut der
Universität Freiburg
Freiburg i. Br. (Germany)

Lawrence Goodfriend
Associate Professor
McGill University
Division of Immunochemistry and Allergy
Royal Victoria Hospital
Montreal, P.Q. (Canada)

Bernard Halpern
(Chairman, The antibody in anaphylaxis)
Professor of Experimental Medicine
College de France
Institut d'Immuno-Biologie
Hôpital Broussais
Paris (France)

Peter M. Henson
Post-doctoral Fellow
Department of Experimental Pathology
Scripps Clinic and Research Foundation
La Jolla, Cal. (USA)

KIMISHIGE ISHIZAKA
Professor of Microbiology
University of Colorado
Children's Asthma Research
Institute and Hospital
Denver, Colo. (USA)

JOERG A. JENSEN
Professor of Microbiology
Department of Microbiology
School of Medicine
University of Miami
Coral Gables, Fla. (USA)

ALICE R. JOHNSON
Instructor
Department of Pharmacology
Division of Basic Health Sciences
Woodruff Medical Center
of Emory University
Atlanta, Ga. (USA)

ELVIN A. KABAT
(Chairman, The antibody in anaphylaxis)
Professor of Microbiology
Department of Microbiology
College of Physicians and Surgeons
of Columbia University
New York, N.Y. (USA)

IRWIN H. LEPOW
Professor and Head
Department of Pathology
The University of Connecticut
School of Medicine
Hartford, Conn. (USA)

LAWRENCE M. LICHTENSTEIN
Assistant Professor of Medicine
and Microbiology
Department of Medicine
Division of Allergy and Infectious Diseases
The John Hopkin's University
School of Medicine
Baltimore, Md. (USA)

KENNETH L. MELMON
Chief, Division of Clinical Pharmacology
Department of Medicine
University of California
San Francisco Medical Center
San Francisco, Cal. (USA)

IVAN MOTA
Professor of Histology
Department of Histology
University of Sao Paulo
Sao Paulo (Brazil)

HENRY Z. MOVAT
Professor and Chairman
Division of Experimental Pathology
Department of Pathology
University of Toronto
Toronto, Ont. (Canada)

J. FRASER MUSTARD
Professor and Chairman
Department of Pathology
Faculty of Medicine
McMaster University
Hamilton, Ont. (Canada)

BRIDGET M. OGILVIE
National Institute for Medical Research
Medical Research Council
Mill Hill,
London (England)

ABRAHAM G. OSLER
(Chairman, Anaphylatoxin and
biologically active fragments of
complement)
Member, Public Health Research
Institute of the City of New York
Professor, Department of Microbiology
New York University School of Medicine
New York, N.Y. (USA)

KAREL W. PONDMAN
Chief, Department of Immunochemistry
Central Laboratorium van de
Bloedtransfusiedienst
van Het Nederlandsche Roode Kruis
Amsterdam (The Netherlands)

JOHN J. ROCKEY
Assistant Professor of Microbiology
Department of Microbiology
University of Pennsylvania
The School of Medicine
Philadelphia, Pa. (USA)

GILL STREJAN
Assistant Professor
Department of Bacteriology and
Immunology
University of Western Ontario
London, Ont. (Canada)

W. VOGT
Professor of Pharmacology
Abteilung Biochemische Pharmakologie
Max-Planck-Institut für
Experimentelle Medizin
Göttingen (Germany)

PETER A. WARD
Chief, Immunology Branch
Armed Forces Institute of Pathology
Washington, D.C. (USA)

MARION E. WEBSTER
Biochemist
Experimental Therapeutics Branch
National Heart Institute
Bethesda, Md. (USA)

Cellular and Humoral Mechanisms in Anaphylaxis and Allergy, pp. 1–12
(Karger, Basel/New York 1969)

The Antibody in Anaphylaxis

KURT J. BLOCH[1]

Department of Medicine Harvard Medical School, and the Arthritis Unit of the Medical
Services, Massachusetts General Hospital
Boston, Mass.

Concepts of the biologic functions of antibodies have evolved through
several stages. Initially, the pluralistic view held that each of the diverse
activities displayed by an antiserum could be attributed to a different molecular form named agglutinin, precipitin, opsonin, skin-sensitizing or protective antibody. This view was subsequently replaced by a unitarian
hypothesis which held that a given population of antibodies could, on
combining with antigen, produce any of the diverse consequences of antigen-
antibody interaction depending on circumstances, i.e., precipitation, if the
antigen was soluble and multivalent; agglutination, if the antigen was part
of the surface of a particulate carrier; protection against infection, if the
antigen was part of the cell wall of a bacteria. The modern concept of antibody activity is a synthesis of both views; accordingly an antibody molecule
is competent to elicit some, but not necessarily all of the various reactions
cited [15]. Reassessment of the biologic function of antibodies has been
especially helpful in understanding the various anaphylactic syndromes of
mammals.

Homocytotropic Antibodies of the Guinea Pig

The modern concept of the biologic functions of antibodies is based in
considerable part on studies of guinea pig antibodies initiated by OVARY,
BENACERRAF and their associates [4, 7, 36] and WHITE, JENKINS and WILKIN-

[1] Publication No. 471 of the Robert W. Lovett Memorial Group for the Study of
Diseases Causing Deformities, Harvard Medical School at the Massachusetts General
Hospital.

Preparation of this report was supported by Grant AM-5067 from the National
Institute of Arthritis and Metabolic Diseases, U.S.P.H.S.

SON [52]. These investigators observed that guinea pigs injected with various protein antigens or hapten-protein conjugates emulsified in complete Freund's adjuvant produced two populations of precipitating antibodies directed against the same antigenic determinant, but differing in their electrophoretic mobility on agar gel or starch block electrophoresis. The rapidly migrating antibody population was identified as $\gamma1$, the more slowly migrating antibody population as $\gamma2$. Both were found to have sedimentation coefficients of approximately 7S [4]. Guinea pig gamma −1, but not gamma −2 antibodies, were found to sensitize guinea pigs for passive cutaneous (PCA) and systemic anaphylaxis [36], and to sensitize washed guinea pig lung slices for antigen-induced release of histamine *in vitro* [1]. Gamma −2 antibodies were able to specifically block PCA reactions provoked by $\gamma1$ antibodies, presumably by competing for antigen [36].

Guinea pig $\gamma2$, but not $\gamma1$, antibodies were able to fix complement in the presence of antigen and sensitized antigen-coated erythrocytes for lysis by complement [7]. In the reverse passive Arthus reaction, guinea pig $\gamma2$ antibodies were considerably more efficient in provoking hemorrhagic lesions than were equal amounts of $\gamma1$ antibodies which primarily provoked edema.

Guinea pig 7S$\gamma1$ and $\gamma2$ immunoglobulins were shown to have identical Fab [50] and Fd fragments [32], but to differ in antigenic properties of their Fc fragments. It was suggested that $\gamma1$ antibodies possessed a site or configuration on the Fc portion of the molecule which allowed for interaction with guinea pig mast cells, so that subsequent union with antigen led to degranulation and histamine release. To date this postulated interaction is based on indirect evidence: (a) guinea pig mesentery sensitized with $\gamma1$ antibody showed disappearance of mast cells following contact with antigen; (b) histamine was the chief pharmacologic agent released from guinea pig lung slices sensitized with $\gamma1$ antibody and exposed to specific antigen [1]; and, (c) antihistamines blocked PCA reactions mediated by $\gamma1$ antibodies [23, 30].

It was similarly suggested that guinea pig $\gamma2$ antibodies lack the site for attachment to mast cells, but possess instead, a site or configuration which permits the attachment of complement components under appropriate conditions. The mechanism of tissue injury provoked by precipitating, complement-fixing guinea pig $\gamma2$ antibodies may be assumed to resemble that by which rabbit antibodies provoke Arthus reactions. Thus, antigen and guinea pig 7S$\gamma2$ antibodies interact and precipitate in, and about, the walls of small blood vessels; complement is fixed, leading to the formation of the C′5–6–7 leukotactic complex. Polymorphonuclear leukocytes accumulate at the site and in the process of phagocytosis release proteolytic

Table I. Characteristics of the homocytotropic antibodies of mammals

Homocytotropic antibody of the	Guinea pig	Mouse		Rat	Rabbit	Dog	Man
	Type I	Type I	Type II	Type II	Type II	Type II	Type II
Reactions mediated in species of origin	PCA; SA; *in vitro*	PCA; *in vitro*	PCA; *in vitro*	PCA; SA; *in vitro*	PCA	PCA; SA;	PK; SA; *in vitro*
Amount of antibody present in serum after immunization	++++	++++	tr.	tr.	tr.	tr.	tr.
Electrophoretic mobility	γ1	γ1	?	β	β	β	γ1
Sedimentation coefficient	6.5S	7S	?	sl. > 7S	sl. > 7S	?	8S
Heat lability	±	—	+	+	+	+	+
Sulfhydryl lability	±	±	+	+	+	?	+
Ability to fix complement	—	—	?	—	—	?	—
Optimum latent period for PCA	4–6 h	1–2 h	72 h	24–72 h	60–84 h	24–48 h	24–48 h
Persistence at passively sensitized skin site	> 2– < 4 d.	< 1 d.	10 d. or >	31 d. or >	17 d. or >	14 d. or >	28 d. or >
Transfer across maternal-fetal membranes	+	?	?	—	?	?	—
Immunoglobulin class	7Sγ1	7Sγ1	?	?	?	?	γE

enzymes and certain cationic proteins. The proteolytic enzymes attack vascular basement membrane with loss of integrity of the vessel walls, resulting in edema and hemorrhage [13].

Guinea pig 7Sγ1 antibodies constitute one type of homocytotropic antibody (Type I). The term 'homocytotropic' antibody was introduced by BECKER and AUSTEN [3], in 1966, to describe a specialized immunoglobulin capable of attaching to certain target cells of the same species, so that subsequent contact with antigen leads to the release of pharmacologic agents from the target cell. Certain physico-chemical properties of these antibodies are summarized in table I. In addition to the properties already listed, it should be noted that heating at 56° C for 4 h had little effect on the ability of the 7Sγ1 homocytotropic antibody of the guinea pig to mediate PCA, and reduction and alkylation only slightly reduced the skin-sensitizing activity of purified anti-hapten antibodies[2]. A relatively brief latent period of 4 to 6 h between intradermal injection of γ1 antibodies and intravenous injection of antibody and dye, was sufficient to produce optimum PCA reactions. Homocytotropic antibody persisted at a passively sensitized skin site for over two, but less than four days; it was transferred across maternal-fetal membranes.

A second type of homocytotropic antibody has been observed by several investigators but details have not been published [11, 35]. This antibody is

[2] References pertinent to these and subsequent statements, unless specifically indicated herein, may be found in the appropriate section of reference [5].

said to appear in serum in low concentration for a brief period during initial immunization. It is reported to be heat-labile; and to persist at a passively sensitized homologous skin site for long periods.

Finally, although several hundred guinea pig γ2 anti-hapten, anti-protein, and anti-E. coli antibody preparation failed to produce PCA reactions in Hartley and Rice strain guinea pigs after a latent period of 2 to 6 h [7, 8, 36] and an observation period of up to 4 h after injection of antigen and dye, [6] such reactions have been reported with guinea pig γ2 anti-Ascaris, anti-hemocyanin and anti-egg albumin antibody preparations [14, 45, 46, 47]. In contrast to the usual PCA reactions mediated by guinea pig γ1 antibodies which become evident within minutes of the intravenous injection of antigen and dye, reactions provoked by γ2 anti-Ascaris and anti-hemocyanin antibodies tended to appear 45 min to 2 h after injection of antigen. The immunologic mechanism involved in these reactions remain to be determined.

Homocytotropic Antibodies of the Mouse

Four major classes of mouse immunoglobulins 7Sγ2, 7Sγ1, γ1A, and γ1M and two subclasses 7Sγ2a and 7Sγ2b have been identified and shown to have distinctive immunochemical and physicochemical properties [16]. In addition, preliminary evidence exists for a new class of immunoglobulins [25, 28, 29, 40] provisionally termed mouse 'early' or reagin-like antibody.

Mouse 7Sγ1 antibody, but not 7Sγ2, γA or γM, prepared mouse skin for PCA after a short latent period; following preparation, skin reactions could be elicited for more than 6, but less than 24 h. Mouse 7Sγ1 antibody appeared in serum early in the course of immunization and persisted in high titer. It was not heat labile; treatment with mercaptoethanol and iodoacetamide reduced, but did not abolish its activity. 7Sγ1 antibody did not mediate the lysis of antigen-coated erythrocytes in the presence of complement.

Unfractionated hyperimmune ascitic fluid [38] as well as purified mouse anti-hapten antibody preparations containing 7Sγ1 and 7Sγ2 immunoglobulins [51], have been used to prepare mouse peritoneal cells *in vitro* for antigen-induced release of histamine and serotonin. It is assumed, that 7Sγ1 antibody is the mediator of these reactions, and that the mast cell, rather than another type of cell present among the peritoneal cell population, is being directly acted upon in these experiments. Preparation of mast cells with 7Sγ1 antibody was rapidly effected, and could be reversed by a single washing [38]. The release of histamine from mouse mast cells was critically dependent on the proportion of antigen to 7Sγ1 antibody (presumably) and could be provoked by freshly prepared antigen-antibody complexes [38, 51].

Mouse 'early' or reagin-like antibody appeared in the circulation early in the course of immunization with protein or hapten-protein conjugates and persisted for a few days to several weeks. The serum titer of this antibody, as measured by PCA in the same species, tended to be low. The antibody was heat-labile, required a prolonged latent period for optimal sensitization of homologous skin for PCA, and persisted at a passively sensitized site for at least 10 days [25, 28, 29, 40]. The time course of appearance of this antibody in the circulation and of the ability to achieve antigen-induced release histamine from peritoneal mast cells obtained from the same animals, were roughly similar [40].

Despite repeated washing, mast cells obtained from mice early in the course of active immunization, as well as from mice passively sensitized by intravenous administration of serum containing the second type of homocytotropic antibody, released histamine on contact with antigen. The release of histamine from mast cells sensitized with this antibody was considerably less dependent on the proportion of antigen to antibody [39, 41].

Homocytotropic Antibodies of the Rat

Four classes of immunoglobulins have been identified in the rat on the basis of immunochemical and physicochemical differences, γG_a, γG_b, γA and γM [9]. There is considerable evidence favoring an additional class comprising certain of the homocytotropic antibodies of the species. The homocytotropic antibody of the rat appeared in the serum early in the course of primary immunization with conventional antigens and either *Bordetella pertussis* or complete Freund's adjuvant; and disappeared by about 30 days; a secondary response could not be demonstrated. Serum titers seldom exceeded 1:100. In contrast, rats infected with the nematode, *Nippostrongylus brasiliensis* produced high titers of homocytotropic anti-worm antibodies, and a secondary response was demonstrated on reinfection [33, 53].

Rat homocytotropic antibody to conventional or worm antigens had similar characteristics [10, 21]. On electrophoresis in agar at pH 8.6, homocytotropic antibody migrated faster than the bulk of γG, $-\gamma A-$ and γM globulins. The molecular size of homocytotropic antibody was intermediate between that of 7S and 19S globulins. On diethylamminoethyl cellulose chromatography, this antibody activity was eluted with the peak of γA globulins, but homocytotropic antibody was not removed by absorption with rabbit antiserum to rat γA. Rat homocytotropic antibody was heat-labile and susceptible to inactivation by 2-mercaptoethanol. A prolonged latent period of 24 to 72 h was required for optimal PCA reactions, and the antibody persisted at passively sensitized skin sites of normal rats for at least 31 days. Rat homocytotropic antibody was not transferred across maternal-fetal membranes.

Rat antisera, devoid of homocytotropic antibody, were able to elicit PCA reactions after an interval of 2 to 4, but not 24 h. This activity has been found to be attributable to a heat-stable antibody of the 7S γG$_a$ class [6]. Antibodies of this class have also been shown to prepare the rat peritoneal cavity for the antigen-induced release of SRS-A^{rat} and histamine [26, 27, 44]; the presence of the polymorphonuclear leukocytes was required for the former [34], and mast cells for the latter reaction [27]. Although γG$_a$ antibodies activate the complement sequence in the presence of antigen, complement did not appear to be required for the antigen-induced release of histamine in rats prepared with γG$_a$ antibodies [27]. These results suggest that, rat γG$_a$ antibody may interact directly with mast cells so as to prepare these cells for antigen-induced release of histamine; γG$_a$ would thus qualify as a second homocytotropic antibody. However, further studies of histamine release by γG$_a$ antibody are required to firmly establish a direct cytotropic mechanism.

Homocytotropic Antibody of the Rabbit

ZVAIFLER and BECKER [54] demonstrated that homocytotropic antibody appeared in the circulation of about fifty per cent of rabbits 6–7 days after immunization with hapten-conjugates emulsified in complete Freund's adjuvant and usually disappeared by the third week. The antibody was present in low concentration; serum titres as measured by PCA after a long latent period seldom exceeded 1:81 [2, 55]. The antibody persisted at passively sensitized skin sites for at least 17 days. It was heat labile and susceptible to inactivation by 2-mercaptoethanol; indirect evidence suggested that it did not activate the serum complement sequence [54].

In rabbits infected with *Schistosoma mansoni*, homocytotropic antibody was detected in serum of nearly all animals, frequently in appreciable titer. Furthermore there was an increase in titer following reinfection [56].

Homocytotropic Antibody of the Dog

Characteristics of the homocytotropic antibody of the dog with spontaneous hypersensitivity to ragweed are summarized in table I.

Homocytotropic Antibody of Man

Human homocytotropic antibody has in the past been referred to as reaginic or skin-sensitizing antibody. It was found in serum after development of spontaneous or induced hypersensitivity to various antigens and appeared to mediate Prausnitz-Küstner (P-K) reactions, certain systemic anaphylactic reactions, as well as *in vitro* antigen-induced release of histamine from actively or passively sensitized leukocytes. Human homocytotropic antibody was capable of sensitizing tissues of monkeys and chimpanzees but not those of the guinea pig. This antibody had the electrophoretic mobility of a $\gamma1$ globulin and a sedimentation coefficient of approximately 8S. It was heat-labile and susceptible to inactivation by sulfhydryl reagents. It did not require complement to mediate antigen-induced release of histamine in *in vitro* tests. Optimum P-K reactions were obtained after a latent period of 24–48 h and the antibody persisted at passively sensitized normal human skin for at least 28 days.

Based on the studies of ISHIZAKA, ISHIZAKA and their associates, human homocytotropic antibody has been assigned to a new immunoglobulin class, γE [19]. The discovery of a myeloma protein, ND, belonging to this class, has permitted the development of quantitative assays for γE globulins [20]. These tests have shown elevated levels of γE globulin in serum from patients with asthma or hayfever secondary to known allergens [20].

Several investigators have reported the isolation of human skin-sensitizing activity in serum fractions which apparently contained only γG globulins [17, 25, 37, 42, 49]. Although it seems unlikely that these fractions were contaminated with γE homocytotropic antibody in each case, this possibility was not rigorously excluded. γG antibody fractions with skin-sensitizing activity varied in heat-stability and susceptibility to inactivation with sulfhydryl reagents [24, 42, 46]. Whether skin-sensitizing activity of γG antibodies is a function of a subclass of γG globulins, and whether this activity is mediated via a direct cytotropic or indirect mechanism, remains to be determined.

Heterocytotropic Antibodies

The term heterocytotropic antibody refers to an antibody which is capable of sensitizing the target cells of a foreign species. Our knowledge of heterocytotropic antibodies is largely based on studies in the guinea pig. These studies have shown that, in general, only the γG antibodies of certain foreign

Table II. Immunoglobulin class of certain heterologous antibodies capable of eliciting PCA in the guinea pig, presumably by a cytotropic mechanism

Species	Immunoglobulin class	
	PCA +[1]	PCA −[1]
Mouse	$7S\gamma_{2a}$	$7S\gamma_{2b}$, $7S\gamma1$, γA, γM
Rabbit	γG	γA, γM, γA (incl. HA)
Dog	γG	HA
Monkey	γG	
Man	γG1, γG3, γG4	γG2, γA, γM, γE, γD

[1] Or results obtained by reverse passive cutaneous anaphylaxis where antibodies belonging to diverse immunoglobulin classes have not been tested directly.

species can sensitize the guinea pig for PCA, and that this capacity may be further restricted to some of the subclasses of γG globulins (table II). It is assumed that heterologous immunoglobulins mediate PCA reactions in the guinea pig by the same cytotropic mechanism used by the guinea pig's own γ1 homocytotropic antibody. This assumption is based on indirect evidence which includes: (a) following exposure to rabbit antibody (mainly γG), mast cells present in guinea-pig mesenteries showed loss of granules on content with antigen [18]; (b) the histologic picture of PCA reactions provoked in guinea pigs with rabbit γG and guinea pig γ1 antibodies were similar [23]; (c) both reactions were inhibited to the same degree by the antihistamine pyrilamine [23]; (d) the presence of non-specific rabbit γG globulin together with specific guinea pig γ1 antibody in the incubation mixture decreased the antigen-induced release of histamine from guinea pig mesenteries following exposure to antigen, suggesting that rabbit γG globulins might be competing for sensitization sites on guinea pig mast cells [6], and (e) specifically purified rabbit γG anti-hapten antibodies prepared washed guinea pig lung slices for antigen-induced release of histamine in the absence of complement in the fluid phase [43].

However, certain *in vivo* experiments suggest that in the guinea pig, PCA reactions mediated by rabbit γG antibodies may involve more than one mechanism of tissue injury. Thus, Taichmann and Movat demonstrated that PCA lesions mediated by rabbit γG antibodies were inhibited by rendering guinea pigs leukopenic with anti-leukocyte antisera or nitrogen mustard [48]. LIEBERMAN and OVARY [23] failed to note any difference in the extent to which PCA reactions mediated by either guinea pig γ1 or rabbit antibodies were inhibited by depletion of polymorphonuclear leukocytes. Pending the resolution of these conflicting findings, it may be appropriate to consider cross species 'sensitization' for anaphylactic reactions in intact animals as a complex phenomenon involving cytotropic, as well as non-cytotropic mechanisms.

Aggregate Anaphylaxis

Aggregate anaphylaxis refers to the clinical syndromes developing within minutes after the combination of antigen with large amounts of (circulating) antibody or after the injection of preformed antigen-antibody complexes. In animals passively prepared with antiserum, no latent period is required prior to eliciting the reaction with antigen. Antigen-antibody complexes may interact directly with certain target cells so as to release their content of vasoactive amines by mechanisms analogous to those employed by homocytotropic antibodies, or indirectly via complement fragments or other complement-mediated reactions, such as cytotoxic injury. Some of the participants in aggregate anaphylaxis have been recognized including vasoactive amines, platelets, polymorphonuclear leukocytes and leukocyte lysosomal enzymes but the details of their interaction and the precise identification of the antibodies involved remain to be established [12, 22, 31].

Analysis of Systemic Anaphylactic Reactions in Intact Animals

Although recognition of the specialized biologic functions of certain antibodies has defined one parameter of the anaphylactic syndromes, there is as yet insufficient information to permit a complete account of the multiple immunologic reactions involved in the systemic anaphylactic reactions of most, if not all mammals. Further information is needed of: 1. the biologic properties of all the antibodies produced against a given antigenic determinant; 2. their possible modes of interaction with target cells; 3. the types of target cells available; 4. the types and properties of the pharmacologic agents released; 5. the role of serum factors, of complement sequences, complement fragments, and the kinin system; and 6. the inhibitors of each of these systems. Information is needed of the dynamic inter-relationship of these mechanism and of the importance of the contribution of each to the total anaphylactic syndrome of a given animal. The following papers and discussions may be expected to contribute to each of these areas and to greatly enhance our understanding of the anaphylactic syndromes of mammals, including man.

References

1. BAKER, A. R.; BLOCH, K. J. and AUSTEN, K. F.: *In vitro* passive sensitization of chopped guinea pig lung by guinea pig 7S antibodies. J. Immunol. *93:* 525–531 (1964).
2. BARBARO, J. F. and ZVAIFLER, N. J.: Antigen-induced histamine release from platelets of rabbits producing homologous PCA antibody. Proc. Soc. exp. Biol., N.Y. *122:* 1245–1247 (1966).
3. BECKER, E. L. and AUSTEN, K. F.: Mechanisms of immunologic injury of rat peritoneal mast cells. I. The effect of phosphonate inhibitors on the homocytotropic antibody-mediated histamine release and the first component of rat complement. J. exp. Med. *124:* 379–395 (1966).
4. BENACERRAF, B.; OVARY, Z.; BLOCH, K. J. and FRANKLIN, E. C.: Properties of guinea pig 7S antibodies I. Electrophoretic separation of two types of guinea pig 7S antibodies. J. exp. Med. *117:* 937–949 (1963).
5. BLOCH, K. J.: The anaphylactic antibodies of mammals including man. Progr. Allergy (Karger, Basel/New York) *10:* 84–150 (1967).
6. BLOCH, K. J. Personal observations, 1968.
7. BLOCH, K. J.; KOURILSKY, F. M.; OVARY, Z. and BENACERRAF, B.: Properties of guinea pig 7S antibodies. III. Identification of antibodies involved in complement fixation and hemolysis. J. exp. Med. *117:* 965–981 (1963).
8. BLOCH, K. J.; KOURILSKY, K. M.; OVARY, Z. and BENACERRAF, B.: Properties of guinea pig 7S antibodies. IV. Antibody response to *E. coli* bacteria. Proc. Soc. exp. Biol., N.Y. *114:* 52–56 (1963).
9. BLOCH, K. J.; MORSE, H. C. III and AUSTEN, K. F.: Biologic properties of rat antibodies. I. Antigen-binding by four classes of anti-DNP antibodies. J. Immunol., *101:* 650–657 (1968).
10. BLOCH, K. J. and WILSON, R. J. M.: Homocytotropic antibody response in the rat infected with the nematode, *Nippostrongylus brasiliensis*. III. Characteristics of the antibody. J. Immunol. *100:* 629–636 (1968).
11. CATTY, D.: Personal communication, 1968.
12. COCHRANE, C. G.: The role of immune complexes and complement in tissue injury. J. Allergy *42:* 113–129 (1968).
13. COCHRANE, C. G. and AIKIN, B. S.: Polymorphonuclear leukocytes in immunologic reactions. The destruction of vascular basement membrane *in vivo* and *in vitro*. J. exp. Med. *124:* 733–752 (1966).
14. COLQUHOUN, D. and BROCKLEHURST, W. E.: Passive sensitization of skin and lung by guinea pig immunoglobulins. Immunology *9:* 591–611 (1965).
15. EISEN, H. N.: in Microbiology; DAVIS, B. D., DULBECCO, R., EISEN, H. N., GINSBERG, H. S. and WOOD, W. B. eds., p. 411 (Hoeber Medical Division, Harper & Row. Publishers, 1967).
16. FAHEY, J. L.; WUNDERLICH, J. and MISCHELL, R.: The immunoglobulins of mice. II. Two subclasses of mouse 7Sγ_2-globulins: $\gamma2_a$ and $\gamma2_b$-globulins. J. exp. Med. *120:* 243–251 (1964).
17. FIREMAN, P.; BOESMAN, M. and GITLIN, D.: Heterogeneity of skin-sensitizing antibodies. J. Allergy *40:* 259–274, 1967.
18. HUMPHREY, J. H. and MOTA, I.: The mechanism of anaphylaxis: Specificity of antigen-induced mast cell damage in anaphylaxis in the guinea pig. Immunology *2:* 31–43 (1959).
19. ISHIZAKA, K.; ISHIZAKA, T. and HORNBROOK, M. M.: Physicochemical properties of reaginic antibody. V. Correlation of reaginic activity with γE-globulin antibody. J. Immunol. *97:* 840–853 (1966).

20. JOHANSSON, S. G. O. and BENNICH, H.: Studies on a new class of human immuno-globulins. I. Immunological properties in 'Gamma Globulins', Proceedings of the Third Nobel Symposium, June 12–17, 1967, ed. J. KILLANDER (Interscience Publishers, 1967).
21. JONES, V. E. and OGILVIE, B. M.: Reaginic antibodies and immunity to *Nippostrongylus brasiliensis* in the rat. II. Some properties of the antibodies and antigens. Immunology *12:* 583–597 (1967).
22. KNIKER, W. T. and COCHRANE, C. G.: The localization of circulating immune complexes in experimental serum sickness. The role of vasoactive amines and hydrodynamic forces. J. exp. Med. *127:* 137–154 (1968).
23. LIEBERMAN, M. K. and OVARY, Z.: Histology of PCA reactions in guinea pigs. A comparison of reactions produced by guinea pig γG1 and rabbit antibodies. J. Immunol. *100:* 159–168 (1968).
24. MALLEY, A. and PERLMAN, F.: Isolation of a reaginic antibody fraction with properties of γG-globulin. Proc. Soc. exp. Biol., N.Y. *122:* 152–156 (1966).
25. McCAMISH, J.: A heat-labile skin sensitizing antibody of mous serum. Nature *214:* 1228–1229 (1967).
26. MORSE, H. C. III; BLOCH, K. J. and AUSTEN, K. F.: Biologic properties of rat antibodies. II. Time course of appearance of antibodies involved in antigen-induced release of slow reacting substance of anaphylaxis (SRS-A^{rat}); association of this activity with rat IgG$_a$ J. Immunol. (in press) 1968.
27. MORSE, H. C. III; AUSTEN, K. F. and BLOCH, K. J.: Biologic properties of rat antibodies. III. Histamine release mediated by two classes of antibodies. J. Immunol. (submitted) 1968.
28. MOTA, I.: Biological characterization of mouse 'early' antibodies. Immunology *12:* 343–348 (1967).
29. MOTA, I. and PEIXOTO, J.: A skin-sensitizing and thermolabile antibody in the mouse. Life Sci. *5:* 1723–1728 (1966).
30. MOVAT, H. Z.; DiLORENZO, N. L.; TAICHMAN, N. S.; BERGER, S. and STEIN, H.: Suppression by antihistamine of passive cutaneous anaphylaxis produced with anaphylactic antibody of the guinea pig. J. Immunol. *98:* 230–235 (1967).
31. MOVAT, H. Z.; URIUHARA, T.; TAICHMAN, N. S.; ROWSELL, H. C. and MUSTARD, J. F.: The role of PMN-leukocyte lysomes in tissue injury inflammation and hypersensitivity. VI. The participation of the PMN-leukocyte and the blood platelet in systemic aggregate anaphylaxis. Immunology *14:* 637–648 (1968).
32. NUSSENZWEIG, V. and BENACERRAF, B.: Presence of identical antigenic determinants in the Fd fragments of γ1- and γ2-guinea pig immunoglobulins. J. Immunol. *97:* 171–176 (1966).
33. OGILVIE, B. M.: Reagin-like antibodies in rats infected with the nematode parasite *Nippostrongylus brasiliensis*. Immunology *12:* 113–131 (1967).
34. ORANGE, R. P.; VALENTINE, M. D. and AUSTEN, K. F.: Antigen-induced release of slow reacting substance of anaphylaxis (SRS-A^{rat}) in rats prepared with homologous antibody. J. exp. Med. *127:* 767–782 (1968).
35. OVARY, Z.: Personal communication, 1968.
36. OVARY, Z.; BENACERRAF, B. and BLOCH, K. J.: Properties of guinea pig 7S antibodies. II. Identification of antibodies involved in passive cutaneous and systemic anaphylaxis. J. exp. Med. *117:* 951–964 (1963).
37. PERELMUTTER, L.; FREEDMAN, S. O. and SEHON, A. H.: Fractionation of sera from ragweed-sensitive individuals by chromatography on DEAE-cellulose. Int. Arch. Allergy *19:* 129–144 (1961).
38. PROUVOST-DANON, A.; QUEIROZ JAVIERRE, M. and SILVA LIMA, M.: Passive anaphylactic reaction in mouse peritoneal mast cells *in vitro*. Life Sci. *5:* 1751–1760 (1966).

39. PROUVOST-DANON, A.; PEIXOTO, J. M. and QUEIROZ JAVIERRE, M.: Reagin-like antibody mediated passive anaphylactic reaction in mouse peritoneal mast cells *in vitro*. Life Sci. *6:* 1793–1801 (1967).

40. PROUVOST-DANON, A.; PEIXOTO, J. M. and QUEIROZ JAVIERRE, M.: Antigen induced histamine release from peritoneal mast cells of mice producing reagin-like antibody. Immunology *15:* 271–286 (1968).

41. PROUVOST-DANON, A.; SILVA LIMA, M. and QUEIROZ JAVIERRE, M.: Active anaphylactic reaction in mouse peritoneal mast cells *in vitro*. Life Sci. *5:* 289–297 (1966).

42. REID, R. T.; MINDEN, P. and FARR, R. S.: Differences among proteins having reaginic activity. J. Allergy *41:* 326–337 (1968).

43. SPUZIC, I.; BLOCH, K. J. and AUSTEN, K. F.: Effect of non-specific gamma globulin on passive sensitization in vitro at different temperatures. J. Allergy *37:* 75–83 (1966).

44. STECHSCHULTE, D. J.; AUSTEN, K. F. and BLOCH, K. J.: Antibodies involved in antigen-induced release of slow reacting substance of anaphylaxis (SRS-A) in the guinea pig and rat. J. exp. Med. *125:* 127–147 (1967).

45. STREJAN, G. and CAMPBELL, D. H.: Hypersensitivity to ascaris antigens. I. Skin-sensitizing activity of serum fractions from guinea pigs sensitized to crude extracts. J. Immunol. *98:* 893–900 (1967).

46. STREJAN, G. and CAMPBELL, D. H.: Hypersensitivity to ascaris antigens. II. The skin-sensitizing properties of 7Sγ2 antibody from sensitized guinea pigs as tested in guinea pigs. J. Immunol. *99:* 347–356 (1967).

47. STREJAN, G. and CAMPBELL, D. H.: Skin-sensitizing properties of guinea pig antibodies to keyhole limpet hemocyanin. J. Immunol. *100:* 1245–1254 (1968).

48. TAICHMAN, N. S. and MOVAT, Z.: Do polymorphonuclear leukocytes play a role in passive cutaneous anaphylaxis in the guinea pig? Int. Arch. Allergy *30:* 97–102 (1966).

49. TERR, A. I. and BENTZ, J. D.: Skin-sensitizing antibodies in serum sickness. Association of reaginic activity with γ2- and γ1M-globulins. J. Allergy *36:* 433–445 (1965).

50. THORBECKE, G. J.; BENACERRAF, B. and OVARY, Z.: Antigenic relationship between two types of 7S guinea pig γ-globulins. J. Immunol. *91:* 670–676 (1963).

51. VAZ, N. M. and OVARY, Z.: Passive anaphylaxis in mice with γG antibodies. III. Release of histamine from mast cells by homologous antibodies. J. Immunol. *100:* 1014–1019 (1968).

52. WHITE, R. G.; JENKINS, G. C. and WILKINSON, P. C.: The production of skin-sensitizing antibody in the guinea pig. Int. Arch. Allergy *22:* 156–165 (1963).

53. WILSON, R. J. M. and BLOCH, K. J.: Homocytotropic antibody response in the rat infected with the nematode, *Nippostrongylus brasiliensis*. II. Characteristics of the immune response. J. Immunol. *100:* 622–628 (1968).

54. ZVAIFLER, N. J. and BECKER, E. L.: Rabbit anaphylactic antibody. J. exp. Med. *123:* 935–950 (1966).

55. ZVAIFLER, N. J. and BARBARO, J.: The demonstration of anaphylactic antibody in the primary response of rabbits. Int. Arch. Allergy *31:* 465–474 (1967).

56. ZVAIFLER, N. J.; SADUN, E. H.; BECKER, E. L. and SCHOENBECHLER, M. J.: Demonstration of a homologous anaphylactic antibody in rabbits infected with *Schistosoma mansoni*. Exp. Parasit. *20:* 278–287 (1967).

Author's address: KURT J. BLOCH, M.D., Department of Medicine, Harvard Medical School and the Arthritis Unit of the Medical Services, Massachusetts General Hospital, *Boston, Mass.* (USA).

Cellular and Humoral Mechanisms in Anaphylaxis and Allergy, pp. 13–22
(Karger, Basel/New York 1969)

Reaginic Antibodies and Helminth Infections

BRIDGET M. OGILVIE and VALERIE E. JONES

National Institute for Medical Research
London

Antibodies which give homologous passive cutaneous anaphylaxis (PCA) have been given various names in the past few years and the confusing nomenclature which has resulted will persist until they have been investigated fully. There are two major classes of antibodies which may be involved in homologous PCA. These can be differentiated by various means, at present most easily and specifically by their differing persistence in the skin. In this paper the antibodies which persist for at least 72 h in skin are called reagins, by analogy with human reagins. This accords with the practice in which antibodies are designated by terms already in common usage until they are properly identified (Bull. WHO, 1964).

Occurrence

Helminth-induced reagins have long been known in man (see reviews by ANDREWS [1], BLOCH [4]) and it is now clear that the formation of reaginic antibodies is a general phenomenon in helminth-infected animals. Originally, it was shown that rats, monkeys and sheep infected with helminths respond by forming reaginic antibodies [21] and subsequent investigations showed that rabbits [11, 36] and mice [19] produce similar antibodies in response to helminth infections. It seems likely, as suggested originally [21] that most if not all species of animals infected with helminths form reaginic antibodies as part of their immune response. All reports so far have been of a reaginic response to helminths in mammals: it would be interesting to investigate the response to helminths in birds and cold blooded vertebrates.

Reaginic antibodies are produced *in vivo* by cells from the spleen, mesenteric lymph nodes and the peritoneum of rats infected with the intestinal nematode *Nippostrongylus brasiliensis* [23] and *in vitro* by fragments of spleen and lymph nodes [35]. However, 7S immunoglobulins but no reagins have been detected in extracts of the gut from infected rats (JONES, unpublished, and WILSON and BLOCH [35]). Although circulating reagins were detected in isologous recipients of cells taken from rats immune to *N. brasiliensis*, these recipients rarely exhibited any acquired immunity to the parasite [23].

In contrast with attempts to stimulate reagin production with defined antigens or worm extracts [4, 22, 19], helminth infections stimulate high titres of reagins and a rapid anamnestic response follows re-infection. An anamnestic response can be achieved even after 3 to 5 infections of *Nippostrongylus*, but it is important to remember that the antigenic stimulus will decline with successive infections, unless these are much larger than the earlier infections, because the life cycle is shortened by the development of acquired immunity and thus the allergen output is reduced. Moreover, animals which have been immunised with extracts of *Nippostrongylus* and then given an infection of *Nippostrongylus* sometimes respond to this infection with an anamnestic rise of reagins [22]. Therefore the reagins stimulated by helminth infections are not formed solely by initial contact with the antigen. The amount of reagins produced by individual animals after several infections with *N. brasiliensis* varies enormously and a few animals never produce high titres.

Therefore, the reaginic response to a particular allergen varies widely between individual animals, just as the antibody responses to other antigens vary.

Properties

The properties of reagins induced by helminth infections are similar to those induced by defined antigens. In this paper, only the properties not discussed in the review by BLOCH [4] will be reported. In rats infected with *N. brasiliensis*, reagins appear in the milk in low titre (relative to the level in the serum of the mother) throughout lactation. However, they are not absorbed through the intestine of suckling rats [18]. In man, reagins have been associated with the γE immunoglobulin class [13], so it was not surprising to find that γE levels are elevated in human populations exposed to helminths [15]. In all animals, the immunoglobulin class of reagins remains to be determined. It has been suggested that the reagins in patients sensitive to more than one allergen may be found in more than one immunoglobulin class [30, 25, 10]. No such variation has been reported yet with helminth induced reagins, probably because animals infected with only a single worm species have been studied and because pooled rather than individual sera have been examined. For example, the physico-chemical properties of the reagins in pooled serum taken from rats given a single *N. brasiliensis* infection do not differ from those in serum from multiply infected rats (JONES and OGILVIE [17] and unpublished results).

Nature of the Allergen

The 3 major classes of helminths (cestodes, trematodes and nematodes) all stimulate reagin formation, although they differ both structurally and biochemically. Helminth allergens are released into culture fluid *in vitro* in large amounts and provide a useful marker antigen for assessing the success of *in vitro* culture techniques [34]. The best way to obtain worm allergen relatively free of other worm material is to incubate worms in phosphate buffered saline (pH 7.0) for 2–5 h at 37°. With *Nippostrongylus*, often as much allergen is released after incubation in saline as can be obtained by extracting a similar number of adult worms before incubation, and the total protein content of this saline culture fluid is as much as one hundred fold less than that of adult worm extract (table I). Our definition of 1 unit of allergen is the amount which, having been injected intravenously into a 150 g rat will demonstrate the maximum PCA titre of a standard antiserum. Fractionation of saline culture fluid on G-100 Sephadex gave a component which contained only 1 μg of protein per unit of allergen but even this relatively pure component still contained other antigenic material.

Allergen is apparently actively released by feeding worms. It is difficult to culture helminths *in vitro* and therefore the amounts of allergen released are probably far less than the amounts released *in vivo*. A massive release of allergen *in vivo* could explain the special ability of living infections to induce reagin formation.

The molecular size of allergens from several nematodes is similar (10,000–20,000) [17, 12, 34]. The *Nippostrongylus* allergen is primarily protein and there may be a carbohydrate moiety [17, 34]. Most of the allergens from helminths are antigenically distinct but there is some cross reaction between allergens of related species [11, 26]. Presumably systemic anaphylaxis and PCA induced by *Nippostrongylus* are both induced by the same allergen, because the fractions of saline culture fluid containing allergen are the only ones which induced systemic anaphylaxis (unpublished).

Table I. A comparison of the allergenic content of adult worm extracts, saline culture fluids and fractions of these preparations: the total protein and numbers of worms giving a unit of allergen

Antigenic Material	Protein (μg) from 1,000 worms	Protein (μg) in 1 unit of allergen[1]	No. worms producing 1 unit of allergen
Worm extract	5,200	520	100
	7,400	740	100
	3,300	330	100
Fraction of worm extract from G-200 Sephadex		35	
		190	
		246	
Culture fluid	167	7.5	45
	46	6.0	295
	85	17	195
	37	5.9	145
	250	10	40
Fraction of culture fluid from G-100 Sephadex		1.0	
		5.0	
		<2.9	

[1] For definition see text.

Besides allergen, nematodes release a substance which degranulates mast cells directly. For *Ascaris*, this has been shown to be a polypeptide, MW 2–3,000 [31]. There is indirect evidence that *N. brasiliensis* also releases a mast cell degranulating agent [14].

We have made a single attempt to determine whether allergen and the protective antigen(s) are identical. The saline culture fluid from 5×10^5 adult worms was collected as described above, concentrated by negative pressure dialysis and separated on a G-100 Sephadex column into 5 fractions. Antiserum known to contain protective antibodies was mixed with each fraction and the mixtures injected into groups of rats. Control rats were given antiserum alone and other rats were left untreated. The following day, all rats were infected with adult worms to test the protective capacity of each antiserum/culture fluid mixture, as described elsewhere [23]. When the worms were recovered 6 days later, all rats given antiserum or antiserum/culture fluid mixtures were passively protected except those rats given antiserum mixed with the fraction of culture fluid which contained material in the MW range 15–30,000. This material which appeared to contain the protective antigens was eluted from the G-100 column between the bulk of the precipitating antigens and the allergen. This (as yet unconfirmed) experiment suggests that the allergen is not the protective antigen.

γG Antibodies

In guinea pigs and mice anaphylactic antibodies associated with the $7S\gamma_1$ class are formed following helminth infection [33, 19]. These are differentiated from reagins by their ability to induce homologous PCA at 4 but not at 72 h after their introduction into the skin. In rabbits and rats infected with helminths, only anaphylactic antibodies of the reaginic type have been detected ([11, 27], and unpublished results) but 4 h PCA antibodies occur in rats immunised with *Nippostrongylus* worm extract (unpublished work). These rats producing 4 hour PCA antibodies were immunised in the same way as the guinea pigs immunised with *Ascaris* which formed 4 h PCA antibodies of the $7S\gamma_2$-type [28]. From the literature it is not always clear whether anaphylactic antibodies of this type have been actively sought in, for example, rabbits or man after helminth infections. Mice are the only species in which both 4 and 72 h PCA antibodies have been reported after helminth infections and it is not known whether these antibodies are directed at the same antigen [19]. Reaginic antibodies have been detected in all helminth infected animals so far investigated with the single exception of guinea pigs. There is, however, no conclusive evidence as yet that guinea pigs cannot produce reaginic antibodies. For example, there is no evidence in the literature that all helminth-induced anaphylactic antibodies can be absorbed from guinea pig serum by an antiserum to guinea pig $7S\gamma_1$-immunoglobulin. It appears that the occurrence of anaphylactic antibodies following helminth infections would reward further investigation. Blocking antibodies occur in rats infected with *N. brasiliensis* or immunised with worm extracts [17, 22]. They are associated with γM immunoglobulin after one infection, γG after multiple infections [17]. The occurrence of these antibodies may explain the lack of correlation between circulating reagin titre and sensitivity to systemic anaphylaxis which is especially evident following reinfection [22].

Desensitisation treatment is used clinically in atopic allergy and can be mimicked using helminth-infected rats. Rats were given a series of injections of worm extract after an initial infection of *N. brasiliensis*. Following reinfection, the anamnestic rise in reagins was almost completely suppressed. These results cannot be explained by the presence of circulating allergen originating from the worm extracts as the amount of allergen released by worms in the reinfection was almost certainly much greater than that in the total worm extract. Presumably, allergen released by the reinfection was neutralised by blocking antibodies before it could restimulate cells forming reagins.

Mast Cells in Helminth Infections

The occurrence of large numbers of mast cells in organs affected by atopic allergy is well known. Mast cells in different organs vary in their response to histological fixatives and histochemical tests [8, 9]. Is it possible that the relationship between antibodies and mast cells may vary in different organs? If so, antibodies which cause anaphylaxis in the skin may be less active in anaphylactic reactions in other organs, e.g. the gut of rats.

JARRETT et al. [14] have demonstrated recently that, coincidently with the onset of worm expulsion, mast cells accumulate rapidly in the intestine of rats at the sites parasitised by *N. brasiliensis*. Immediately following the increase in mast cells and in parallel with worm expulsion, there is an increase in cells known as globular leucocytes. MURRAY et al. [20] provide strong evidence that globular leucocytes are mast cells which have discharged some of their amine content and not immunoglobulin containing cells as suggested by others [7, 32]. Like the occurrence of reaginic antibodies, an accumulation of mast cells is a common feature in helminth infections [20].

Are mast cells actively involved in worm expulsion? Although the sudden rise in mast cell numbers is closely associated with worm expulsion in nippostrongylosis, and although histamine release from mast cells of actively infected rats can first be detected at about the same time that worms begin to be damaged by host immunity [35, 24] direct evidence that these cells are essential for worm damage or expulsion is lacking. Mast cells occur in situations where neither helminths nor reagins are present [5]. Also, many of the other changes in the gut in nippostrongylosis are similar to those found in pathological conditions of varying etiology [29] and the appearance of mast cells could be a result of mechanical damage by living worms rather than a manifestation of acquired immunity.

Reagins and Protective Immunity to N. brasiliensis

After infection with *N. brasiliensis*, reaginic antibodies and sensitivity to anaphylaxis can be detected in the rat concurrently with active protective immunity to the parasite. This correlation led to the concept that reagins might be an essential component of protective immunity to helminths [21, 4].

Anaphylaxis induced by the interaction of an antigen and its antibody which were unrelated to parasites, had no effect on the expulsion of worms from the host [3, 22]; but, when this 'unrelated' anaphylaxis was induced in the presence of passively administered protective antiserum, the worms were expelled more rapidly than worms expelled by protective antiserum alone [3]. However there was no increase in the rate of worm expulsion from the host when anaphylaxis was induced instead with a complex mixture of *N. brasiliensis* antigens and passively administered protective antiserum. In this experiment, the parasite antigens presumably neutralised protective antibodies in the antiserum and the anaphylactic shock alone was unable to affect the worms [17]. These results suggested that protective antibodies in an antiserum were needed to damage the worms before an anaphylactic reaction could affect the rate of worm expulsion. Indeed, damage to *N. brasiliensis* worms by active immunity has been detected several days before the worms were expelled from the host [24].

We now have evidence however that reaginic antibodies, and thus an anaphylactic mechanism, are not essential components of protective immunity to *N. brasiliensis*. Therefore, enhancement of worm expulsion by anaphylaxis with an 'unrelated' antigen-antibody interaction may have little relevance to the mechanism of worm expulsion in protective immunity. This evidence is derived from three separate experiments:

a) A pool of antiserum was taken from rats a few days after they had expelled an infection of *N. brasiliensis*. This pool had good passive protective activity although it contained no reagins and could not passively sensitise rats for systemic anaphylaxis.

Pools of protective rat antisera have been fractionated to determine the immunoglobulins responsible for protective activity. The nomenclature for rat immunoglobulins has been revised [16]; rat IgG is classed as $7S\gamma_2$-globulin and the immunoglobulin previously called rat IgA [2] is $7S\gamma_1$-globulin.

b) Separation of antiserum on DEAE cellulose (by stepwise elution with the buffers described by STECHSCHULTE, AUSTEN and BLOCH [27]) gave a component which consisted almost wholly of $7S\gamma_2$-globulin. This component contained less than 0.5% of $7S\gamma_1$-globulin, no reagins nor PCA activity of the $7S\gamma_2$-type and yet gave good protective immunity.

c) A further antiserum pool was taken from donors 19 days after a primary infection and separated on G-200 Sephadex. One of the fractions from the 7S peak contained no reagins nor PCA activity of the $7S\gamma_2$-type but only a mixture of $7S\gamma_1$- and γ_2-globulins with other serum proteins. This fraction was partially protective (demonstrated by suppression of reproductive capacity of the worms but not shown by their more rapid expulsion).

These results show that passive protection against *N. brasiliensis* adults can be equally effective whether reagins are absent or present in the antiserum. Definite conclusions however about the mechanisms of worm damage and worm expulsion cannot be drawn from passive immunisation experiments until the possibility of an active contribution by the recipients has been eliminated.

References

1. ANDREWS, J. M.: Parasitism and allergy. J. Parasit. *48:* 3–12 (1962).
2. ARNASON, B. G.; DE VAUX ST. CYR, C. and RELYVELD, E. H.: Role of the thymus in immune reactions in rats. IV. Immunoglobulins and antibody formation. Int. Arch. Allergy *25:* 206–224 (1964).
3. BARTH, E. E. E.; JARRETT, W. F. H. and URQUHART, G. M.: Studies on the mechanism of the self-cure reaction in rats infected with *Nippostrongylus brasiliensis*. Immunology *10:* 459–464 (1966).
4. BLOCH, K. J.: The anaphylactic antibodies of mammals including man. Progr. in Allergy *10:* 84–150 (Karger, Basel/New York 1967).
5. BLOOM, G. D.: Structural and biochemical characteristics of mast cells; in The Inflammatory Process, Ed. by B. W. ZWEIFACH, L. GRANT and R. T. McCLUSKEY, pp. 355–388 (Academic Press, New York/London 1965).
6. Bulletin of World Health Organisation: Nomenclature for human immunoglobulins. Bull. World. Hlth Ass. *30:* 447–450 (1964).
7. DOBSON, C.: Immunofluorescent staining of globule leucocytes in the colon of the sheep. Nature, Lond. *211:* 875 (1966).
8. ENERBÄCK, L.: Mast cells in rat gastrointestinal mucosa. I. Effects of fixation. Acta path. microbiol. scand. *66:* 289–302 (1966).
9. ENERBÄCK, L.: Mast cells in rat gastrointestinal mucosa. 2. Dye-binding and metachromatic properties. Acta path. microbiol. scand. *66:* 303–312 (1966).
10. FIREMAN, P.; BOESMAN, M. and GITLIN, D.: Heterogeneity of skin sensitising antibodies. J. Allergy *40:* 259–268 (1967).
11. HOGARTH-SCOTT, R. S.: Rabbit reagin-like antibodies. Int. Arch. Allergy *32:* 201–207 (1967).
12. HOGARTH-SCOTT, R. S.: The molecular weight range of nematode allergens. Immunology *13:* 535–537 (1967).
13. ISHIZAKA, K.; ISHIZAKA, T. and HORNBROOK M.: Physico-chemical properties of human reaginic antibody. IV. Presence of a unique immunoglobulin as a carrier of reaginic activity. J. Immunol. *97:* 75–85 (1966).
14. JARRETT, W. F. H.; JARRETT, E. E.; MILLER, H. R. P. and URQUHART, G. M.: Quantitative studies on the mechanism of self-cure in *Nippostrongylus brasiliensis* infections; in The Reaction of the Host to Parasitism, ed. by E. J. L. SOULSBY, p. 55 (Academic Press, New York/London 1968

15. JOHANSSON, S. G. O.; MELLBIN, T. and VAHLQUIST, B.: Immunoglobulin levels in Ethiopian preschool children with special reference to high concentrations of immunoglobulin E (IgND). Lancet *i:* 1118–1121 (1968).
16. JONES, V. E.: Rat 7S immunoglobulins: characterisation of γ_2- and γ_1-anti-hapten antibodies. Immunology *16:* 589–599 (1969).
17. JONES, V. E. and OGILVIE, B. M.: Reaginic antibodies and immunity to *Nippostrongylus brasiliensis* in the rat. II. Some properties of the antibodies and antigens. Immunology *12:* 583–597 (1967).
18. JONES, V. E. and OGILVIE, B. M.: Reaginic antibodies and immunity to *Nippostrongylus brasiliensis* in the rat. III. Passive immunity in the young rat. Int. Arch. Allergy *31:* 490–504 (1967).
19. MOTA, I.; SADUN, E. H.; BRADSHAW, R. M. and GORE, R. W.: The immunological response of mice infected with *Trichinella spiralis*. Biological and physico-chemical distinction of two homocytotropic antibodies. Immunology *16:* 71–82 (1969).
20. MURRAY, M.; MILLER, H. R. P. and JARRETT, W. F. H.: The globule leucocyte and its derivation from the subepithelial mast cell. Lab. Invest. *19:* 222–234 (1968).
21. OGILVIE, B. M.: Reagin-like antibodies in animals immune to helminth parasites. Nature, London *204:* 91–92 (1964).
22. OGILVIE, B. M.: Reagin-like antibodies in rats infected with the nematode parasite *Nippostrongylus brasiliensis*. Immunology *12:* 113–131 (1967).
23. OGILVIE, B. M. and JONES, V. E.: Passive protection with cells or antiserum against *Nippostrongylus brasiliensis* in the rat. Parasitology *58:* 939–949 (1968).
24. OGILVIE, B. M. and HOCKLEY, D. J.: Effects of immunity on *Nippostrongylus brasiliensis* adult worms. Reversible and irreversible changes in infectivity, reproduction and morphology. J. Parasit. *54:* 1073–1084 (1968).
25. REID, R. T.; MINDEN, P. and FARR, R. S.: Reaginic activity associated with IgG immunoglobulin. J. exp. Med. *123:* 845–858 (1966).
26. SADUN, E. H.; MOTA, I. and GORE, R. W.: Demonstration of homocytotropic reagin-like antibodies in mice and rabbits infected with *Trichinella spiralis*. J. Parasit. *54:* 814–821 (1968).
27. STECHSCHULTE, D. J.; AUSTEN, K. F. and BLOCH, K. J.: Antibodies involved in antigen-induced release of slow reacting substance of anaphylaxis (SRS-A) in the guinea pig and rat. J. exp. Med. *125:* 127–147 (1967).
28. STREJAN, G. and CAMBPELL, D. H.: Hypersensitivity to *Ascaris* antigens. I. Skin-sensitising activity of serum fractions from guinea pigs sensitised to crude extracts. J. Immunol. *98:* 893–900 (1967).
29. SYMONS, L. E. A. and FAIRBAIRN, D.: Pathology, absorption, transport and activity of digestive enzymes in the rat jejunum parasitized by the nematode *Nippostrongylus brasiliensis*. Fed. Proc. *21:* 913–918 (1962).
30. TERR, A. and BENTZ, J.: Skin-sensitizing antibodies in serum sickness. J. Allergy *36:* 433–445 (1965).
31. UVNÄS, B. and WOLD, J. K. Isolation of a mast cell degranulating polypeptide from *Ascaris suis*. Acta physiol. scand. *70:* 269–276 (1967).
32. WHUR, P. and JOHNSTON, H. S. Ultrastructure of globule leucocytes in immune rats infected with *Nippostrongylus brasiliensis* and their possible relationship to the Russell body cell. J. Path. Bact. *93:* 81–85 (1967).
33. WILSON, R. J. M.: γ_1-antibodies in guinea pigs infected with the cattle lungworm. Immunology *11:* 199–209 (1966).
34. WILSON, R. J. M.: Homocytotropic antibody response to the nematode *Nippostrongylus brasiliensis* in the rat – studies on the worm antigen. J. Parasit. *53:* 752–762 (1967).

35. WILSON, R. J. M. and BLOCH, K. J.: Homocytotropic antibody response in the rat infected with the nematode *Nippostrongylus brasiliensis*. II. Characteristics of the immune response. J. Immunol. *100:* 622–628 (1968).
36. ZVAIFLER, N. J.; SADUN, E. H.; BECKER, E. L. and SCHOENBECHLER, M. J.: Demonstration of a homologous anaphylactic antibody in rabbits infected with *Schistosoma mansoni*. Exp. Parasit. *20:* 278–287 (1967).

Authors' address: BRIDGET M. OGILVIE, Ph.D., and VALERIE E. JONES, Ph.D. National Institute for Medical Research, *London, N.W.7* (England).

Cellular and Humoral Mechanisms in Anaphylaxis and Allergy, pp. 23–36
(Karger, Basel/New York 1969)

Mouse Homocytotropic Antibodies[1]

I. MOTA, D. WONG, E. H. SADUN and R. W. GORE

Departments of Immunochemistry and Medical Zoology
Walter Reed Army Institute of Research
Washington, D.C.

Recent observations on the ability of mouse antiserum to induce homologous passive cutaneous anaphylaxis (PCA) have indicated that mice can also produce a homocytotropic antibody similar in its properties to human reagins [18, 16, 10]. The mouse reagin-like antibody is produced in high levels by mice infected with parasites [26, 19]. The production and properties of mouse reagin as well as its relationship to and differentiation from mouse $7S\gamma1$ antibody is the subject of our presentation.

Materials and Methods

Animals. ICR, Bagg and hairless mice weighing 20–30 g and Walter Reed strain albino male rats weighing 150–250 g were used throughout. All animals were reared at Walter Reed Army Institute of Research Animal Farm. The principles of animal care as promulgated by the National Society for Medical Research were observed.

Antigens. Five times crystallized ovalbumin (Ea) obtained from Pentex Inc., (Kankakee, Ill.) and an extract of *Trichinella spiralis* larvae were used as antigen. A lipoid-free somatic extract of *T. spiralis* larvae was prepared at 4°C in anhydrous ether [6]. Lyophilized aliquots of the finished product were sealed in vials and stored at 4°C. Solutions were made when necessary by dissolving the dry extract in saline (0.85% NaCl).

Preparation of antisera. Anti-Ea. Antisera containing antibodies to Ea were obtained by injecting mice (Bagg) subcutaneously with 0.5 ml aluminum hydroxide gel containing 50 μg Ea. Starting from the 13th day after the first dose of antigen the animals were injected intradermally every week with 50 μg Ea in 0.1 ml saline for a period of 20 weeks. Blood was collected at different times by puncture of the ophthalmic plexus and the individual sera obtained at each time were pooled. Seven pools were obtained: Ea I and Ea II obtained respectively 10 and 12 days after the first dose of antigen; Ea III obtained

[1] This investigation was supported in part by USPHS, NIH Grant AI-07444.

one week after the third dose of antigen; Ea X obtained one week after the 10th dose of antigen; Ea HH obtained a week after the 15th dose of antigen; Ea 1415 obtained a week after the 16th dose of antigen and Ea HL obtained a week after the 20th dose of antigen.

Anti-trichinella spiralis. Mice (ICR) were infected with 100 washed *T. spiralis* larvae and reinfected with the same number 9 weeks later. Ten days after the secondary infection the animals were bled by cutting the brachial plexus under ether anesthesia and collecting the extravasated blood. After allowing the blood to clot in an ice-bath, the serum was separated by centrifugation in a refrigerated centrifuge, and kept at $-20°$ C until used.

Block electrophoresis. Antiserum (1.6 to 2.0 ml) was fractionated on Pevikon C-870 (Mercer Chemical Corp. N.Y.) according to previously described procedures [21, 5] with slight modification. Block dimensions measured $30 \times 2 \times 6$ cm and electrophoresis was carried out in 0.1 μ Veronal Buffer, pH 8.55 with 340 v, 40 mAmps for 24 h at 5°C. After the electrophoretic separation the entire block was cut in 0.5 cm wide sections which were transferred to 15 ml coarse Labpor plastic funnels. Each section was then eluted under negative pressure with 5 ml phosphate buffer to achieve a final pH of 7.0–7.5. The protein content of the eluates was determined by the method of LOWRY [9].

Passive cutaneous anaphylaxis (PCA). Mice. Hairless mice were used as recipients for PCA. Ovary's technique for PCA [23] utilizing a two hour sensitization period was employed for detecting and estimating antibody; in addition, a sensitization period of 72 h was also used [13]. The animals were sensitized with 2 or 3 intradermal injections of 0.05 ml antiserum or antiserum dilution made at different sites on each side of the dorsal skin with a microliter syringe (Hamilton Co., Whittier, California) attached to a hypodermic needle. They were then challenged 2 or 72 h later by injecting intravenously 0.5 ml of a 0.25% solution of pontamine sky blue in saline containing 0.5 mg Ea or 0.5 mg *T. spiralis* antigen. Fifteen to 30 min later the animals were killed with a blow on the head and the lesion diameters measured. *Rats.* These animals were shaved with an electric clipper 24 h in advance and prepared for PCA by injecting 0.05 ml of mouse antiserum or antiserum dilution in each side of the dorsal skin. They were then challenged 2 or 72 h later with an intravenous injection of 1 ml of a 0.25% pontamine sky blue containing 2 mg Ea or 2 mg *T. spiralis* antigen. Twenty to 30 min later they were killed and the lesions measured.

Rabbit Anti-mouse immunoglobulins. Highly specific rabbit anti-mouse 7Sγ1 and 7Sγ2 were prepared and kindly provided to us by Dr. F. Hymes, Melpar Laboratories, Va. When tested by immunoelectrophoresis against a pool of mouse normal sera it produced a single sharp line indicating its monospecificity.

Absorption of antiserum. For absorption experiments the antisera were first diluted with saline in a proportion of 1 to 5 or higher depending on their PCA activity. Rabbit anti-mouse 7Sγ1 was then added to the antiserum and the mixture was allowed to react for 15 min in an ice-bath. After centrifugation the precipitate was discarded and the supernatant was used for PCA reactions. Rabbit normal serum or rabbit anti-mouse 7Sγ2 instead of rabbit anti-mouse γ1 added to aliquots of the same antiserum served as controls.

Preparations for mast cell observation. The response to antigen of mouse and rat mast cells sensitized with mouse antisera was studied. Mouse mast cells were observed in skin preparations obtained from sites prepared for PCA 2 or 72 h earlier. Five to 15 min after antigen injection, the skin site showing a PCA reaction was carefully dissected and fixed. Skin obtained from contiguous nonsensitized sites served as a control. Rat mast cells were observed in the mesentery. Two or 3 pieces of rat mesentery were incubated with mouse antiserum at 37°C for 5 min and then transferred to Tyrode's solution containing 1 mg/ml antigen for 15 min at 37°C. The histological techniques used for mouse and rat tissues have been described [15].

Results

Ability of mouse antiserum to induce PCA in rats. The ability of mouse antisera to induce PCA in rats was studied simultaneously with their activity in mice using a sensitization period of 2 and 72 h in both species. The results of these experiments shown in table I indicated that mouse antiserum was able to induce PCA in rats. Furthermore, inspection of the same table also showed that whereas the 2 h PCA activity in mice increased steadily during the course of immunization, the rat PCA activity did not increase at the same rate and indeed decreased after repeated antigenic stimulations. It is also worth noting the fact that there was a positive correlation between the 2 h PCA titer in rats and the 72 h PCA titer in mice. This correlation however, was not apparent when hyperimmune sera having very high 2 h PCA activities were used. In this regard it must be explained that when mice were sensitized for PCA with these antisera challenging of the animals 72 h later resulted in a generalized blueing of the entire skin when low dilutions of the antiserum

Table I. Effectiveness of mouse antiserum obtained at different times during the course of immunization to induce PCA reactions in mice and rats

Pool	Antisera obtained at	PCA Titer[1] Mice		Rats	
		2 h	72 h	2 h	72 h
Ea I	10 days after 1 antigenic stimulation	80	80	80	80
Ea II	12 days after 1 antigenic stimulation	80	40	40	40
Ea III	1 week after 3 antigenic stimulations	400	100	100	100
Ea X	1 week after 10 antigenic stimulations	800	100	100	100
Ea HH	1 week after 15 antigenic stimulations	1,000	< 100	40	20
Ea 1415	1 week after 16 antigenic stimulations	1,000	< 100	50	10
Ea HL	1 week after 20 antigenic stimulations	1,600	< 100	80	5

[1] Reciprocal of the highest antiserum dilution giving a skin reaction. Each value is the mean of six animals.

were used (< 100) and no localized or generalized blueing when higher (> 100) dilutions were used. Under these circumstances the PCA titer could not be determined (probably due to excess of $\gamma 1$) and so it was assumed to be less than the highest dilution of the antiserum producing completely negative skin reactions after 72 h.

Effect of heating on the homologous and heterologous PCA activity of mouse antiserum. The results of the previous experiments suggested that the antibody responsible for PCA activity of mouse antisera in rats might also be the same antibody responsible for the 72 h PCA in mice. Since it has previously been observed that the antibody responsible for the 72 h PCA in mice is heat labile [18], the rat PCA activity of mouse antisera if due to the same antibody should also be destroyed by heat. Accordingly mouse antisera were heated at 56° C for a time sufficient to abolish the 72 h PCA activity in mice and then tested for PCA activity in rats. In fact, as can be seen in table II heating of mouse antisera completely destroyed their ability to induce PCA in rats in most antisera. However, when hyperimmune antisera were heated different results were obtained when a 2 or 72 h sensitization period was employed. Heating of hyperimmune sera for a time long enough to destroy the highest 72 h homologous PCA activity of an 'early' antiserum was sufficient to destroy the 72 h rat PCA activity of all hyperimmune sera studied. However, heating of the same antisera for a time 4 or 8 times longer never resulted in a complete inactivation of the 2 h rat PCA activity as shown in table II. Nevertheless heating always produced a reduction in the 2 h rat

Table II. Homologous and heterologous PCA activity of mouse antisera before and after heating at 56° C for 60 min

	PCA Titer Mice				PCA Titer Rats			
	2 h		72 h		2 h		72 h	
Pool	Control	Heated	Control	Heated	Control	Heated	Control	Heated
Ea I	80	80	80	0	80	0	80	0
Ea II	80	40	40	0	40	0	40	0
Ea III	400	400	100	0	100	0	100	0
TB 2	400	400	400	0	400	0	400	0
TB 4	200	200	200	0	200	0	200	0
Ea HH[1]	1,000	1,000	–	–	40	5	20	0
Ea 1415[1]	1,000	1,000	–	–	50	5	10	0
Ea HL[1]	1,600	1,600	–	–	80	40	5	0

[1] Antisera heated for an additional 3 h.

PCA activity of these sera as can be seen in the same table. This reduction tended to be greater in those hyperimmune antisera having higher 72 h rat PCA activity.

Effect of absorbing mouse antiserum with rabbit anti-mouse 7Sγl on homologous and heterologous PCA. The known increase of 7Sγ1 antibody after repeated antigenic stimulation [2, 7, 3] probably explains the increase in homologous PCA activity of mouse antisera during the immunization process. Furthermore, since the rat PCA activity of the same antisera decreased during the same process it was assumed that the PCA activity of mouse antisera in rats was probably not due to mouse 7Sγ1. To test this a specific rabbit anti-mouse 7Sγ1 was used. Preliminary experiments were performed to find out the minimal amount of this preparation to completely remove the ability of mouse antiserum to induce PCA after a sensitization period of 2 h. This amount of rabbit anti-mouse γ1 was then used for absorption and the ability of the absorbed sera to induce PCA in rats and mice was then tested. The results of these experiments (table III) showed that absorption of mouse antisera with an amount of rabbit anti-mouse γ1 sufficient to completely abolish the 2 h PCA activity in mice did not decrease either their PCA activity in rats or their 72 h PCA activity in mice. The possibility remained that the mouse serum PCA activity in rats could be due to mouse 7Sγ2 which is responsible for the heterologous PCA activity of mouse antisera in guinea pigs [22, 1]. However, absorption of mouse antisera with rabbit anti-mouse 7Sγ2 did not decrease the PCA activity of these antisera either in mice or rats.

Absorption of hyperimmune serum. Since there was a large difference between the homologous and heterologous PCA activity of hyperimmune sera the absorption experiments with such antisera had to be done using different antisera dilutions for mice and rats. Thus anti-Ea HL (homologous PCA titer 1,600; heterologous PCA titer 80) was diluted 1 to 40 with saline and absorbed with enough rabbit anti-mouse γ1 to cause a 50% decrease in the homologous PCA activity. The PCA activity of the absorbed serum was then tested in mice and rats. The results of this experiment (table IV) show that although absorption with anti-γ1 resulted in a 57% decrease in the homologous 2 h PCA activity, the heterologous PCA activity was increased.

Distribution of the homologous and heterologous PCA activity after Electrophoresis. The PCA activities of the electrophoretic samples obtained from

Table III. Effect of absorbing mouse antiserum with rabbit anti-mouse 7Sγ1 on PCA reactions induced in mice and rats

Anti-serum	PCA Titer[1]					
	Mice 2 h PCA Before absorption	After absorption	72 h PCA Before absorption	After absorption	Rats 2 h PCA Before absorption	After absorption
Ea I	80	0	80	80	80	80
Ea II	80	0	40	40	40	40
Ea III	400	0	100	100	100	100
TB 2	400	0	400	400	400	400
TB 4	200	0	200	200	200	200

[1] Reciprocal of the highest antiserum dilution giving a skin reaction. Each value is the mean of six animals.

Table IV. Homologous and heterologous (rat) PCA activity of mouse hyperimmune serum[2] after absorption with rabbit anti-mouse 7Sγ1 antiserum

Antiserum dilution	Heterologous PCA activity [2 h] Control serum	Absorbed serum	Antiserum dilution	Homologous PCA activity [2 h] Control serum	Absorbed serum
40	15[1]	13	400	15	15
50	12	13	500	13	14
60	±	10	600	12	10
70	0	12	700	11	8
80	0	10	800	12	0
100	0	0	1,300	10	0
200	0	0	1,600	8	0

[1] Diameter of the lesion in mm. Each figure is the mean of 6 animals.
[2] Anti-Ea HL.

Table V. Homologous and heterologous PCA activity of mouse antiserum fractions obtained after 24 h electrophoresis with pevikon and barbital buffer pH 8.6

		Pevikon Block Fractions																													
		-4	-3	-2	-1	1°	2	3	4	5	6	7	8	9	10	11	12	13	14	15	16	17	18	19	20	21	22	23	24	25	26
2 h PCA Early serum (Ea I)	Mouse	O	O	O	O	O	+	+	+	+	+	+	+	+	+	+	+	+	+	+	O	O	O	O	O	O	O	O	O	O	O
	Rat	O	O	O	O	+	+	+	+	+	+	+	+	+	+	+	+	+	+	+	O	O	O	O	O	O	O	O	O	O	O
72 h PCA Early serum (Ea I)	Mouse	O	O	O	O	O	+	+	+	+	+	+	+	+	+	+	+	+	+	+	O	O	O	O	O	O	O	O	O	O	O
	Rat	O	O	O	+	+	+	+	+	+	+	+	+	+	+	+	+	+	+	+	O	O	O	O	O	O	O	O	O	O	O
2 h PCA Hyperimm. serum (Ea X)	Mouse	O	+	+	+	+	+	+	+	+	+	+	+	+	+	+	+	+	+	+	+	+	+	+	+	+	O	O	O	O	O
	Rat	O	O	O	O	+	+	+	+	+	+	+	+	+	+	+	+	+	+	+	O	O	O	O	O	O	O	O	O	O	O
72 h PCA Hyperimm. serum (Ea X)	Mouse	O	O	O	O	O	+	+	+	+	+	+	+	+	+	+	+	+	+	+	O	O	O	O	O	O	O	O	O	O	O
	Rat	O	O	O	O	+	+	+	+	+	+	+	+	+	+	+	+	+	+	+	O	O	O	O	O	O	O	O	O	O	O

1° = Origin.
340 v, 40 mAmps.

early and hyperimmune sera is shown in table V. When 'early' anti-Ea or anti-*Trichinella spiralis* sera were used, both homologous and heterologous PCA activities were present in the same electrophoretic samples extending from the origin up to the 15th fraction. No activity was found in the pre-origin samples. When hyperimmune sera containing reaginic antibody in relatively low levels were used 3 regions could be differentiated as shown in table V. A pre-origin region able to induce 2 h PCA in mice but unable to induce either homologous 72 h PCA or heterologous PCA; an intermediary region extending from the first 0.5 cm after the origin up to the 15th fraction in which both rat and mice activities were found; and a final fast migrating region showing only 2 h homologous PCA activity.

Mast cell changes. Mouse mast cells showed 2 types of alteration after induction of PCA. One type of alteration was represented by granule extrusion similar to that already described in rat anaphylaxis [12]. The other type was characterized by complete loss or great diminution in the staining of the granules. This change was similar to that presented by guinea pig mast cells in anaphylaxis [20]. Both types of changes may be present after induction of PCA when either a 2 or 72 h sensitization period was used. However, in some instances one of these changes would predominate over the other. Whether these differences in mast cell changes are due to different antibodies or to variation in the response of the sensitized cells is not yet known.

Rat mast cells were very efficiently sensitized with mouse antiserum containing reagin-like antibody. Incubation or rat mesenteric mast cells for a few minutes followed by contact with the specific antigen resulted in mast cell damage identical to those presented by these cells after passive anaphylaxis with rat 'mast cell sensitizing' antibody [14]. The ability of mouse antisera to sensitize rat mast cells was completely destroyed by heating and decreased during the course of immunization. Attempts to sensitize rat mast cells with mouse hyperimmune sera resulted in slight or no damage to these cells when they were subsequently incubated with antigen.

Discussion

The term homocytotropic antibody was given by BECKER and AUSTEN [4] to some antibodies capable of transferring PCA to the same species that produce them. In contrast heterocytotropic antibodies are not able to sensitize the same species from which they originate. A typical example of these antibodies is provided by guinea pig 7Sγ1 and 7Sγ2 of which only the first has homocytotropic activity. Although 5 different immunoglobulins are produced by mice [8] only the 7Sγ1 was shown to have homocytotropic activity [22, 1]. However, there was some indirect evidence for the existence of more than one homocytotropic antibody in the mouse. Thus McCAMISH and her colleagues [11] observed 2 distinct phases in active cutaneous hypersensitivity reactions in mice. A transient phase characterized by an immediate edematous response detectable within 6–9 days after a single sensitizing dose of ovalbumin and a later and long lasting phase starting 12 days after sensitization characterized by a response resembling an Arthus reaction. Further indirect evidence also suggesting the existence of an early transient mouse homocytotropic antibody arose from a completely different line of study. PROUVOST-DANON and her collaborators [24] working with isolated mouse peritoneal mast cells observed that the ability of these cells to release histamine upon addition of antigen rose early after immunization and disappeared soon afterwards. Direct evidence for the existence of such an antibody was provided by MOTA and PEIXOTO [18] who were able to detect in serum of mice immunized with a single dose of antigen a skin-sensitizing, long lasting and heat labile antibody that disappeared from about one month after antigen administration. Later these findings were further studied by MOTA [16] who suggested the simultaneous presence of γ1 antibody in mouse early antisera based on the ability of such antisera to produce a heat resistant 4 h PCA in addition to the heat labile 72 h PCA. Furthermore it was suggested that in some cases γ1 was the only PCA antibody present in the antiserum. The presence of a heat labile antibody in mouse early antisera was soon after confirmed by McCAMISH [10] who also indicated that the mouse reagin antibody may or may not occur simultaneously with γ1 antibody. Later these findings were also confirmed by PROUVOST-DANON and collaborators [25] who in addition were able to show the identity between the serum heat labile antibody and the antibody responsible for the early anaphylactic response of mouse peritoneal mast cells.

The mouse reagin-like antibody is of an unknown nature. It was first differentiated from mouse γ1 due to its skin-sensitizing property and its heat lability. Previous attempts to isolate these antibodies by using gradient chromatography on DEAE-cellulose resulted in initial eluates inducing PCA only after 4 h and late eluates inducing PCA after 4 and 72 h [17]. However, whether the PCA activity present in the last eluates was due to one or two antibodies was still undetermined. Our present experiments although resulting in no separation of the two antibodies reinforce our previous conclusion that the 2 h PCA is due to γ1 whereas the 72 h PCA is due to mouse reaginic antibody. Furthermore, they also indicate that the activity of mouse antisera in rats is due to the reagin-like antibody.

As shown in table I the ability of mouse antiserum to induce PCA in rats decreased during the course of immunization whereas its activity in mice increased. This seems to indicate that the mouse antibody able to induce PCA in rats disappeared gradually during the immunization procedure whereas the antibody responsible for PCA reactions in mice increased. The same Table shows that the decrease in the ability of mouse antiserum to transfer PCA to rats parallelled the decrease in the ability of the same antisera to induce homologous PCA after 72 h. This observation added to the fact that heating of mouse antisera suppressed both the ability to induce 72 h PCA reactions in mice and the ability to transfer PCA to rats (table II) also suggested that the mouse antibody responsible for rat PCA is the same one responsible for the 72 h PCA in mice. Furthermore, these same observations indicated that the mouse antibody able to induce PCA reactions in mice after a short sensitization was not capable of inducing PCA in rats. Since there is ample evidence showing that mouse 7Sγ1 is responsible for homologous PCA induced after a short latent period [22, 1] and since mouse 7Sγ1 is known to increase after additional injections of antigen [2, 7, 3] it was considered reasonable to conclude that mouse γ1 was either unable or very inefficient in its ability to transfer PCA to rats. This conclusion is consistent with the results of our experiments showing that absorption of mouse antisera with rabbit antimouse 7Sγ1 completely removed the 2 h homologous PCA activity of mouse antisera without decreasing rat PCA activity. This same result also indicates that mouse 7Sγ1 is not responsible for the homologous 72 h PCA activity of mouse antiserum. The fact that the 2 h PCA titer in mice was not changed by heating whereas the 72 h homologous PCA and the rat activity were both suppressed implies that reagin does not contribute to the 2 h PCA. Thus mouse reagin would behave like rabbit PCA antibody which requires a long sensitization period to produce a PCA reaction [27]. However, this does not necessarily imply that a purified mouse reagin would not be able to induce homologous PCA within a short sensitization period.

The results reported here suggest that PCA reactions induced in rats with mouse antisera may be used as a specific measurement of mouse reagin-like antibody. However, when hyperimmune mouse antisera are used for PCA reactions in rats some discrepancies appear which do not seem to agree with this conclusion (see antisera HH, 1415 and HL in tables I and II). Thus when these antisera were used the 72 h homologous PCA titer was not identical to the 2 h PCA in rats and the 2 h PCA in rats was only partially destroyed by heating. Two facts seem to explain the dissociation between the 2 h PCA in rats and the 72 h PCA in mice in these antisera. On one hand there is a difference in the amounts of reagin and $\gamma1$ antibody present in hyperimmune sera. Consequently injection of the antisera in the level of dilution adequate to show reagin activity results unavoidably in the simultaneous application of high amounts of $\gamma1$ which prevents or masks the reagin activity. In this situation challenge of the animals 72 h later results in a generalized blueing of the skin. On the other hand the 2 h PCA activity of these hyperimmune sera in rats seems to be due to another antibody in addition to the reagin antibody. It is possible that some other mouse antibody present in insufficient amounts in earlier antisera to induce PCA in rats may attain a concentration in hyperimmune sera high enough to sensitize these animals for PCA. This would explain the partial heat resistance of 2 h PCA reactions induced in rats with mouse hyperimmune sera. However, the 72 h PCA induced in rats with these antisera is probalby due to mouse reagin since it is completely abolished by heating. This implies that the 72 h PCA induced in rats with mouse hyperimmune sera is a more specific measure of mouse reagin than the 2 PCA. The heat stable mouse antibody present in hyperimmune sera able to induce 2 h PCA in rats does not seem to be $\gamma1$ antibody for otherwise it would be difficult to explain the increase in rat PCA activity when mouse hyperimmune serum was absorbed with rabbit anti-mouse $\gamma1$ (table IV). This increase may be due to the existence of a possible competition between mouse $\gamma1$ and reagin so that removal of a portion of $\gamma1$ would cause an increase of the reagin PCA activity. However the possibility cannot be ruled out that mouse $\gamma2$ antibody may be the antibody responsible for the 2 h rat PCA activity of mouse hyperimmune antisera. In this case removal of $\gamma1$ could by the same mechanism postulated above result in an increase in the PCA activity of the antiserum after absorption with anti-$\gamma1$.

The fact that mouse early antiserum is very efficient in passively sensitizing rat mast cells and that heating at 56°C results in a complete loss of this ability strongly suggests that the mouse antibody responsible for the sensitization of rat mast cells is the reagin-like antibody. Furthermore the observation that mouse hyperimmune sera is practically devoid of this property also indicates that mouse $\gamma1$ antibody is not able to sensitize the rat mast cell. The preliminary attempts to separate mouse reagin from $\gamma1$ antibody with Pevikon block electrophoresis were not successful as indicated in table V. This seems to indicate that the electrophoretic mobilities of mouse $\gamma1$ and reaginic antibody are very close. We have not yet determined whether the homocytotropic activities present in the pre-origin and in the fast migrating regions are due to the same or 2 different antibodies. Electrophoretic fractions obtained from early antisera and containing rat activity were completely inactivated by heat in contrast to fractions obtained from hyper-immune sera in which only a small amount of activity was heat labile. This confirms our earlier results found with crude serum which suggested that the rat PCA activity in early sera was due primarily to mouse reaginic antibody and that as immunization was continued a stable antibody appeared in sufficient concentration to cause PCA in rats. Further experimental data are required for an adequate interpretation of the serum fractions obtained by block electrophoresis.

Acknowledgments

We thank Dr. J. L. Fahey and Dr. F. Hymes for a generous gift of rabbit anti-mouse immunoglobulin preparations and Dr. E. L. Becker for fruitful discussions during this work. The technical assistance of Mrs. J. Chandler is gratefully acknowledged.

Summary

A study was made of the ability of mouse antisera obtained at different times during the course of immunization with ovalbumin to induce homologous and heterologous (rat) PCA. Antisera obtained from *Trichinella spiralis* infected mice containing high levels of reaginic antibody were also used. The following observations were made: (a) The 2 h homologous PCA activity increased during immunization where as the 72 h homologous and the heterologous PCA activity decreased; (b) in antisera obtained after the initial antigenic stimulations the 72 h PCA titer in mice was the same as the 2 h PCA titer in rats; (c) the 72 h PCA activity in mice and the PCA activity in rats were both heat labile; (d) absorption of mouse early antisera or anti-*T. spiralis* sera with rabbit anti-mouse 7Sγ1 removed the 2 h homologous PCA activity but neither the 72 h homologous PCA nor the heterologous PCA activity was changed; (e) hyperimmune antisera with very high 2 h PCA activity in mice had very low 2 and 72 h PCA activity in rats and very low 72 h PCA activity in mice; (f) the 2 h PCA activity of hyperimmune antisera in rats was partially heat stable whereas the 72 h PCA activity was completely heat labile; (g) absorption of hyperimmune antisera with rabbit anti-mouse γ1 induced a reduction in the 2 h homologous PCA activity and an increase in the heterologous 2 h PCA activity; (h) mouse antisera containing reagin-like antibody were very efficient in sensitizing rat mast cells; (i) this ability was completely destroyed by heating; (j) hyperimmune mouse antisera caused no or very little sensitizing of rat mast cells; (k) pevikon block electrophoresis with barbital buffer pH 8.6 was not able to separate γ1 antibody from the reagin-like antibody.

These results are discussed and the suggestion is made that the 72 h homologous PCA activity and the heterologous activity of mouse early anti-Ea and anti-*T. spiralis* antisera are due to mouse reagin-like antibody. The nature of the heat stable activity of mouse hyperimmune antisera in rats is discussed.

References

1. BARTH, W. F. and FAHEY, J. L.: Heterologous and homologous skin-sensitizing activity of mouse 7Sγ1- and 7Sγ2-globulins. Nature 206: 730 (1965).
2. BARTH, W. F.; McLAUGHLIN, C. L. and FAHEY, J. L.: The immunoglobulins of mice. IV. Response to immunization. J. Immunol. 95: 781 (1965).
3. BAZIN, H.: Les immunoglobulines de la souris. II. Etude des anti-corpes synthétisés dans les différentes classes d'immunoglobulines en réponse à l'injection de deux antigènes protéiques solubles. Ann. Inst. Pasteur 112: 162 (1967).
4. BECKER, E. L. and AUSTEN, K. F.: Anaphylaxis; in Immunopathology. MÜLLER-EBERHARD and MIESCHER, eds. (in press).
5. BOCCI, V.: Protein fractionation by zone electrophoresis on Pevikon C-870. Sci. Tools 11: 7 (1964).
6. CHAFFEE, E. F.; BAUMAN, P. M. and SHAPILLO, J. J.: Diagnosis of schistosomiasis by complement fixation. Amer. J. trop. Med. Hyg. 3: 905 (1954).
7. COE, J. E.: 7Sγ1 and 7Sγ2 antibody response in the mouse. I. Influence of strain antigen and adjuvant. J. Immunol. 96: 744 (1966).
8. FAHEY, J. L.; WUNDERLICH, J. and MISHELL, R.: The immunoglobulins of mice. I. Four major classes of immunoglobulins: 7Sγ2, 7Sγ1, γ1A (2A) and 18Sγ1M-globulins. J. exp. Med. 120: 223 (1964).
9. LOWRY, O. H.; ROSEBROUGH, N. J.; FARR, A. L. and RANDALL, R. J.: Protein measurement with the folin phenol reagent. J. biol. Chem. 193: 265 (1951).
10. McCAMISH, J.: A heat-labile skin-sensitizing activity of mouse serum. Nature 214: 1228 (1967).
11. McCAMISH, J. and BENEDICT, A. A.: Studies on immediate cutaneous hypersensitivity in mice. J. Immunol. 91: 65 (1963).
12. MOTA, I.: Action of anaphylactic shock and anaphylatoxin on mast cells and histamine in rats. Brit. J. Pharmacol. 12: 453 (1957).
13. MOTA, I.: Passive cutaneous anaphylaxis induced with mast cell sensitizing antibody. The role of histamine and 5-hydroxytryptamine. Life Sci. 1: 917 (1963).
14. MOTA, I.: Biological characterization of 'mast cell sensitizing' antibodies. Life Sci. 1: 465 (1963).
15. MOTA, I.: Release of histamine from mast cells; in Hdb. der experimentellen Pharmakologie (Springer, Berlin 1966).
16. MOTA, I.: Biological characterization of mouse 'early' antibodies. Immunology 12: 343 (1967).
17. MOTA, I.: Early mouse homocytotropic antibodies. Fed. Proc. 27: 367 (1968).
18. MOTA, I. and PEIXOTO, J. M.: A skin-sensitizing and thermolabile antibody in the mouse. Life Sci. 5: 1723 (1966).
19. MOTA, I.; SADUN, E. H.; BRADSHAW, R. M. and GORE, R. W.: The immunological response of mice infected with Trichinella spiralis. Biological and physico-chemical distinction of two homocytotropic antibodies. Immunology (in press).
20. MOTA, I. and VUGMAN, I.: Effects of anaphylactic shock and compound 48/80 on the mast cells of the guinea pig lung. Nature 177: 427 (1956).
21. MÜLLER-EBERHARD, H. J.: A new supporting medium for preparative electrophoresis. Scand. J. clin. Lab. Invest. 12: 33 (1960).
22. NUSSENZWEIG, R. S.; MERRYMAN, C. and BENACERRAF, B.: Electrophoretic separation and properties of mouse antihapten antibodies involved in passive cutaneous anaphylaxis and passive hemolysis. J. Immunol. 120: 315 (1964).
23. OVARY, Z.: Passive cutaneous anaphylaxis in the mouse. J. Immunol. 81: 355 (1958).

24. Prouvost-Danon, A.; Lima, M. S. and Javierre, M. Q.: Active anaphylactic reaction in mouse peritoneal mast cells *in vitro*. Life Sci. *5:* 289 (1966).
25. Prouvost-Danon, A.; Peixoto, J. M. and Javierre, M. Q.: Reagin-like mediated passive anaphylactic reaction in mouse peritoneal mast cells *in vitro*. Life Sci. *6:* 1793 (1967).
26. Sadun, E. H.; Mota, I. and Gore, R. W.: Demonstration of homocytotropic reagin-like antibodies in mice and rabbits infected with *Trichinella spiralis*. J. Parasit. *54:* 814 (1968).
27. Zvaifler, N. J. and Becker, E. L.: Rabbit anaphylactic antibody. J. exp. Med. *123:* 935 (1966).

Authors' addresses: I. Mota, M.D., Department of Histology, University of São Paulo, *São Paulo* (Brazil); D. Wong, M.D., E. H. Sadun, M.D. and R. W. Gore, Departments of Immunochemistry and Medical Zoology, Walter Reed Army Institute of Research, *Washington D.C.* (USA).

Cellular and Humoral Mechanisms in Anaphylaxis and Allergy, pp. 37–45
(Karger, Basel/New York 1969)

Induction of Anti-dinitrophenyl Reaginic Antibody in the Atopic Dog[1]

John H. Rockey and Robert M. Schwartzman[2]

Department of Microbiology, School of Medicine and School of Veterinary Medicine,
University of Pennsylvania Philadelphia, Pa.

The atopic dog offers a unique opportunity to study a spontaneous disease process which closely parallels human atopic allergic disease [16, 10, 15] and to characterize the antibodies produced in an atopic animal under a variety of experimental conditions. Atopic canine reaginic (homocytotropic skin-sensitizing) anti-ragweed antibody has been found to be similar to atopic human reaginic antibody in all parameters thus far investigated: the antibodies of both species are capable of sensitizing homologous recipients for cutaneous and systemic anaphylaxis, are incapable of inducing a passive cutaneous anaphylactic (PCA) reaction in the guinea pig, are inactivated by heat and upon exposure to 2-mercaptoethanol, have a rapid electrophoretic mobility and a sedimentation coefficient of approximately 8–9 S, and are recovered upon Sephadex G-200 gel filtration in an intermediate region after the recovery of γM-macroglobulins and polymeric γA-globulins but before the recovery of the 7 S γG-globulins [12, 14]. A number of advantages for antibody purification and for the study of antibody specificity and molecular structure are afforded by antibody directed against small haptenic groupings. A previous attempt to produce homocytotropic skin-sensitizing anti-DNP (2,4-dinitrophenyl) antibody in the non-atopic dog met with only limited success [9]. In the present report we describe the induction of homocytotropic skin-sensitizing anti-DNP antibody in an atopic dog, immunized with dinitrophenylated ragweed pollen, and show that the induced anti-DNP antibody is similar in heat-lability, charge and molecular size to the spon-

[1] This investigation was supported by Public Health Service Research Grants AI–05305 and AI–07512 from the National Institute of Allergy and Infectious Diseases.

[2] Recipient of a Public Health Service Research Career Award (5–K3–AM–16, 606) from the National Institute of Arthritis and Metabolic Diseases.

taneous anti-ragweed homocytotropic skin-sensitizing antibody of the same serum.

Materials and Methods

Preparation of antigens. Canine and equine serum albumins were isolated by Pevikon block zone electrophoresis [7] at 4° in a barbital-buffered solution of $\tau/_2$ 0.05, pH 8. Bovine gamma globulin (Fraction II, Armour Pharmaceutical Co., Kankakee, Illinois) was used as purchased. Short ragweed *(Ambrosia artemisifolia)* pollen was obtained from Hollister-Stiers Laboratories (Spokane, Washington). Sodium 2,4-dinitrobenzenesulfonate (Eastman Organic Chemicals, Rochester, N.Y.) was dissolved in boiling 95% ethanol containing charcoal (Norite A), and recrystalized from the cooled filtrate. The recrystalization was repeated 3 times. Proteins and crude ragweed pollen were dinitrophenylated by the method of EISEN [3]. One g of protein or ragweed pollen and 1 g of potassium carbonate were dissolved or suspended in 50 ml of distilled water. One g of sodium 2,4-dinitrobenzenesulfonate was added and the mixture was stirred overnight at room temperature. The reaction products were dialyzed exhaustively at 4° against distilled water. Soluble antigens were precipitated by adjusting the pH of the solution to 2–3 with 1 N hydrochloric acid. The precipitates were centrifuged, washed twice with 0.25% (v/v) acetic acid, taken up in 0.2 M sodium chloride, 0.01 M sodium phosphate buffer, pH 8, and filtered through columns of Sephadex G-25 in the same solvent. The following dinitrophenylated antigens were prepared: DNP-CA (canine albumin), DNP-EA (equine albumin), DNP-BγG (bovine gamma globulin), and DNP-RWP (ragweed pollen). Antigens were stored at minus 20° until used.

Preparation of DNP-EA-cellulose immunoabsorbent. DNP-EA (equine albumin) was coupled to cellulose by bromoacetyl bromide linkage according to the method of ROBBINS, HAIMOVICH and SELA [13]. Whatman cellulose powder was washed with acetone and distilled water and dried to a constant weight *in vacuo* over phosphorus pentoxide. Bromoacetyl cellulose was prepared by reacting 10 g of cellulose with 75 ml of bromoacetyl bromide (Eastman Organic Chemicals) in a solution of 40 ml of dioxane containing 100 g of bromoacetic acid. The reaction was carried out at room temperature in a closed flask. The hydrobromic acid formed was removed by a continuous stream of dry air admitted through a sodium hydroxide trap and removed through a second sodium hydroxide trap. After 12–24 h, the reaction mixture was cooled and poured slowly into a large volume of distilled water in an ice bath. The bromoacetyl cellulose was washed with distilled water, 0.1 M sodium bicarbonate, again with distilled water, and then suspended in 0.15 M sodium phosphate citrate buffer, pH 3.2. Five hundred mg of DNP-EA was added to 1 g of bromoacetyl cellulose in the above solvent and the suspension was stirred for 48 h at room temperature. The reaction mixture was centrifuged and the precipitate was resuspended in 50 ml of 0.1 M sodium bicarbonate buffer, pH 8.9. The suspension was stirred at 4° for 48 h, centrifuged, and the precipitate resuspended in 0.05 M 2-aminoethanol, 0.1 M sodium bicarbonate buffer, pH 8.9. After remaining for 24 h at 4°, the material was again centrifuged and washed exhaustively with distilled water and 0.15 M sodium chloride, 0.01 M sodium phosphate buffer, pH 8.0. A solution of 8 M urea (3 X recrystalized from ethanol) was prepared and passed over a mixed bed resin (AG 501-X8 (D), Bio Rad Laboratories, Richmond, California) column immediately prior to use, and was used to wash the DNP-EA-cellulose. The immunoabsorbent finally was washed exhaustively with distilled water, and with 0.15 M sodium chloride, 0.01 M sodium phosphate buffer, pH 8. The moist immunoabsorbent (250–500 mg dry weight) was added to 25–50 ml of canine anti-DNP serum. The mixture was incubated at 37° for 1 h and then at 4° for 3 days with constant stirring. The immunoabsorbent was centrifuged, washed exhaustively with 0.15 M sodium chloride, 0.01 M sodium phosphate buffer, pH 8, and anti-DNP antibody then was eluted with 0.1 M 2,4-dinitrophenol in the phosphate buffer of pH 8. The eluted proteins were concentrated by negative pressure ultrafiltration and examined by immunoelectrophoresis.

Immunization. An atopic dog manifesting spontaneous hypersensitivity to short ragweed pollen was exposed to DNP-CA by nebulization at bi-weekly intervals for 32 weeks. The animal then received 10 mg of DNP-RWP in Alginate (Hollister-Stier Laboratories) injected subcutaneously. A non-atopic dog was immunized repeatedly at bi-weekly intervals with 5–10 mg of DNP-BγG suspended in an equal volume of complete Freund's adjuvant (Difco Laboratories, Detroit, Michigan). The animals were bled at weekly intervals after each antigen administration, and the sera were stored either at 4° or at minus 20° until used. Rabbit antisera specific for canine serum proteins were prepared as previously reported [14].

Passive transfer reactions. Canine homocytotropic skin-sensitizing antibody was assayed by the Prausnitz-Küstner (PK) reaction in normal homologous recipients. Dermal sites were sensitized with 0.1 to 0.2 ml of serum or serum fraction and challenged 1–15 days later by intradermal injections of antigen. The dermal reactions were observed for 30 to 60 min after antigen administration and reactions were graded on an arbitrary negative to 4 plus positive scale. Passive cutaneous anaphylactic (PCA) reactions were performed in the guinea pig according to the method of OVARY [8].

Agar electrophoresis. Immunoelectrophoresis was accomplished by the microtechnique as described by HEREMANS [4]. Preparative agar electrophoresis was carried out on immunoelectrophoresis slides as described by OVARY, BLOCH and BENACERRAF [9].

Gel filtration. Canine serum proteins were fractionated at room temperature by filtration through 3 in-series 4 × 60 cm columns of Sephadex G-200 in sterile 0.2 M sodium chloride, 0.002 M ethylenediaminetetraacetic acid (EDTA), 0.01 M sodium phosphate buffer, pH 8. Proteins were passed through a sterile bacterial filter (Swinney Filter, Becton, Dickinson and Co., Rutherford, N.J.) before application to the first column. The column effluent was monitored at 280 mμ, and periodically cultured on blood agar plates to ascertain that gross bacterial contamination had not occurred. Canine γG-globulins were isolated from serum by DEAE (diethylaminoethyl)-cellulose column chromatography [14]. A pathologic human γM-macroglobulin was precipitated from serum by dilution with 15 vol of distilled water, taken up in 0.15 M sodium chloride, subjected to Sephadex G-200 gel filtration and finally to Pevikon block zone electrophoresis. The γG- and γM-globulins were used as standards for the Sephadex G-200 column sets.

Sucrose density gradient ultracentrifugation. Diluted antiserum or a mixture of antisera (0.1–0.2 ml) was layered on a 4.8 ml linear gradient of 10 to 25 % sucrose in 0.2 M sodium chloride, 0.01 M sodium phosphate buffer, pH 8, and centrifuged for 8–15 h in an SW65 swinging bucket rotor at either 50,000 or 65,000 rpm in a Beckman Model L 2-65 ultracentrifuge at 4°. The concentration of protein in the serially-collected fractions from the gradient was determined by measuring the optical density at 280 mμ in microcells (Type 17, 10-mm light path, Precision Cells, Inc., New York, N.Y.) in a Zeiss PMQ II spectrophotometer.

Results

Induction of reaginic anti-DNP antibody. The atopic dog failed to produce passively-transferable homocytotropic skin-sensitizing antibody after repeated exposure to DNP-CA by nebulization. In contrast, two weeks after a single subcutaneous injection of DNP-RWP, the atopic dog serum was capable of transferring a strongly-positive PK reaction to normal canine recipient skin sites. The dermal PK reactions could be elicited in passively-sensitized sites by injecting either DNP-BγG or DNP-CA, but could not be elicited with either bovine gamma globulin or canine albumin alone. The dermal reactions obtained varied widely with different normal canine recipients. The urticarial reactions frequently developed pseudopodia, and in some recipients the acute dermal anaphylactic reactions were extremely large. The reciprocal titer of the skin-sensitizing activity was determined in one recipient, and was found to be 640. The PK activity of sequentially-obtained sera gradually diminished, and activity was absent from serum obtained 6 weeks after the initial DNP-RWP immunization. A second immunization with DNP-RWP again produced a high titer of PK activity in serum obtained 1 week after antigen administration.

The non-atopic dog, repeatedly immunized with DNP-BγG in complete Freund's adjuvant, failed to produce homocytotropic skin-sensitizing anti-DNP antibody.

Duration of dermal sensitization. The duration of fixation of the canine anti-DNP skin-sensitizing antibody to homologous skin sites was determined by injecting serum at dermal sites in 2 normal dogs every other day for 2 weeks. The sites were challenged with DNP-BγG 15 days after the initial serum injection. An immediate urticarial reaction was observed at all sites, including the sites sensitized 15 days previously.

Heat-lability of PK activity. Atopic anti-DNP serum samples from a number of bleedings were heated in a water bath at 56° for 2, 3 and 4 h. The anti-DNP PK activity was destroyed after exposure of sera to 56° for 3–4 h. Exposure of sera to 56° for 2 h resulted in an estimated 60% reduction in PK skin-sensitizing activity. Similar results were obtained when the anti-ragweed PK activity of the same serum was studied.

Electrophoretic mobility of anti-DNP skin-sensitizing antibody. The results obtained upon agar electrophoresis of the atopic canine anti-DNP serum are presented in figure 1. The homocytotropic skin-sensitizing anti-DNP activity had a γ_1 (β) electrophoretic mobility. A similar result was obtained when the electrophoretic distribution of the anti-ragweed skin-sensitizing activity, present in the same serum, was determined.

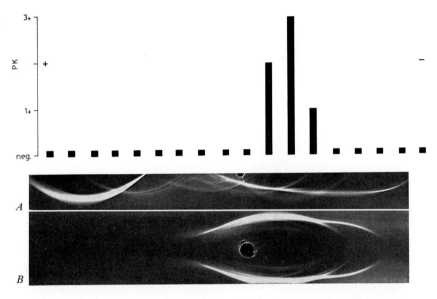

Fig. 1. A. Agar electrophoresis of canine homocytotropic skin-sensitizing anti-DNP serum. The upper half of the agar slide was cut into small fractions, and the proteins in each fraction were eluted with 0.15 M sodium chloride and used for passive transfer reactions. The distribution of the anti-DNP PK activity in the electrophoretic fractions is illustrated in the upper part of figure. The remaining half of the agar slide was developed with rabbit antiserum, prepared against canine serum proteins, and is presented in the lower part of the figure. *B.* Immunoelectrophoresis of anti-DNP antibodies isolated from a non-atopic antiserum, lacking homocytotropic skin-sensitizing antibody activity, by use of a solid immunoabsorbent (DNP-EA-cellulose).

Sucrose Density Gradient Ultracentrifugation. The canine homocytotropic skin-sensitizing anti-DNP antibody sedimented on sucrose density gradient ultracentrifugation in a manner similar to the skin-sensitizing anti-ragweed antibody of the same serum. Both activities sedimented more rapidly than the 7 S γG-globulins of the same serum and the PCA (guinea pig) activity contained in isolated γG-globulins ($s^\circ_{20,w}$ = 6.8 S) from non-atopic canine anti-hemocyanin antiserum [14]. The results of a representative experiment are presented in figure 2. The sedimentation coefficient of the skin-sensitizing antibody was estimated as a linear function of its position in the density gradient, employing canine γG-globulins (6.8 S), canine albumin (4.5 S) and a polymeric canine γA myeloma protein (9.8 S) [14] as reference markers. The homocytotropic skin-sensitizing anti-DNP antibody had a sedimentation coefficient of approximately 8 S.

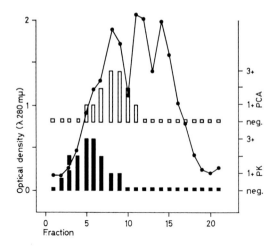

Fig. 2. Sucrose density gradient ultracentrifugation of a mixture of atopic canine anti-DNP serum and the γG-globulins isolated from the serum of a non-atopic dog immunized with hemocyanin [15]. The distribution of the homocytotropic skin-sensitizing anti-DNP antibody activity (PK) and of the anti-hemocyanin PCA (guinea pig) antibody activity in the density gradient fractions is illustrated. The homocytotropic skin-sensitizing activity sedimented more rapidly than the heterocytotropic skin-sensitizing activity.

Sephadex G-200 Gel Filtration. When the atopic canine antiserum containing anti-DNP and anti-ragweed homocytotropic skin-sensitizing antibodies was subjected to Sephadex G-200 gel filtration, both activities were recovered in a similar distribution at a volume greater than those at which γM-macroglobulins and a canine 10 S γA myeloma protein [14] were recovered, but at a volume less than that at which the 7 S γG-globulins eluted. A representative experiment is presented in figure 3.

Anti-DNP antibody of non-atopic serum. Anti-DNP antibody, isolated from non-atopic sera lacking homocytotropic skin-sensitizing activity by use of the DNP-EA-cellulose solid immunoabsorbent, was found to be antigenically heterogeneous when examined by immunoelectrophoresis. These findings are illustrated in the lower portion of figure 1.

Discussion

The immunoglobulins of the dog have been shown to be composed of a number of related, but not identical, classes of protein. PATTERSON and co-

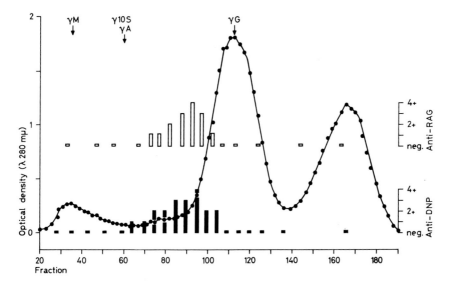

Fig. 3. Sephadex G-200 gel filtration of an atopic canine antiserum, containing both anti-DNP and anti-ragweed (RAG) homocytotropic skin-sensitizing antibody activities. The distribution of the 2 activities in the gel filtration fractions is illustrated. The positions at which γM-macroglobulins (γM), a polymeric canine γA myeloma protein (10 S γA), and canine γG-globulins were recovered from the same 3 (4 × 60 cm) column set also are recorded.

workers have described precipitating canine anti-protein antibodies of low electrophoretic mobility and non-precipitating antibodies of higher electrophoretic mobility [11]. Neither antibody possessed homocytotropic skin-sensitizing activity. Johnson and Vaughan have defined 6 antigenically distinct classes of canine immunoglobulins: 7 S γ_{2a}, 7 S γ_{2b}, 7 S γ_{2c}, 7 S γ_1, Int. S γ_1 and γM [5]. An antibody activity has been identified in each immunoglobulin class [6]. A γ_{2c} canine myeloma protein has been described, and the non-precipitating anti-protein antibody of PATTERSON and co-workers has been shown to be a 7 S γ_1 protein [5]. We have studied a polymeric canine myeloma protein of γ_1 (β) electrophoretic mobility [14] and have classified the protein as a canine γA-globulin on the basis of the following criteria: the myeloma protein consisted of a principal component with a sedimentation coefficient ($s^\circ_{20,w}$) of 9.8 S together with a number of higher polymeric species, and analytical ultracentrifugation of the myeloma serum gave a picture closely similar to that typical for polymeric human γA myeloma proteins; mild reduction and alkylation reduced the polymers to monomers with sedimentation coefficients ($s°_{20,w}$) of 6.8 S; an antigenically related protein was present in higher concentration in colostrum than in serum; the optical rotatory dispersion (ORD) curve of the polymeric canine myeloma protein was similar to the ORD curves of human γA myeloma proteins and lacked the Cotton effect at 240 mμ typical of γG-globulins [2][1]. The Int. S γ_1 protein described by JOHNSON and VAUGHAN also may be the canine equivalent of the γA-globulins of other species [5].

A comparison of the findings of JOHNSON and VAUGHAN [5] with our results for canine anti-ragweed and anti-DNP antibodies indicated that the canine homocytotropic skin-sensitizing (atopic reaginic) antibodies may be physically separated from the 7 S γ_{2a}, 7 S γ_{2b}, 7 S γ_{2c}, 7 S γ_1 and γM proteins either by density gradient ultracentrifugation or by Sephadex G-200 gel filtration. The 7 S γ_{2a}, 7 S γ_{2b}, 7 S γ_{2c} and 7 S γ_1 proteins were recovered in the major second peak on Sephadex G-200 gel filtration [5] in a region which we have found to be devoid of homocytotropic skin-sensitizing antibody activity [14]. The reaginic antibody activity was recovered from Sephadex G-200 columns after the γM-macroglobulins and also after polymeric canine γA proteins [14]. Human atopic reaginic antibody activity has been associated with a unique class of immunoglobulins γE(IgE) [1]. The canine reaginic antibody also may represent a new class of canine immunoglobulin analogous to the human γE protein. We now are employing techniques which have been used successfully to isolate other anti-hapten antibodies with the hope that the canine anti-DNP reaginic antibody may be specifically purified and its immunoglobulin class and molecular structure defined.

Summary

Canine homocytotropic skin-sensitizing anti-DNP (2,4-dinitrophenyl) antibody has been induced in an atopic dog, manifesting spontaneous hypersensitivity to ragweed pollens, by immunization with dinitrophenylated short ragweed pollen *(Ambrosia artemisifolia)*. The induced antibody elicited strongly positive PK reactions in normal canine skin sites, passively sensitized as long as 2 weeks previously, when challenged with either DNP-bovine γG-globulin or DNP-canine albumin. Exposure of the anti-DNP serum to 56° for 4 h destroyed the skin-sensitizing activity. The anti-DNP skin-sensitizing antibody has a γ_1 (β) electrophoretic mobility, and sedimented on sucrose density gradient ultracentrifugation more rapidly than the 7 S γG-globulins, with an approximate sedimentation coefficient of 8 S. The antibody was recovered upon Sephadex G-200 gel filtration in an intermediate region after the canine γM-macroglobulins and a polymeric (10 S) canine

[1] The canine γA myeloma protein and the related proteins in serum and colostrum also were specifically precipitated with a rabbit antiserum prepared against a human γA myeloma protein and absorbed with the serum of an individual lacking γA-globulins.

γA myeloma protein, but before the 7 S γG-globulins. Anti-DNP antibody lacking homocytotropic skin-sensitizing activity has been isolated from non-atopic dogs for comparative studies with the atopic anti-DNP reaginic antibody.

References

1. BENNICH, H.H.; ISHIZAKA, K.; JOHANSSON, S.G.O.; ROWE, D.S.; STANWORTH, D.R. and TERRY, W.D.: Immunoglobulin E. A new class of human immunoglobulin. J. Immunol. *10:* 1143 (1968).
2. DORRINGTON, K.J. and ROCKEY, J.H.: Studies on the conformation of purified human and canine γA-globulins and equine γT-globulin by optical rotatory dispersion. J. biol. Chem. *243:* 6511 (1968).
3. EISEN, H.N.: Preparation of purified anti-2,4-dinitrophenyl antibodies. Methods Med. Res. *10:* 94 (1964).
4. HEREMANS, J.: Les Globulines sériques du système gamma (Arscia S.A., Bruxelles 1960).
5. JOHNSON, J.S. and VAUGHAN, J.H.: Canine immunoglobulins. I. Evidence for six immunoglobulin classes. J. Immunol. *98:* 923 (1967).
6. JOHNSON, J.S.; VAUGHAN, J.H. and SWISHER, S.N.: Canine immunoglobulins. II. Antibody activities in six immunoglobulin classes. J. Immunol. *98:* 935 (1967).
7. MÜLLER-EBERHARD, H.J.: A new supporting medium for preparative electrophoresis. Scand. J. clin. Lab. Invest. *12:* 33 (1960).
8. OVARY, Z.: Immediate reactions in the skin of experimental animals provoked by antibody-antigen interaction. Progr. Allergy vol. 5, p. 459 (Karger, Basel/New York 1958).
9. OVARY, Z.; BLOCH, K.J. and BENACERRAF, B.: Identification of rabbit, monkey, and dog antibodies with PCA activity for guinea pigs. Proc. soc. exp. Biol., N.Y. *116:* 840 (1964).
10. PATTERSON, R.: Investigations of spontaneous hypersensitivity of the dog. J. Allergy *31:* 351 (1960).
11. PATTERSON, R.; PRUZANSKY, J.J. and JANIS, B.: Biologic activity of canine nonprecipitating and precipitating antibody. J. Immunol. *93:* 51 (1964).
12. PATTERSON, R.; TENNENBAUM, J.I.; PRUZANSKY, J.J. and NELSON, V.L.: Canine anti-ragweed serum. Demonstration of 'blocking' activity by *in vivo* and *in vitro* techniques. J. Allergy, vol. 36 p. 138 (Karger, Basel/New York 1965).
13. ROBBINS, J.B.; HAIMOVICH, J. and SELA, M.: Purification of antibodies with immunoadsorbents prepared using bromoacetyl cellulose. Immunochemistry *4:* 11 (1967).
14. ROCKEY, J.H. and SCHWARTZMAN, R.M.: Skin sensitizing antibodies: a comparative study of canine and human PK and PCA antibodies and a canine myeloma protein. J. Immunol. *98:* 1143 (1967).
15. SCHWARTZMAN, R.M. and ROCKEY, J.H.: Atopy in the dog. Arch. Derm. *96:* 418 (1967).
16. WITTICH, F.W.: Spontaneous allergy (atopy) in the lower animal. J. Allergy, vol. 12, p. 247 (Karger, Basel/New York 1941).

Authors' address: JOHN H. ROCKEY, M.D., and ROBERT M. SCHWARTZMAN, V.M.D., Department of Microbiology, School of Medicine and School of Veterinary Medicine, University of Pennsylvania, *Philadelphia, Pa.* (USA).

Cellular and Humoral Mechanisms in Anaphylaxis and Allergy, pp. 46–62
(Karger, Basel/New York 1969)

Skin Sensitizing Antibodies in the Guinea Pig[1]

Karel W. Pondman, H. J. den Harink and L. van Es

Central Laboratory of the Netherlands Red Cross Blood Transfusion Service, Amsterdam
(Director: Prof. Dr. J. J. van Loghem)

The statement has been made that there are only two types of 7 S immuno-globulins produced in the guinea pig after antigenic stimulation [1, 2, 6].

These immunoglobulins have distinct H chain antigenic determinants as well as a different characteristic electrophoretic mobility. By immunoelectro-phoretic analysis of guinea pig antibodies the 7 S immunoglobulins are recognized as fast moving γ_1 and slow moving γ_2 components.

See for instance the study of Nussenzweig and Benacerraf on the properties of guinea pig γ_1 and γ_2 antibodies and antibody fragments with special reference to figure 1 in that publication [4].

We would like to present another view point by discussing some of our experimental data which convinced us that the guinea pig also produces two immunoglobulins other than γ_1 that have an electrophoretic mobility equal to that of γ_1. In this electrophoretically defined area we noted – probably two – immunoglobulins that have H chain antigenic determinants in common with γ_2. These three immunoglobulins nearly always occur simultaneously in our preparations.

Since the capacity to provoke anaphylaxis is believed to be a unique property of the electrophoretically fast moving γ_1 immunoglobulin, it is almost natural that we investigated the anaphylactic properties of accom-panying guinea pig IgG in the γ_1 preparations.

Figure 1 gives an example in precipitation and autoradiography of the antibodies that present themselves in immunoelectrophoresis. The anti-guinea pig precipitation pattern at left shows the presence of γ_1 as well as of γ_2 (note also the presence of an unidentified guinea pig protein above

[1] Supported by financial aid of the Netherlands Organization for the Advancement of Pure Research (ZWO), The Hague, The Netherlands (grant no. 91–5).

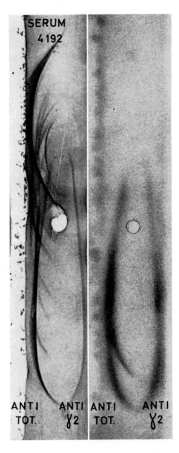

Fig. 1. Guinea pig immunoglobulins bearing antibody activity. At left immunoelectrophoresis of guinea pig anti-insulin serum using rabbit anti-guinea pig serum (extreme left) and rabbit anti-guinea pig IgG γ_2 in right trough. The autoradiogram is made of the same slide after diffusion of I^{131} labeled insulin from the troughs.

the γ_1 precipitation line. The rabbit anti-guinea pig IgG (γ_2) serum made against intact γ_2 globulins precipitates nothing else but IgG. It does not show a distinct difference between γ_1 and γ_2 guinea pig immunoglobulins. The autoradiogram at right of the same slide presents the specific anti-insulin antibodies present in the various immunoglobulin populations. Attention should be paid to the fact that IgG antibody is seen to be accumulated in two spots, in IgG γ_2 and in fast moving antibody of the same immunochemical specificity.

In order to differentiate among the various guinea pig immunoglobulin populations as presented in the previous paper of Dr. BLOCH, we keep to a slightly different nomenclature. We continued to use the original notation for differentiation of IgG into two immunochemical identical populations. These are γ_1 for fast moving IgG and γ_2 for slow IgG. The statement about the H chain differences in electrophoretically fast moving IgG as mentioned above in the introductory note is not yet expressed in this nomenclature. The immunoglobulin with distinct H chain specificity known from the work of BENACERRAF and associates as γ_1 is tagged γ_1A in our work. This serves the purpose of better identification during the following discussions and these labels will be used hereafter.

The next relevant experiment to be quoted here gives information about the antibody specificity of guinea pig immunoglobulins in about 20 sera with reference to the PCA activity of the same sera. The sera were taken from guinea pigs at different times after immunization had started using insulin in incomplete Freund's adjuvants. Variations in immunoglobulin types and concentration bearing anti-insulin specificity were expected.

The results are summarized and tabulated in figure 2. The specific antibody activity was recognized by means of autoradiography, since all guinea

code	duration of immun. in months	gp anti-insulin sera[1] in radio-immunoassay			PCA			comments
		slow IgG	fast IgG[2]	γ_1A[2]	serum	fraction 1	fraction 2	
4192	> 2	+ + +	+ + +	+ + +	+⁺			
500	5	+ + +	+ + +	+	+ +⁺			
65	> 2	+ +	+ +	+	+ + + +	−	+ + +	+ 1/2056
501	12	+ + + +	+ + +	+	+ + + +	−	+ + + +	
4201	> 2	+ +	+	+ + +	−			
4168	1½–2	+ + +	+ + +	+ + +	−			
263	2	−	+ +	+ + +	+ + + +			
14	> 2	+	+ +	*	+ + + +	−	+ + + +	+ 1/1024
516	3/4	+ +	+ +	*	+ + + +			

* = doubtful

[1] Guinea pigs were immunized by weekly injections of 10 U of insulin in incomplete Freund's adjuvants.

[2] Gradient first peak fractions from column chromatographic fractionation of antisera on DEAE cellulose using the method of YAGI et al. [9]; see also fig. 4.

Fig. 2. Immunoglobulins and homologous PCA activity in gp anti-insulin sera.

pig sera contain equally normal levels of precipitating IgG and γ_1A immuno-globulins without specific antibody activity. It was demonstrated here that there exists no correlation between PCA activity and presence or absence of immunoglobulin bearing specific antibody activity. This result becomes manifest from the following observations: It is shown that some of the guinea pig sera that are very weak in γ_1A antibody contents, give excellent PCA activity up to a serum dilution of 1 over 1024 (serum no. 14). Compare this with an anti-insulin serum of equal sensitivity in PCA having much more antibody activity in γ_1A (serum no. 65). Serum 516 of which the antibody activity in γ_1A is doubtful is also giving a strong anaphylactic response in guinea pig skin.

In addition there are anti-insulin sera shown with strong antibody activity in γ_1A as well as in IgG γ_1, that do not elicit skin anaphylaxis.

Since there is no correlation between PCA and γ_1A activity it seems likely that the PCA activity is a function of another immunoglobulin.

Figure 3 reproduces examples of the sera discussed above thereby demonstrating the specific antibody contents by means of autoradiography with I^{131} labeled insulin and antiguinea pig serum.

Actually all of the sera shown here are weak in γ_1A antibody concentration; this point can be verified by re-examination of the autoradiogram of antiserum 4192, in figure one, a typical example, which shows strong insulin binding in γ_1A immunoglobulin.

Of the sera 14 and 516 with excellent PCA the antibody activity in γ_1A is doubtful.

Not relevant for the discussion but an interesting observation is the absence of γ_2 antibody specificity in an antiserum of early bleeding, no. 263.

In the next series of experiments we shall describe the purification procedures used and the results obtained to date. In early work isolating the antibodies with DEAE cellulose in Tris phosphate buffer we obtained data that – serving as representative information – are graphically reproduced in figure 4.

This demonstrates that with the chromatography method used in our work we separated from the guinea pig anti-insulin serum slow and fast moving immunoglobulins containing specific antibody. The immuno-electrophoretic identification of the charge characteristic is noted in figure 5.

The first eluate, obtained before the salt/pH-gradient is started, is noted to be homogeneous. This contains the complement binding and electro-phoretically slow moving guinea pig IgG population with anti-insulin spec-ificity. The fast moving immunoglobulins that are distributed in the second protein peak are shown here already to form a rather inhomogeneous mixture of specific antibodies. There are actually two protein maxima under the gradient each containing specific antibody. Since the first protein peak of these fast moving immunoglobulins contains most antibody that has the capacity to elicit homologous PCA with antigen, we went into eleborate experimental work to isolate and define immunochemically the immunoglobulin types bearing this capacity. As was already demonstrated before, the antibody in this fraction did not bind complement [8]. The CH_{50} titer did not decrease in ordinary complement binding tests. By means of the C_2 titration technique of AUSTEN and associates [0], there was no significant uptake of complement indicated. Finally, using pancreatic cells, fast moving

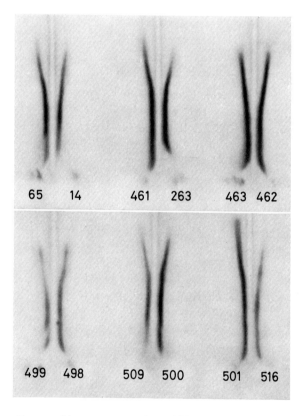

Fig. 3. Autoradiogram of immune sera against rabbit anti-guinea pig serum fortified with radiolabeled insulin using the isotope I^{131}, 1 atom per insulin molecule and adding 100.000 counts/min to the troughs.

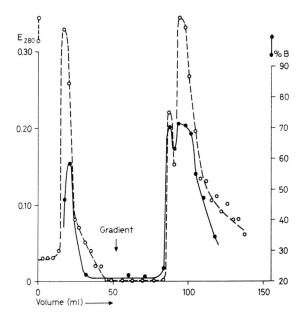

Fig. 4. Chromatographic isolation of anti-insulin antibodies on DEAE cellulose, Eastman Kodak type, in Tris-phosphate buffer. The method used is described in [9]. Specific activity (–––) as well as protein (————) is recorded. For detailed information see [8].

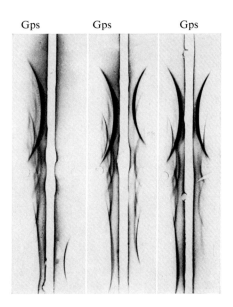

Fig. 5. Immunoelectrophoresis against rabbit anti-guinea pig serum of purified guinea pig IgG γ_2 (left side), proteins of first antibody protein maximum (center slide) containing PCA active antibody and second antibody protein maximum (right slide). Left side of each slide shows immunoprecipitation pattern of normal guinea pig serum.

antibody and serum complement no fluorescence appeared upon addition of fluorescent anticomplement serum. The experimental results to be demonstrated next serve to show the protein and immunoglobulin composition of the peak fractions isolated as discussed above. Figure 5 is a composition of three immunoelectrophoresis slides. Each slide shows the immunoprecipitation pattern of guinea pig serum on the left side. Rabbit anti-guinea pig serum is in the troughs. Again the IgG γ_2 is presented as a homogeneous population of guinea pig immunoglobulins.

The column eluate with PCA active anti-insulin antibodies is shown to contain two immunoglobulins. It was established that one of these is a fast moving IgG, the other being identified as γ_1A. Both of these two immunoglobulins contained antibody activity as was concluded from autoradiography with radiolabeled antigen.

In further experiments the polyacrylamide gel electrophoresis technique was used in efforts to separate the mixture of fast moving immunoglobulins. A typical result is noted in figure 6. It was noted that the PCA activity is a

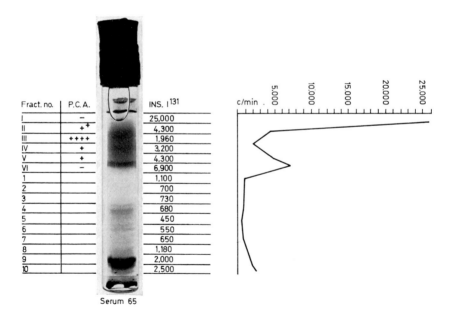

Serum 65

Fig. 6. Localization of PCA active antibody in electrophoretically fast moving antibody protein, first gradient peak protein shown in fig. 4 and 5. Main contaminant is albumen in fractions IX and X that also carries radioactivity aspecifically.

property of only a small portion of immunoglobulins, located at an intermediate electrophoretic position within the area shown to contain specific antibody. More than one amido black stained protein band can be noted in this immunoglobulin area. The specific activity curve also demonstrates that there is more than one population of specific antibody present. The PCA activity is maximal in eluates of gel cut no. III which binds a minimum of antigen as is noted in the accompanying curve covering the amount of radioactive insulin bound in the antibody fraction. Since data on radioactive counts of gel cuts were obtained by incubation of the whole gel after electrophoresis with radioactive insulin and subsequent washing of the gel, it might well be that this curve expresses the binding force between antigen and antibody and that the PCA activity is retained in a low avidity antibody.

At least of equal interest in this respect is the experimental result noted in figure 7, which has been designed to isolate and identify the PCA active antibody. The insulin binding capacity of acrylamide fractions is noted. Also shown in this figure is the immunoglobulin precipitation pattern, simultaneously with the localization of specific antibody in autoradiography. The fraction used in acrylamide gel electrophoresis is peak protein that does not contain IgG γ_2, the first peak under the gradient shown earlier in this work in figure 4. PCA activity is present in eluates of segment III, all other fractions being devoid of skin sensitizing capacity. The PCA active antibody is once again associated with relatively low binding capacity. Once more is shown the intermediate position of skin sensitizing antibodies among the entire population of specific antibodies. Disregarding at this moment the immunoglobulin specificity of the anaphylactic antibody it looks as if this biological property belongs to only as small portion of the entire antibody population of the immunoglobulin in question.

Description of the immunoglobulin specificity with antibody activity in the conjunction with skin sensitizing capacity is the result of experiments of which a typical one is given in figure 8.

Using the method of LEVY and SOBER [3] slightly modified with the pH of the starting buffer changed to 8.5 in chromatographic isolation of guinea pig antibodies on DEAE cellulose we obtained antibody containing fractions of which the immunoglobulin composition is given. $\gamma_1 A$ antibody activity of the colum fractions is noted in the autoradiogram at left together with the IgG subpopulations present in the same fractions at the right side in this figure.

Shown is the presence of strong $\gamma_1 A$ antibody activity in one fraction (fraction 47) that is inactive in PCA.

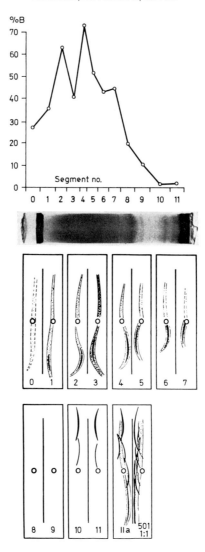

Fig. 7. Localization of PCA active antibody in electrophoretically fast moving antibody protein simultaneously with insulin binding curve and distribution of immunoglobulins in eluates of the acrylamide gel cuts. Insulin binding is expressed in % bound versus free antibody according to YALOW and BERSON [10]. Numbers of autograms refer to gel cut numbers. Last slide shows original fast moving antibody protein fraction (left). Right pattern is antiserum from which the antibody fractions are derived.

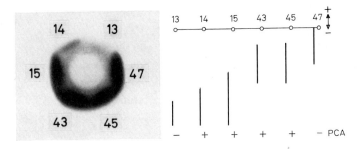

Fig. 8. Autoradiographic representation of γ_1A anti-insulin antibody simultaneously with graphic representation of IgG of various electrophoretic mobility and PCA activity. Numbers refer to eluates from DEAE cellulose column chromatographic isolation of guinea pig antibodies. At left anti γ_1A + Insulin S^{125} in centerwell.

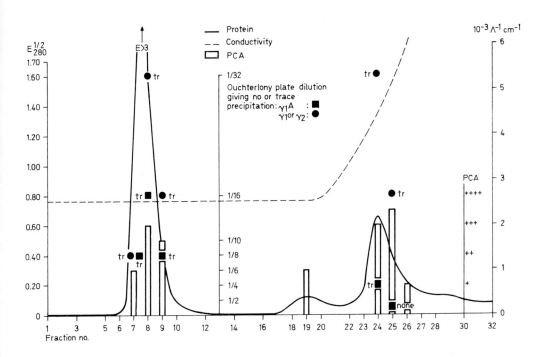

Fig. 9. Isolation of guinea pig antibodies on carboxymethyl cellulose type Serva Heidelberg. Starting buffer 0.01 M NaH_2PO_4 pH 6.8; gradient buffer 0.25 M NaH_2PO_4 + 0.1 M NaCl, pH 7.2. Gradient: 300 ml starting buffer and dropwise addition of gradient buffer. Column size 20/1.5 cm using 1½ ml of dialyzed immune serum.

Demonstrated is further that extremely fast moving IgG also present in this fraction 47 does not bear skin sensitizing capacity either.

Fraction 14, showing only very low antibody activity in γ_1A comparable to 0.5γ of antibody protein, provokes an anaphylactic response in guinea pig skin.

Examination of the fast moving immunoglobulin protein patterns shows that all PCA positive fractions contain medium speed moving IgG.

If γ_1A is really homogeneous with respect to its biological properties it is clear from this experiment that this immunoglobulin does not mediate skin anaphylaxis.

Further attempts to localize and identify the PCA active antibody are shown in the next figure 9. This is an experiment the results of which were obtained using carboxymethyl cellulose as an adsorbent for isolation of antibodies from guinea pig anti-insulin serum. Shown is that the PCA active antibodies appear in two populations with different binding capacity as characterized by the conductivity of the buffer with which the proteins are removed from the cellulose.

The immunoglobulins in the PCA active fractions are γ_1 and γ_1A on the left side and medium speed IgG at right together with IgG γ_2.

The fractions are checked on the immunoglobulin contents by serial dilutions in Ouchterlony plates. This way is demonstrated that fraction 25 with none or virtually no γ_1A is very active in PCA showing that the medium speed Ig is bearing the capacity to sensitize guinea pig skin. The amount of γ_1A in this fraction is calculated to be less than $0.1\ \gamma$ antibody protein.

The PCA active eluates from the CMC isolated guinea pig immune serum were tested for the heat stability of the anaphylactic antibody.

While in earlier work PCA active antibody in guinea pig serum withstood an incubation period of 24 hours at $56°C$, all active column fractions in this case were warmed up to $56°C$ and left for 2 hours at that temperature. There was no change in the ability to sensitize the skin of any of the fractions. Using a four hour lag time period in demonstrating the skin sensitizing capacity of the guinea pig antibodies the anaphylactic antibodies were shown to be heatstable in the homologous skin test.

In the experiment to be described next we attempted again to define the PCA active antibody. A different column chromatographic method in isolating the guinea pig antibodies was used. Figure 10 is the first of a series of figures representing the results obtained using a discontinuous gradient system and Cellex type of DEAE cellulose.

Using 6 Tris-phosphate buffers of increasing molarity and decreasing pH, essentially the same buffer system as used in the column chromatography experiments described in the first paragraph of this paper, we prepared eleven pool fractions, combined as noted in figure 10. These fractions were investigated with respect to immunoglobulin composition and concentration, to specific antibody contents and capacity to provoke anaphylaxis. The location in the effluent of PCA active antibody is already indicated in the protein elution pattern.

The specific antibody contents is demonstrated in figure 11. This is an autoradiograph of the pool fractions I thru XI using radiolabeled antigen (insulin I[125]) together with rabbit anti-guinea pig serum in the troughs.

The result notes the sole presence of guinea pig γ_2 anti-insulin in the first four fraction pool and immunoglobulins bearing anti-insulin specificity of increasing electrophoretic mobility in the later pool fractions.

The presence in type and concentration of immunoglobulin together with the location and magnitude of PCA is tabulated in figure 12. The

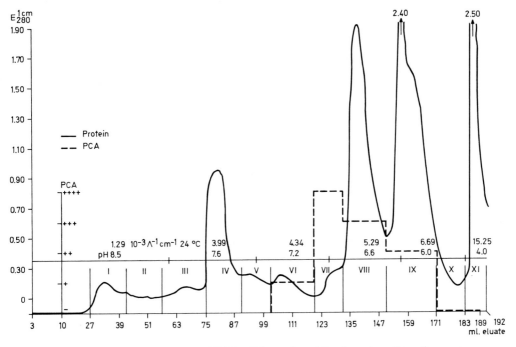

Fig. 10. Fractionation on Cellex DEAE cellulose of pool I guinea pig anti-insulin serum in discontinuous gradient system with Tris-phosphate buffers (# LE 229).
protein: ⎯⎯⎯
Localization of PCA activity: ⎯ ⎯ ⎯

Buffers were prepared by mixing starting buffer of pH 8.5 and gradient buffer of pH 4 until the desired pH value was reached.

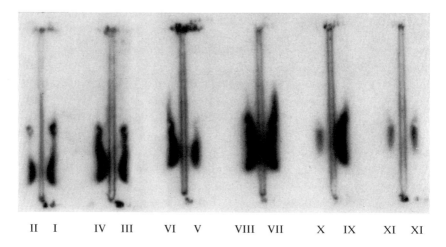

II I   IV III   VI V   VIII VII   X IX   XI XI

Fig. 11. Autoradiogram of immunoglobulin fraction pools I–XI from experiment of fig. 10, using anti-guinea pig serum and insulin I^{125} (# LE 229).

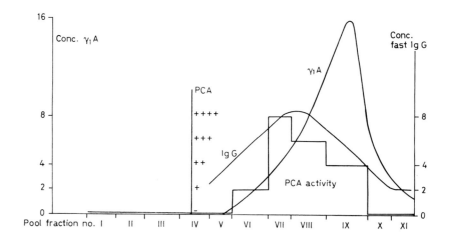

Fig. 12. PCA activity in relation to the concentration of fast IgG and γ_1A. The immunoglobulin concentration given is the serial fraction dilution giving minimal precipitation in Ouchterlony plates with specific anti-immunoglobulin sera. The fraction numbers refer to the fraction pools from experiment reproduced in fig. 10. Fraction XI contains sufficient anti-insulin antibody to give PCA activity if there were antibodies bearing sites for sensitization.

immunoglobulin concentration was estimated in Ouchterlony plates, noting the dilution of minimal precipitation from serial fraction dilutions around a single central well containing specific anti-guinea pig IgG γ_2 and anti-guinea pig γ_1A sera.

This experimental result serves to prove that maximal PCA is located somewhere in the IgG population near maximal IgG γ_1 concentration, while the anaphylactic response rapidly decreases with concomitant decrease of this immunoglobulin concentration. The PCA active antibody concentration is in full return while γ_1A immunoglobulins still rise to their maximum. The main point is the evidence that the skin sensitizing capacity resides with IgG γ_1 or with other antibody type, not with γ_1A.

The next two figures 13 and 14 are Ouchterlony plates demonstrating the specificity of the immunoglobulins present in the pool fractions. Figure 13 shows the presence of γ_1A using a rabbit anti-guinea pig immunoglobulin serum[2] which we had previously absorbed with purified guinea pig γ_2. Noted is the presence of γ_1A in the fractions VI, VII, VIII, IX and XI; IgG γ_2 (in fraction I) is not precipitated as expected.

Figure 14 demonstrates the results obtained when using the same fractions and L chain absorbed rabbit anti-guinea pig IgG γ_2 made against native γ_2. Noted is the presence of two immunoglobulins in the pool fractions containing electrophoretically fast moving immunoglobulins, id est the fractions VII, VIII and IX. One of the two precipitation lines of fraction VII merges with γ_2 in fraction I. IgG γ_2 cross reacts with the immunoglobulin precipitated nearest to the center well. The suggestion is further that this immunoglobulin lacks certain H chain antigenic determinants of γ_2. The anti-γ_2 has never caused γ_1A to precipitate and therefore the second precipitation line probably represents an immunoglobulin of the IgG category. Since the antiserum used is prepared by immunization with native IgG γ_2, the L chain absorbed antiserum may however lack antibodies characteristic for the H chain of this new immunoglobulin.

There is some evidence that γ_1A and γ_2 have antigenic determinants of the Fd fragment of the heavy chain in common [5]. This has not yet been proven for IgG γ_1. While it is unlikely that the L chain absorbed anti-γ_2 contains sufficient antibodies against antigenic determinants of the Fd fragment of the heavy chain, experiments are being made to eliminate the possibility that these anti Fd antibodies cause precipitation of IgG γ_1 and γ_1A.

    [2] We gratefully acknowledge the gift of the rabbit anti-immunoglobulin serum used in this experiment from Dr. G. J. THORBECKE.

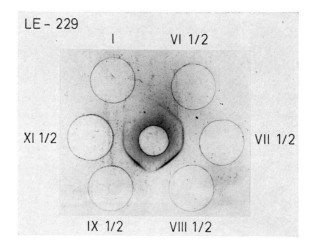

Fig. 13. Ouchterlony plate showing immunoglobulin precipitation in fraction pools of column chromatography experiment of fig. 10. Shown is the γ_1A activity of the fraction pools (#LE 229). Antiserum in central well is anti-immunoglobulin serum absorbed with pure IgG γ_2. Fraction pool I that contains IgG γ_2, guinea pig IgG γ_2 is used as a control.

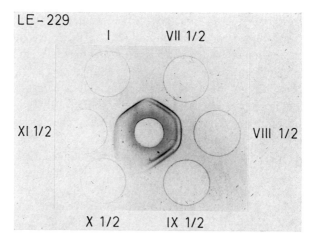

Fig. 14. Ouchterlony plate showing immunoglobulin precipitation in fraction pools of column chromatography experiment of fig. 10. Shown is the IgG activity of the fraction pools (# LE 229). Antiserum in central well is rabbit anti-guinea pig IgG γ_2 serum absorbed with guinea pig L chains obtained from IgG γ_2.

Renewed definition of the IgG γ_1 molecules is necessary since there are shown to be two types which crossreact with each other, while one of these does not differ antigenically from guinea pig IgG γ_2.

In return now to the question again about the specificity of the anaphylactic antibody.

Precise information about the molecular structure of the anaphylactic group in the antibody molecule is not available. While it seems accepted that antibody is homogeneous with respect to its biological properties, this is by no means proven. It may be that the capacity to elicit an anaphylactic response is reserved for a restricted population of immunoglobulin molecules that are immunochemically indistinguishable with the present means. The most acceptable alternative hypothesis is that the capacity to sensitize homologous skin remains a property of a unique heat stable immunoglobulin an anaphylactic, homocytotropic antibody which espaces detection by means of the antisera used in this work.

References

0. AUSTEN, F. K.; BEER, F.: The measurement of second component of human complement (C′2^{h4}) by its interaction with EAC′la^{9p}, 4^{9p} cells. J. Immun. 92: 946–957 (1964).
1. BENACERRAF, B.; OVARY, Z.; BLOCH, K. J. and FRANKLIN, E. C.: Properties of guinea pig 7S antibodies. I. Electrophoretic separation of two types of guinea pig 7S antibodies. J. exp. Med. 117: 937–949 (1963).
2. BLOCH, K. J.; KOURILSKY, F. M.; OVARY, Z. and BENACERRAF, B.: Properties of guinea pig 7S antibodies. III. Identification of antibodies involved in complement fixation and hemolysis. J. exp. Med. 117: 965–981 (1963).
3. LEVY, H. B. and SOBER, H. A.: A simple chromatographic method for preparation of gamma globulin. Proc. Soc. exp. Biol. and Med. 103: 250–252 (1960).
4. NUSSENZWEIG, V. and BENACERRAF, B.: Studies on the properties of fragments of guinea pig γ_1 and γ_2 antibodies obtained by papain digestion and mild reduction. J. Immunol. 93: 1008–1014 (1964).
5. NUSSENZWEIG, V. and BENACERRAF, B.: Presence of identical antigenic determinants in the Fd fragments of γ_1- and γ_2-guinea pig immunoglobulins. J. Immunol. 97: 171–176 (1966).
6. OVARY, Z.; BENACERRAF, B. and BLOCH, K. J.: Properties of guinea pig 7S antibodies. II. Identification of antibodies involved in passive cutaneous and systemic anaphylaxis. J. exp. Med. 117: 951–964 (1963).
7. PONDMAN, K. W.; VAN ES, L. and SCHUURS, A.: The relationship between complement, the heterogeneity of antibody and anaphylaxis. Proc. 10th Congr. int. Soc. Blood Transf., Stockholm 1964, pp. 825–828 (1965).
8. SCHUURS, A. H. W. M.; VAN ES, L. and PONDMAN, K. W.: Separation of skin-sensitizing and complement-fixing antibodies from guinea pig anti-bovine insulin sera. Int. J. Immunochem. 2: 67–70 (1965).

9. YAGI, Y.; MAIER, P. and PRESSMAN, D.: Two different anti-insulin antibodies in guinea pig antisera. J. Immunol. *89:* 442–451 (1962).
10. YALOW, R. S. and BERSON, S.: Immuno assay of endogenous plasma insulin in man. J. clin. Invest. *39:* 1157–1175 (1960).

Authors' address: KAREL W. PONDMAN, Ph.D., H. J. DEN HARINK and L. VAN ES, Central Laboratory of the Netherlands Red Cross Blood Transfusion Service, *Amsterdam* (The Netherlands).

Cellular and Humoral Mechanisms in Anaphylaxis and Allergy, pp. 63–89
(Karger, Basel/New York 1969)

Characterization of Human Reaginic Antibodies and Immunoglobulin E[1]

KIMISHIGE ISHIZAKA

Children's Asthma Research Institute and Hospital, Denver, Col.

Since PRAUSNITZ and KÜSTNER discovered reaginic activity in atopic patients' sera, the nature of the skin-sensitizing antibody has been studied by many investigators using various fractionation methods such as electrophoresis, ion exchange chromatography and ultracentrifugation. In summarizing the findings obtained by the previous investigators (cf. 29), it is apparent that the reaginic antibody is not present in the major components of either γG or γM.

After the third major class of human immunoglobulins, namely γA, was isolated and characterized, evidence has been accumulated which supports the concept that reaginic antibodies may belong to γA immunoglobulin class. For example, HEREMANS and VAERMAN [5] prepared γA globulin fraction from atopic patients' sera and detected reaginic activity in it. FIREMAN, VANNIER and GOODMAN [4] precipitated γA from atopic patients' sera and found that reaginic activity was precipitated as well. In our laboratory, attempts were made to block passive sensitization with reaginic antibody by immunoglobulins of different classes and the results indicated that normal γA fraction but neither γG nor γM fraction blocked the passive sensitization [13]. Finally, YAGI et al. [35] detected γA antibody against ragweed allergen in patients' sera. These findings strongly supported the concept that reaginic antibodies are γA. However, some findings obtained in several places could not be explained by the γA globulin hypothesis. For example, we have been studying on human γA antibody against blood group A substance and found that this γA antibody did not give P-K reactions even with 1μg antibody. So, we went over the previous experiments by others as well as those by our-

[1] This work was supported by Research Grants AI-04985 from the U.S. Public Health Service and GB-4646 from the National Science Foundation.

Table I. Lack of correlation between reaginic antibody and known immunoglobulins

---

1. Lack of parallelism between reaginic activity and γA globulin concentration in chromatographic fractions
2. The reaginic activity is not coprecipitated with any of the γG-anti-γG, γA-anti-γA, γM-anti-γM or γD-anti-γD precipitate
3. γA globulin in fraction contained reaginic activity but the antibody remained in the supernatant after the precipitation of γA globulin
4. Normal γA but not myeloma γA blocked passive sensitization
5. γA antibody in patients' sera did not correlate with reaginic activity

---

selves. The results are summarized in table I. When atopic patients' sera were fractionated by DEAE cellulose column chromatography and gel filtration, the distribution of reaginic activity failed to correlate with γA globulin concentration in the fractions [7]. Similar results were obtained by Perelmutter *et al.* [25] as well as by Reid and Farr [26] in the fractionation under different conditions. Furthermore, reaginic antibodies in atopic patients' sera were not precipitated by anti-γA antibody in our hands [7]. As reported previously [1, 5, 33], reaginic activity was detected in γA globulin fraction of patients' sera and the γA antibody against allergen was detected by radioimmunodiffusion [35]. When anti-γA antibody was added to the fraction, however, γA antibody to ragweed allergen was precipitated, leaving essentially all reaginic activity in the supernatants [18]. It was also found that normal γA fraction blocked passive sensitization whereas A myeloma proteins did not [8]. These observations eliminated the evidence which supported the γA globulin hypothesis. It was also found that reaginic activity in the active fractions was not precipitated by any of the antibodies specific for γG, γM or γD [7, 17, 19] and suggested the possibility that the reaginic activity is associated with a unique immunoglobulin which is different from the 4 known immunoglobulins with respect to antigenic structure.

A. Detection and Characterization of Immunoglobulin E.

In order to prove this hypothesis, we have tried to prepare rabbit antibody which reacts with the carrier of reaginic activity [14, 15]. A rabbit was immunized with a reagin-rich fraction from atopic patients' serum and antiserum was absorbed with normal γG, and A and D myeloma proteins. The supernatant did not give any precipitin band with the four immunoglobulins but gave a γ_1 precipitin band with a reaginrich fraction in immunoelectrophoresis, and the γ_1 precipitin band combined radioactive antigen as shown in the radioautograph (fig. 1 a, b). As the protein forming the γ_1 precipitin band was different from the known immunoglobulins with respect to antigenic structure and possess antibody activity, we tentatively called this protein γE globulin. In fact, the antiserum specific for γE globulin precipitated reaginic activity against ragweed, grass pollen, egg and horse dander in 20 atopic patients' sera so far tested. It was also found that the presence of γE antibodies correlated with the skin-sensitizing activity of atopic patients' sera. As shown in figure 2a, 4 patients' sera having reaginic activity against purified ragweed allergen showed radioactive γE band, whereas the two sera lacking reaginic activity did not.

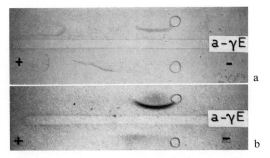

Fig. 1. Radioimmunoelectrophoresis of a reagin-rich fraction. Both the stained slide (a) and the radioautograph (b) are shown. Antibody trough was filled with anti-γE serum. A γ_1 (γE) precipitin band combined radioactive antigen.

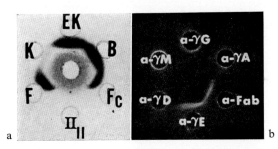

Fig. 2. Radioimmunodiffusion analyses of reaginic sera and a γE fraction. The center well in (a) was filled with a mixture of anti-γE and radioactive antigen E and peripheral wells were filled with reaginic sera. K and II_{11} did not contain reaginic antibody against antigen E. (b) Radioimmunodiffusion of γE fraction placed in the center well. Peripheral wells were filled with the antisera specific for one of the 5 immunoglobulin classes (γG, γA, γM, γD and γE) and the antibody against F_{ab} portion of γG (anti-F_{ab}). After washing, the slide and peripheral wells were filled with radioactive antigen E.

When the patients' sera were fractionated by DEAE cellulose column chromatography and analyzed by gel filtration, sucrose density gradient ultracentrifugation and gel electrophoresis, distribution of reaginic activity paralleled that of γE antibody which was determined by radioimmunodiffusion[15]. No correlation was obtained between the reaginic activity and either γG or γA antibody. Based on these results, attempts were made to purify γE globulin in patients' sera (table II). The sera were fractionated successively by DEAE cellulose chromatography, recycling gel filtration and DEAE Sephadex column chromatography. On a weight basis, reaginic activity in the most active fraction obtained was 150 to 200 times more active than the original serum. However, the fraction still contained γG and γA. These proteins were then absorbed with purified rabbit antibodies specific for the immunoglobulins. In order to avoid contamination with rabbit γ-globulin, the rabbit antibodies were precipitated with goat antibody specific for F_c portion of rabbit γG and the precipitates were added to the reagin-rich fractions. By this procedure, almost all γG and γA were removed leaving reaginic activity in the supernatants. On a weight basis, the final preparation was about 1,000 times more active than the original serum. Only 0.0001 μgN of the preparation gave positive Prausnitz-Küstner reactions and the P-K titer of the preparation was 1:80,000. When the preparation was analyzed by radioimmunodiffusion (fig. 2b), the preparation contained only γE antibody but none of the γG, γA, γM or γD antibody. As will be discussed later, the radioactive band formed by anti-F_{ab} antibody is due to the presence of light chains in γE globulin. Furthermore, both the γE antibody and reaginic activity in the preparation was removed by anti-γE. These results show that γE antibodies have skin-sensitizing activity [9].

In the course of this work, we have postulated that γE globulin is a unique immunoglobulin. More detailed antigenic structure of the protein

Table II. Purification of reaginic antibodies

Procedure	Fraction	Protein concentration mgN/ml	Minimal dose for P-K $\times 10^{-2}$ μgN
None	serum	13.5	9
DEAE cellulose	11	7.0	1
Gel filtration	11_{21}	2.1	0.35
DEAE Sephadex	B	0.44	0.06
Specific absorption	B_{ab}	0.16	0.01

was studied after identification of the protein as a carrier of reaginic activity. First of all, γE globulin possesses antigenic determinants present in κ and λ light chains (fig. 3). The top of this slide shows γE precipitin band formed between a reagin-rich fraction and anti-γE antibody. If one applied radioactively labeled anti-κ antibody to the antibody trough, the radioactive antibody was combined to the γE precipitin band. The combination of the radioactive antibody was blocked by pretreating the slide with cold anti-κ antibody but not with anti-λ antibody. Similarly radioactive anti-λ antibody was specifically combined to the γE precipitin band [19].

It was also found that γE globulin does not have a major antigenic determinant in the known immunoglobulins. When γE fraction from an atopic patient's serum was placed in an Ouchterlony plate against antibodies specific for each immunoglobulin class, only the anti-γE antiserum gave a precipitin band and the precipitin band combined radioactive allergen in the radioautograph of the plate (fig. 4 a, b). Thirdly, the antigenic determinant responsible for the γE precipitin band is not shared by any of the immuno-

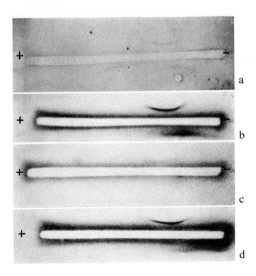

Fig. 3. Radioimmunoelectrophoresis showing the presence of light chains in γE. Both stained slide (top) and radioautographs (a, b, c) are shown. After the γE precipitin band developed, the slides were washed and each slide was treated with normal rabbit serum (a), unlabeled anti-κ (b) or anti-λ antibody (c) followed by application of radioactive anti-κ antibody. The radioactive antibody combined with the γE precipitin band (a, c) and the combination was blocked by unlabeled anti-κ antibody (b).

globulins of known classes and subclasses (fig. 4c, d). In the Ouchterlony plates, monospecific anti-γE antiserum was placed in the center well. The antiserum gave a single precipitin band of identical specificity with the whole serum and γE containing fraction but failed to react with the myeloma proteins of 4 γG subclasses, 3 γA subclasses, γD and γM macroglobulin. The results of antigenic analysis of the γE globulin indicate that γE globulin is composed of light chains common to other immunoglobulins and heavy chains having characteristic antigenic determinants [19]. The protein does not possess any of the antigenic determinants in heavy chains of other immunoglobulins. This information together with the fact that γE globulin has antibody activity is sufficient to conclude that γE globulin represents a distinct immunoglobulin class.

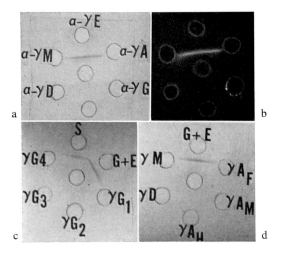

Fig. 4. Antigenic analysis of γE. (a) A γE fraction of a reaginic serum was placed in the center well against the antisera specific for the 5 immunoglobulins placed in peripheral wells. Only the anti-γE serum gave a precipitin band with the fraction. The slide was washed and radioactive antigen E was applied to peripheral wells. Radioautograph (b) of the slide shows that the γE precipitin band combined radioactive antigen. (c) A monospecific anti-γE serum was placed in the center well of the plate against a reaginic serum (S), a fraction composed of γG and γE globulins (G + E) and γG myeloma proteins of 4 subclasses. (d) The center well was filled with the same anti-γE serum and γA myeloma proteins of three subclasses, γD myeloma and γM macroglobulin were placed in peripheral wells. γA$_f$, γA$_m$ represent Fu type and Ma type by TERRY and ROBERT [33]. γA$_h$ represents He type by VAERMAN and HEREMANS [34]. Both Fu and Ma types belong to Le type by the latter investigators. The results in (c) and (d) show that the γE antigenic determinant is not shared by any of the other immunoglobulins of known classes and subclasses.

The conclusion was supported by the presence of E myeloma protein. Drs. JOHANSSON and BENNICH in Sweden found an atypical myeloma protein ND [20]. As the protein did not react with antisera specific for known immunoglobulins and physicochemical properties of the protein were quite similar to γE, we have exchanged antiserum specific for the myeloma protein and for γE globulin to study the relationship. A γE preparation from ragweed sensitive serum was placed in the center well, against the antisera specific for the five immunoglobulins and the antiserum against myeloma ND. As shown in figure 5 a, anti-myeloma ND and anti-γE gave a single precipitin band of identical specificity and the precipitin band combined radioactive antigen in radioautograph (fig. 5 b). It was also found that the myeloma protein gave a precipitin band with anti-γE antiserum and anti-ND serum.

The physicochemical properties of γE globulin are summarized in Table III in comparison with the other immunoglobulins. The figures in parenthesis are those of E myeloma protein. It is clear now that γE globulin is a γ_1 glycoprotein of which sedimentation coefficient is 8 S and the molecular weight of nearly 200,000.

The chromatographic properties of γE in table III represent the molarity of phosphate buffer (pH 8.0) by which the major part of γE is eluted from a DEAE cellulose column. However, γE is chromatographically heterogene-

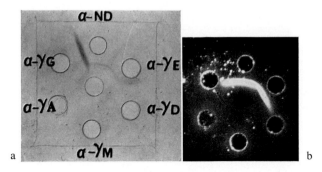

Fig. 5. Radioimmunodiffusion showing the antigenic identity of myeloma protein ND with γE. A reagin-rich fraction was placed in the center well and antisera specific for each of the 5 immunoglobulins and that specific for myeloma ND (a-ND) were placed in center well (a). Anti-γE and anti-ND showed a precipitin band of identical specificity with the reagin-rich (γE) fraction. The slide was washed and radioactive antigen E was applied to peripheral wells. A radioautograph (b) of the slide showed that the precipitin band combined radioactive antigen.

ous. When the γE-rich fraction from a ragweed sensitive serum was applied to a DEAE Sephadex column and eluted by increase of molarity of Tris-HCl buffer, γE antibody was detected in all fractions shown in figure 6. As expected, all fractions had reaginic activity which paralleled the intensity of radioactivity of the γE precipitin band. Precipitation of γE with anti-γE in Frs. A, B and D was accompanied by loss of reaginic activity. The chromato-

Table III. Physicochemical properties of human immunoglobulins

	γG	γM	γA	γD	γE (myeloma ND)	Reagin
Electrophoretic Mobility	$\gamma_1-\gamma_2$	γ_1	γ_1	γ_1	γ_1	γ_1
Sedimentation Coefficient S_{20},W	6.6	18	6.6	7.0	8.0　(8.2)	Ca 7.8
DEAE Cellulose Chromatography (M) a)	0.005	0.15	0.035	0.035	0.02	0.02
Molecular weight	150,000	900,000	180,000	–	(200,000)	–
Carbohydrate %	2.9	11.8	7.5	–	(10.7)	–

( ) = myeloma ND.
　a) Stepwise elution with phosphate buffers, pH 8.0. The numerals indicate molarity of phosphate buffer for elution of the major component.

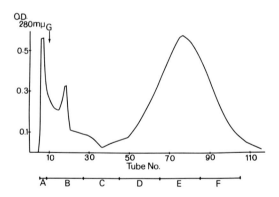

Fig. 6. DEAE Sephadex chromatography of a reagin-rich fraction. The starting buffer was 0.1 M Tris-HCl buffer, pH 8.0. After the first peak was obtained, proteins remaining in the column were eluted with a gradient increase of molarity. G represents the start of gradient elution. The major component in the first and second peaks were γG and γA, respectively. The highest reaginic activity and γE antibody was detected in Fr. B.

graphic heterogeneity of γE might explain heterogeneity of reaginic anti-bodies observed by other investigators [25, 26]. In rabbit, SELA and MOZES [28] have shown that chromatographic distribution of γG antibodies differs depending on antigen for immunization. One can expect that chromato-graphic distribution of γE antibodies may also be different depending on allergen.

As γE concentration in the serum is too low to be isolated for structural studies, all available information on the structure of this protein was obtained with an E myeloma protein. BENNICH and JOHANSSON [2] have reduced the E myeloma protein (myeloma ND) with mercaptoethanol followed by alkyla-tion with iodoacetamide and isolated two components which correspond to heavy and light chains (fig. 7). The yield of light chain was 20% of the total protein and its molecular weight, calculated from the amino acid composi-tion, was 22,500. Since the molecular weight of the original molecule is 200,000, the results indicate that the molecule contained two light chains. Assuming two heavy chains per molecule, the molecular weight of each heavy chain was calculated to be approximately 75,500, which is significantly higher than those of γ, μ and a chains. The myeloma protein was subjected

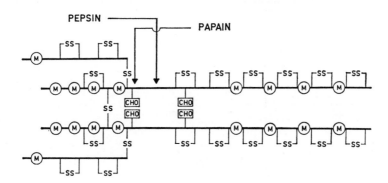

	Molweight	S°_{20w}	Tot. Carbohydrate	1/2 Cystine	Methionine
Myeloma Protein ND	196000	7.9	10.71	42	18
Light chain (λ), 214 aa	22500	—	0	5	1
Heavy chain (ND)	75500	—	14	16	8
(Fab')$_2$	104000	6.1	10.76	18	10
Fd'	29500	—	19	4	4
1/2 'Fc' = (Heavy-Fd')	46000	—	11	12	4

Fig. 7. Scheme of E myeloma protein. M represents methionine and CHO represents carbohydrate.

to papain or pepsin digestion. The papain digestion produced two fragments which correspond to F_c and F_{ab} fragments from γG. The F_{ab} fragment contained λ chain determinants, indicating the presence of λ chain, whereas F_c fragment did not. The γE antigenic determinant(s) were present in F_c but not in F_{ab} fragments. Sedimentation coefficient of the F_c fragment was 5 S and its molecular weight was estimated to be 100,000. These data indicate that F_c fragment of the E myeloma protein represents a portion of heavy (ε) chains. Although the isolated ε chain did not have γE antigenic determinant, the presence of the determinant in F^c fragment indicates that the determinants were originally present in the heavy chains. After pepsin digestion of the protein followed by gel filtration, approximately 52% of the material was recovered as 6 S fragment. The fragment contained λ chains and corresponded to $F(ab)_2$. Distribution of half cysteine and methionine residue in heavy and light chains was estimated from chemical analysis of the isolated heavy and light chains and $F(ab')_2$ fragment. From these findings BENNICH and JOHANSSON [2] proposed a schematic model of the E myeloma protein as shown in figure 8. Apparently, the great number of methionine

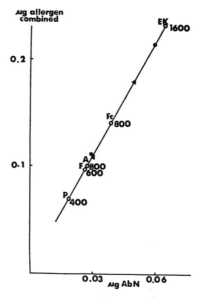

Fig. 8. Relation between antibody concentration and allergen-binding activity of rabbit antibody (●, △ represent two different measurements). The allergen-binding values of γE antibodies in serum EK, F_c, F and P were interpolated. The numerals in the figure represent the Prausnitz-Küstner titer of the serum samples.

residues per heavy chain and of half cysteine residues in the F_c portion of the molecules are characteristics of this immunoglobulin. As will be discussed later, this structure might be related to peculiar biological properties of γE antibodies.

B. Immunochemical Properties of γE Antibodies

Characteristic antigenic structure of γE globulin suggested to us the possibility that quantitation of skin-sensitizing antibody may be estimated *in vitro* by measuring the allergen-binding activity of γE antibody in the serum samples. Attempts were made to measure the activity of anti-ragweed antibodies associated with each immunoglobulin class. An excess amount of radioactively labeled purified ragweed allergen (antigen E) was incubated with patients' sera. Aliquots of the mixture were then incubated with the antibody specific for one of the immunoglobulins or anti-light chain to precipitate each immunoglobulin or all immunoglobulins. Radioactivity in the precipitates represents the amount of allergen combined with the antibody associated with each immunoglobulin class. The dose of antigen specifically bound to γG, γA, γE antibodies and to all antibodies is shown in table IV.

Table IV. Allergen-binding activity of antibodies in patients' sera[1]

Serum	Allergen-binding activity			1G[2]	1G cal[3]	P–K Titer
	γG	γA	γE			
EK	0.40	0	0.23	0.62	0.63	1600
B	0.26	0	0.38	0.66	0.64	3200
F$_c$[4]	0.16	0.082	0.14	0.33	0.38	800
F[4]	0.14	0.016	0.097	0.25	0.27	600
A	0.23	0	0.10	0.34	0.33	800
W	0.61	0.033	0.099	0.79	0.74	600
P	1.8	0	0.07	1.9	1.9	400
I	1.9	0	0	1.9	1.9	0

[1] Numerals in the table indicate μg of antigen E bound by immunoglobulins in 1 ml of serum.
[2] Measured by precipitation of all immunoglobulins with anti-light chain antibodies.
[3] Allergen-binding activities of γG, γA and γE antibodies were added.
[4] Untreated patients, all other patients were treated.

It is apparent that the antigen-binding activity of γE antibody bears no correlation with those of either γG or γA antibodies and that the sum of the antigen bound by γG, γA and γE antibodies in the serum specimens is in agreement with that of total antibody, which was measured by the precipitation with anti-light chain antibodies. An important finding in this experiment was that skin-sensitizing activity of the serum samples correlated with γE antibody concentration as measured by antigen-binding activity [16].

The antigen-binding values of γE antibody in the sera were compared with that of rabbit antibody against antigen E to estimate the concentration of γE antibody in patients' sera. The relation between antibody concentration and antigen-binding values of rabbit antibody is shown in figure 8. The antigen-binding values of γE antibody in patients' sera were interpolated to the relationship to estimate the concentration of rabbit antibody which has the same antigen-binding value as γE antibody and the values are shown in table V. As the antigen-binding activity of antibodies is dependent on their avidity and valency, the concentration of rabbit antibody does not represent the actual concentration of γE antibody but gives some idea on the range of γE antibody concentration in the patients' sera. As P-K titers of these sera are known, one can calculate the dose of rabbit antibody which corresponds to that of γE antibody in the minimum sensitizing dose of the sera. The calculated dose in six different specimens are very close to one another and

Table V. Estimation of the minimum sensitizing dose of γE antibody in Prausnitz-Küstner reactions

Serum specimen	Allergen-binding value of γE antibody μg/ml	Rabbit antibody concentration[1] μgN/ml	Rabbit antibody corresponding to minimum P–K dose $\times 10^{-6}$ μgN
EK	0.23	0.065	2.0
F$_c$	0.14	0.038	2.4
F	0.097	0.026	2.1
A	0.10	0.028	1.8
W	0.099	0.027	2.2
P	0.07	0.019	2.4

[1] The concentration of rabbit antibody which is comparable to γE antibody with respect to allergen-binding activity.

in the range of 2×10^{-6} μgN. If one assumes that the avidity of γE antibody is comparable to that of rabbit antibody, the minimum dose of skin-sensitizing antibody required for giving positive P-K reactions would be in the order of 10^{-6} to 10^{-5} μgN. The results also showed a complete correlation between γE antibody concentration and reaginic activity and support the concept that the skin-sensitizing antibody is γE.

It has been shown by LAYTON and his co-workers [21] that human reaginic sera induced passive cutaneous anaphylaxis (PCA) reactions in the monkey. The previous findings strongly suggest that human reaginic antibody is responsible for the reactions; however, the problem still remained as to whether the reaginic antibody itself or some other antibodies in reagin-rich fraction was involved in the PCA reactions. In order to study this problem, sera from ragweed sensitive individuals were fractionated by DEAE cellulose column chromatography and the γG, γA and γE antibodies against purified ragweed allergen in the fractions were measured using the *in vitro* method. The ability of the same fractions to induce PCA reactions were tested. It became clear that the fractions containing γE antibody induced PCA reactions, whereas the fractions containing γG or γA antibody but no γE antibody, failed to induce the reaction. The γE antibody combining with only 0.0002 μg of purified allergen was enough to give a positive reaction, but 1,000 times as much γG antibody or 20 times as much γA antibody was incapable of inducing a positive reaction. Furthermore, the ability of the reagin-rich fraction or original serum to induce the PCA reaction was absorbed by anti-γE antiserum, but the absorption of γG and γA globulins in the active fraction did not reduce the skin-sensitizing activity. It appears that γE antibody is responsible for the PCA reactions in monkeys [12].

The reaginic antibodies were considered to be univalent because the sera from atopic individuals do not give a precipitin reaction with allergen in spite of high skin-sensitizing activity. However, the problem has to be re-evaluated because the actual concentration of reaginic antibodies in patients' sera is very low on a weight basis. From the measurement of antigen-binding value of γE antibodies, the concentration of γE antibody in a patient's serum having a P-K titer of 1:10,000 seems to be comparable to 0.4 μgN/ml of rabbit antibody. It is possible that the lack of precipitin reaction may be due to low concentration rather than univalent nature of the antibody. In fact, our studies have shown that γE antibodies are capable of agglutinating red cells coated with antigen. In this experiment, the preparations of γE antibodies were obtained by fractionating reaginic sera followed by absorption of immunoglobulins other than γE with rabbit antibodies specific for

Table VI. Effect of anti-immunoglobulin on hemagglutination

Anti-ragweed	Anti-1 g	Antibody concentration[1]						
		0.05	0.025	0.0125	0.006	0.003	0.0015	0
γG	None	3	3	1	0	0	0	0
	Anti-γG	3	3	3	3	2	1	0
	Anti-γA	3	2	1	0	0	0	0
	Anti-γE	3	3	1	0	0	0	0
γE	None	3	2	1	0	0	0	0
	Anti-γG	nd	2	1	0	0	0	0
	Anti-γA	nd	2	1	0	0	0	0
	Anti-γE	nd	3	3	3	2	1	0

[1] Antibody concentration of γG and γE antibodies was estimated by antigen-binding activity and represented by the concentration of rabbit antibody having the comparable antigen-binding activity.

each immunoglobulin class. In radioimmunodiffusion using I^{131}-labeled antigen E, only the γE antibodies were detected in the preparations. After measuring antigen-binding activity of the γE antibodies, serial dilutions of the preparations were incubated with rabbit erythrocytes coated with ragweed allergen. The results showed that the γE antibody preparation agglutinated the cells (table VIII). On the basis of antigen-binding activity, the γE and γG antibodies obtained from the same serum had comparable hemaggluti-nating activity. The reactions by both γG and γE antibodies were completely inhibited if the antibody preparations were incubated with 1 μg/ml of antigen E before the addition of the antigen-coated cells, indicating that the reactions were specific for the antigen. Furthermore, the hemagglutination by γE antibody was enhanced if the sensitized cells were incubated with anti-γE (table VI). The enhancement was specific because both anti-γG and anti-γA failed to enhance the hemagglutination. As expected, the agglutination of the same antigen-coated cells by γG antibody preparation was enhanced by anti-γG but not by either anti-γA or anti-γE. The results showed that γE antibodies were actually responsible for the hemagglutination and indicated that the antibodies are multivalent with respect to their antibody-combining sites. As described before, BENNICH and JOHANSSON [2] indicated that γE is composed of two heavy and two light chains. If the antibody combining sites of γE antibody locate in F_{ab} portion of the molecules, one can speculate that γE antibodies are probably divalent.

C. Molecular Basis of Reaginic Hypersensitivity Reactions by γE Antibodies

In anaphylactic reactions in the guinea pig, it has been shown that guinea pig $γ_1$ and γG globulins from certain animal species nonspecifically block passive sensitization. The mechanisms of the blocking is considered to be due to competition between antibody and nonantibody immunoglobulins for combination with certain guinea pig tissues with which sensitizing antibodies combine upon sensitization [3]. Similar findings were obtained in P-K reactions in humans. Nonantibody γE blocks passive sensitization of human skin, when the protein was mixed with reaginic serum and the mixtures were injected intracutaneously into normal individuals for passive sensitization [19]. The blocking of passive sensitization is one of the characteristic properties of γE immunoglobulin. As shown in table IX, myeloma proteins of the other four classes and subclasses failed to block the passive sensitization. Blocking of passive sensitization by E myeloma protein was also reported [30]. The fact that only γE blocked passive sensitization indicates that the protein has affinity for human skin tissues to which reaginic antibodies combine upon sensitization. Quite recently, STANWORTH et al. [31] have shown that F_c fragment rather than F_{ab} fragment of the E myeloma protein blocked passive sensitization. The findings are in agreement with the fact that F_c fragment of rabbit γG blocked passive sensitization of guinea pig skin with the γG antibody [6].

One of the characteristic properties of human reaginic antibodies is that the sensitizing activity of antibodies is lost by heating at 56°C for 2 to 4 hours. In fact, skin-sensitizing activity of γE antibody was lost by heating. The heat inactivation of the γE antibodies may be explained by the loss of affinity of γE molecules for tissue sites because the blocking activity of nonantibody γE was lost by heating at 56°C for 4 h (table VII) [18]. On the other hand, evidence was obtained that antibody combining sites in γE antibodies remained after heating. When the antigen-binding activity of γG, γA and γE antibodies was measured before and after heating at 56°C for 4 h, more than 50% of the allergen-binding activity of γG and γA antibodies remained after heating, whereas γE antibody was not detected after heat treatment (table VIII). However, the apparent loss of antigen-binding activity of γE antibodies is due to the non-precipitability of heated γE. It was found that γE antigenic determinants are heat labile and heated γE is not precipitated by anti-γE. When antigen-antibody complexes in the same mixture were precipitated by anti-light chain antibody, the antigen-binding value of the heated γE antibody preparation was more than 50% of the

Table VII. Blocking effect of immunoglobulins on passive sensitization with reaginic antibody

Proteins injected with reaginic antibody		μgN	Wheal mm	Erythema mm
γG	γG_1	2.0	8.5	30×32
	γG_2		9.5	35×42
	γG_3		10.5	30×43
	γG_4		10.0	30×49
γA	Fu	2.0	9.5	30×41
	Ma		9.5	34×37
	He		10.0	31×45
γD		1.6	9.5	31×34
γM		2.0	9.5	34×36
γE + γG[1]		0.06	0	0
		0.03	5.0	20×22
		0.015	6.0	21×25
γE + γG (heated)		2.8	9.0	30×32
Saline		0	9.5	36×42

[1] γE globulin comprises 25% or less of total protein.

Table VIII. Effect of heat on antigen-binding activity of γG, γA and γE antibodies

Fraction	Heat	Antibody for precipitation	AgE combined μg $\times 10^{-2}$	Activity remaining %
γG	—	anti-γG	2.0	
	+		1.5	75
γA	—	anti-γA	1.5	
	+		1.2	78
	—	anti-γE	6.0	
	+		0.5	8
Reagin	—	anti-F_{ab}	6.7	
	+		4.4	66
	—	anti-γG	0	
	—	anti-γA	0	

value of the native preparation. As the original preparation did not contain a significant amount of either γG or γA antibody and the antigen-binding value of total antibody was comparable to that of γE antibody in the preparation, almost all antibody in the preparation should by γE immunoglobulin. It seems, therefore, that γE antibody was responsible for the antigen-binding of the heated preparation. In fact, the heated γE preparation showed blocking antibody activity. It is apparent that heat inactivation of reaginic antibody is not due to the loss of antibody combining sites but to degradation of certain structures in the γE molecules, which are involved in the fixation to skin tissues [18].

Another characteristic of reaginic antibodies is the inactivation by reduction and alkylation [27, 22]. In agreement with the previous observations, skin-sensitizing activity of γE antibodies greatly diminished by reduction in 0.1 M mercaptoethanol for one hour followed by alkylation with iodoacetamide, although 0.01 M mercaptoethanol did not change the skin-sensitizing activity. Further studies on the effect of reduction-alkylation on anti-ragweed γE antibodies indicated antigen-binding activity of the antibodies diminished to about $^{1}/_{3}$ by the reduction in 0.1 M mercaptoethanol followed by alkylation. No effect was detected on the γE antigenic determinant. The reduced-alkylated γE maintained affinity for skin tissues to which reaginic antibody combines. However, the affinity of the treated molecules was less than that of native γE. Approximately 5 times as much reduced-alkylated material than untreated sample was required for blocking the passive sensitization with reaginic antibodies against heterologous allergen. It was also found that sensitization with the reduced-alkylated γE antibody did not persist for a long time. The minimum dose of the treated antibody required for giving a positive P-K reaction increases when the sensitization period was changed from 2 h to 48 h. It is apparent that reduction and alkylation affects two different portions of γE antibody molecules, i.e., antibody combining sites and tissue fixation site.

In the anaphylactic reactions in the guinea pig, it is well known that injections of nonantibody rabbit γG into guinea pigs skin followed by anti-rabbit γG gives reversed PCA reactions. As normal individuals have γE, one can expect that the protein is present on target cells to which reagin combines upon sensitization and therefore that an intracutaneous injection of the antibody specific for γE into normal individuals would give a reversed type allergic reaction. In fact, normal individuals give erythema-wheal reactions upon injection of anti-γE. The minimum dose of the antibody for giving the reaction was in the order of 10^{-5} μgN. None of the antibodies specific for other immunoglobulins, i.e., anti-γG, anti-γA, anti-γM and anti-γD, gave reactions even with 10^{-2} μgN (fig. 9) [10]. Anti-light chain antibodies prepared from anti-γG antisera gave a positive reaction with 0.01 μgN. Since anti-γ chains failed to give the reaction, it seems that anti-light chain reacts with γE on the target cells and induces the reaction. Requirement of 1,000-fold more of anti-light chain than anti-γE is probably due to the combination of anti-light chain with immunoglobulins of other classes present in the skin tissues.

The sensitivity of human skin to anti-γE differs depending on the individuals. An atopic patient who has extremely high γE concentration in his serum gave a positive reaction with 10^{-8} μgN of anti-γE, whereas two agammaglobulinemic patients did not react to 10^{-3} μgN of anti-γE. In all of these cases, the sensitivity to histamine was in normal level. It was found that the activity of anti-γE serum was removed by precipitation of anti-γE antibody with γE. The induction of reversed type allergic reactions by anti-γE antibody is a direct proof that normal individuals possess γE on target cells.

It was also found that intracutaneous injection of anti-γE to normal monkeys increased permeability of their skin capillaries. With Evans' blue injected intravenously, skin sites receiving anti-γE showed a blueing reaction. The amount of rabbit anti-γE required for the positive reaction was 10^{-5} μgN. Again, none of the antibodies specific for other immunoglobulins gave the reaction with 0.04 μgN (fig. 10). These findings indicate that the monkey has a protein which cross-reacts with anti-human γE, and that the protein is present on the cells to which human reaginic antibodies are fixed upon passive sensitization. The monkey protein was detected in normal monkey serum. Although the monkey protein has not been isolated, distribution of the protein in chromatographic fractions in normal monkey serum as well as its size was similar to human γE and suggested that the protein is 'γE' immunoglobulin of the monkey [10].

Lichtenstein et al. [24] have observed histamine release from isolated leukocytes of atopic patients upon exposure to allergen to which the donors are sensitive. Their results suggest that reaginic antibodies are involved in the reaction. Levy and Osler [23] succeeded in passively sensitizing leukocytes with the patients' sera for histamine release. If reaginic antibodies are actually involved in the histamine release, γE should be present on leukocytes and therefore one can expect reversed type histamine release from leukocytes by the exposure to anti-γE. In fact, anti-γE released histamine from leukocytes of atopic patients. Similar to the skin reaction, none of the anti-γG, anti-γA, anti-γM and anti-γD released histamine from the cells whereas anti-light chain antibodies did. It was also found that the sensitivity

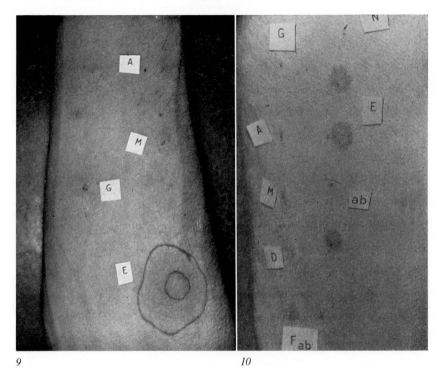

9   10

Fig. 9. Induction of erythema wheal reaction by anti-γE in human skin. Skin sites marked (G, A, M) received 0.01 μgN of anti-γG, anti-γA and anti-γM, respectively. The site E received 10^{-5} μg N of anti-γE antibody.

Fig. 10. Induction of blueing reaction by anti-γE in monkey skin. The sites (G, A, M) received 0.02 μgN of anti-γG, anti-γA and anti-γM. 1:100 dilutions of anti-γD and of a normal rabbit serum were injected into the site D and N. Two sites (F_{ab}) received 0.02 μgN and 0.004 μgN of anti-F_{ab} antibody. 1:8,000 and 1:80,000 dilutions of an anti-γE serum containing 2×10^{-4} μgN and 2×10^{-5} μgN antibody were injected into sites (E). The anti-γE antiserum was absorbed with an equal volume of γE globulin and 1:400 and 1:4,000 dilutions of the supernatant was injected into sites (ab). The site receiving 1:400 dilution gave a negative reaction.

of normal leukocytes to anti-γE for histamine release increased by incubation of leukocytes with a γE-rich serum containing antiragweed reaginic antibody (fig. 11). As demonstrated by LEVY *et al.* [23], the sensitized cells released histamine by exposure to ragweed antigen. It is evident that γE immunoglobulin is fixed to leukocytes and the reaction of the cell-fixed γE with anti-γE is responsible for histamine release. These findings strongly

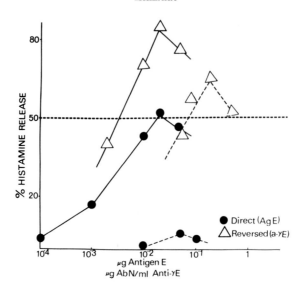

Fig. 11. Histamine release by anti-γE (△) and by ragweed antigen (●) from normal leukocytes before (– – – –) and after passive sensitization (———) with ragweed sensitive serum.

support the hypothesis that γE antibodies are responsible for histamine release from leukocytes by allergen.

In our previous studies on soluble antigen-antibody complexes, it has been shown that preformed antigen-γG-antibody complexes induce an increased permeability of guinea pig skin capillaries. The skin reactivity of the complexes depends on the nature of antibody involved. Only the antibodies having sensitizing activity to guinea pigs formed skin-reactive complexes, indicating that the formation of skin-reactive complexes *in vivo* is responsible for PCA reactions in guinea pigs [6]. The results also showed that the skin reactivity of the complexes differ depending on antigen/antibody ratio in the complexes and indicated requirement of at least two antibody molecules for the formation of a skin-reactive complex. Similarities between PCA reactions in the guinea pig and P-K reactions in humans suggested the possibility that soluble complexes composed of γE antibody may give erythema-wheal reactions in normal human skin. This possibility was therefore studied in the next experiments [11]. The γE-rich fraction containing γE antibody but none of the γG, γA or γM antibody against ragweed allergen was obtained from atopic patients' sera and the antigen-binding activity of the γE antibody in the preparation was measured. The preparation was incubated with varying concentrations of purified ragweed allergen for 15 min at 37°C and the mixtures were injected into normal human skin. The mixture of γE antibody with the ragweed allergen provoked erythema-wheal reactions, whereas those of either γG or γA antibody with the same antigen failed to do so. The intensity of the skin reaction was different depending on the antigen/antibody ratio in the mixture. The maximal reaction was obtained when slightly excess antigen was added and the activity of the mixture became lower by the addition of more antigen (table IX). At the optimal antigen/antibody ratio, the amount of antibody in the minimal skin reactive dose of the complex was approximately 30 to 50 times more than the minimal dose of the same preparation required for a positive P-K reaction at the sensitization period of 24 h. However, the dose of the γE antibody in the mixture was in the same order of magnitude as that required for giving a positive reaction when the skin sites were challenged within 5 min. As the findings strongly suggested that skin reaction by antigen-γE antibody mixtures are due to preformed complexes, experiments were undertaken to prove that γE antibodies actually formed complexes with antigen *in vitro*. Purified ragweed antigen (antigen E) was labeled with I^{131} and added to γE antibody preparation. The antigen/antibody ratio in the mixtures was in extreme antigen excess in a mixture and in moderate antigen excess in the other. The latter mixture gave positive erythema-wheal reaction with a dilution of 1:128, whereas the mixture containing a great excess

Table IX. Skin reactions by γE antibody-antigen complex[1]

Dilution of complex	Antigen (μg/ml)						
	32	10	2	0.5	0.1	0.025	0
Undiluted[2]	5.5 (22)	7.0 (24)	8.0 (27)	9.0 (29)	11.0 (35)	8.0 (30)	0
2×	0	5.5 (20)	7.0 (22)	8.0 (28)	10.5 (33)	7.0 (27)	0
8×	0	0	0	6.5 (22)	9.0 (30)	5.0 (20)	0

[1] Numerals in this table represent average diameters of wheal in mm, and those in parentheses represent average diameters of erythema in mm.

[2] The antigen-binding value of the antibody preparation was 0.09 μg/ml.

antigen did not show the reaction even at a dilution of 1:8. Both of the mixtures were then analyzed by sucrose density gradient ultracentrifugation. As controls, γE antibody preparation or radioactive antigen E was applied to separate tubes and analyzed. After centrifugation, distribution of radioactivity in the gradient fractions was studied. Free antigen gave a single peak of 3.3 S and sedimentation coefficient of γE antibody was 8 S. The mixture of γE antibody with a great excess antigen gave two radioactive peaks. A slower sedimenting peak corresponded to free antigen (3.3 S) and the sedimentation coefficient of the faster component was 9.7 S which was higher than that of γE antibody alone. The mixture with a moderate excess antigen showed three peaks, i.e., 3.3 S, 9.7 S and 13.1 S (table X). The 9.7 S and 13.1 S components represent antigen-antibody complexes because radioactive antigen in the fractions was precipitated by anti-γE whereas free antigen was not. As the antigen-antibody mixture containing 13 S complex had high skin reactivity while the activity of the mixture containing only 9.7 S complex was very low, it seems that 13 S complex has the activity whereas 9.7 S complex does not.

Since γE antibody is probably divalent, one can expect that the major part of complexes formed in great antigen excess are probably composed of two antigen and one antibody molecules (Ag_2Ab complex) of which molecular weight is 270,000. It appears likely that the 9.7 S complex represents an Ag_2Ab complex. As γE antibody is 8 S, the complex should not contain

Table X. Sedimentation coefficient ($S_{20,w}$) of antigen, antibody and antigen-antibody complexes[1]

| Preparations | Sedimentation coefficients | | | |
	Antigen	Antibody	Complex 1	Complex 2
Antigen E	3.3	–	–	–
Reaginic antibody	–	8.0	–	–
Ag-Ab complex Extreme Ag excess	3.4	–	9.7	–
Ag-Ab complex moderate Ag excess	3.4	–	9.7	13.1

[1] The values in the table were calculated in comparison with $S_{20,w}$ of rabbit γG antibody as standard. The $S_{20,w}$ of the antibody was 6.5 S.

more than one γE antibody molecule, whereas 13 S complex is probably composed of two antibody molecules. It seems that two or more γE antibody molecules are required for the formation of a skin reactive complex.

The requirement of two or more γE antibody molecules for the formation of skin reactive complex is comparable to the previous observations on rabbit γG antibody complexes having skin reactivity in the guinea pig. In the case of the γG antibody complexes, it was suggested that an interaction between antibody molecules brought into apposition by antigen and possible consequent structural changes in the F_c portion of the antibody molecules might be involved in the induction of the biological activity [6]. The requirement of two γE antibody molecules for the formation of skin reactive complexes suggested that induction of skin reactive properties by the formation of the complexes may also involve interaction between the γE antibody molecules and/or structural change in the molecules.

Our recent studies on reversed type hypersensitivity reactions supported this idea. As mentioned before, anti-γE antibody induced erythema-wheal reactions in normal individuals and released histamine from leukocytes of atopic patients. In order to study more about the mechanisms of the reactions, 7 S fraction was obtained from anti-γE serum by gel filtration and digested with pepsin. 5 S fraction was obtained by gel filtration and the protein in the fraction was reduced and alkylated. Most of the protein was split to 3.5 S fragments. When the fragments were injected intracutaneously into normal individuals, 5 S fraction gave positive skin reactions and the minimal dose of the fragment required for a positive reaction was less than that of 7 S fraction. Whereas the 3.5 S fraction failed to give a reaction even when 100 times as much preparation was injected. Similarly, both the original antibody and 5 S fragments released histamine from leukocytes, whereas 3.5 S fragment did not. Representative results of histamine release are shown in figure 12. It was also found that reduced-alkylated antibody released histamine. Although we could not measure antigen-binding activity of 3.5 S fragment, the presence of combining site in the fragment was proved by inhibition of precipitin reaction between the original antibody and γE by the 3.5 S fragment. The results showed requirement of divalency for the induction of erythema-wheal reactions and for histamine release, and strongly suggested that bridging of 2 cell-fixed γE molecules by divalent antibody is necessary for reversed type allergy. Induction of erythema-wheal reactions and histamine release by F(ab')$_2$ also indicate that C' is not essential for the reactions and therefore that the reactions are not cytotoxic phenomena in which C' is involved.

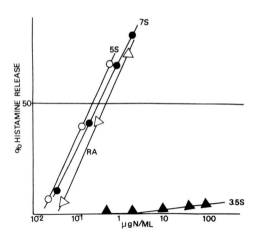

Fig. 12. Histamine release by anti-γE antibody and its fragments from leukocytes. Abscissa represents protein concentration of the antibody preparations. 7 S, 5 S, and 3.5 S represent 7 S fraction of antanti-γE serum, F(ab')₂ fragments and F$_{ab}$' fragments obtained from the 7 S preparation. RA indicates reduced-alkylated preparation.

Summary

Reaginic activity in sera of atopic patients is associated with γE immunoglobulin rather than the other 4 immunoglobulins, i.e., γG, γA, γM and γD. The conclusion is based on the facts that 1. reaginic activity in the patients' sera was precipitated by anti-γE but not by the antibodies specific for heavy chains of the 4 immunoglobulins; 2. distributions of reaginic activity and of γE antibody paralleled with each other when the patients' sera were fractionated by anion exchange column chromatography, gel filtration, density gradient ultracentrifugation and zone electrophoresis; 3. γE fraction of the patients' sera, in which only γE antibody but none of the γG, γA, γM and γD antibodies was detected, possessed high reaginic activity and the activity in the preparation was removed by anti-γE.

The protein has κ and λ light chains of immunoglobulins, possesses characteristic antigenic determinants which are not shared by the other immunoglobulins of known classes and subclasses, and lacks the major antigenic determinants in the other classes. The antigenic structure of γE as well as association of antibody activity with the protein indicate that γE represents a distinct immunoglobulin class. Physicochemically, γE immunoglobulin is a γ_1 glycoprotein with a sedimentation coefficient of 8 S and a molecular weight of 200,000. Structural studies of an E myeloma protein showed that the protein is composed of 2 heavy (ε) and 2 light polypeptide chains. The heavy (ε) chains of the protein have peculiar structure and γE antigenic determinants are present in F$_c$ portion of the heavy chains.

The γE antibodies are responsible for P-K reactions in humans, PCA reactions in the monkey by reaginic sera, and probably for antigen-induced histamine release from leukocytes of atopic individuals. The minimum dose of γE antibody required for giving positive P-K reactions in humans was estimated to be 10^{-6} to 10^{-5} μgN. The γE antibody agglutinated red cells coated with antigen, indicating that the antibody is multivalent (probably divalent). Non-antibody γE and a E myeloma protein blocked passive sensitization of human skin with reagin, indicating that the protein has affinity for the tissue constituents to which reagin combines upon sensitization. Structures of the protein responsible for the affinity were heat labile, whereas antibody combining sites in the γE antibodies remained after heating at 56° C. Reduction of the antibody in 0.1 M mercaptoethanol followed by alkylation partially degraded both antibody combining sites and tissue fixation site in the molecules. It was also found that antibodies specific for γE induced erythema-wheal reactions in normal individuals and monkeys, and released histamine from leukocytes of atopic individuals. Induction of the reversed type reactions by the anti-γE antibody indicated that γE immunoglobulin is present on target cells to which reaginic antibodies combine upon sensitization.

With respect to the immune mechanisms of reaginic hypersensitivity reactions by γE antibodies, it was found that soluble antigen-γE antibody complexes preformed *in vitro* gave erythema-wheal reactions in normal individuals. Analysis of the antigen-antibody complexes strongly suggested requirement of two or more γE antibody molecules for the formation of a skin-reactive complex. This finding indicated that bridging of two cell-fixed γE molecules initiated the hypersensitivity reactions.

References

1. Augustin, R.; Conolly, R.C. and Lloyd, G.M.: Atopic reagin as a protype of cytophillic antibodies; Protide of the Biological Fluids *11:* 56 (1963).
2. Bennich, H. and Johansson, S.G.O.: Studies on a new class of human immunoglobulins. III. Chemical and physical properties, Nobel Symposium III. p. 199, ed. by J. Killander, 1967.
3. Biozzi, G.; Halpern, B.N. and Binaghi, R.: The competitive effect of normal serum proteins from various animal species on antibody fixation in passive cutaneous anaphylaxis in the guinea pig. J. Immunol. *82:* 215 (1959).
4. Fireman, P.; Vannier, W.E. and Goodman, H.C.: The association of skin sensitizing antibody with the β_{2a} globulin in sera from ragweed sensitive patients. J. exp. Med. *117:* 603 (1963).
5. Heremans, J.F. and Vaerman, J.P.: β_{2a} globulin as a possible carrier of allergic reaginic activity. Nature *193:* 1091 (1962).
6. Ishizaka, K.: Gamma globulin and molecular mechanisms in hypersensitivity reactions. Progr. Allergy, Vol. 7, p. 32 (Karger, Basel/New York 1963).
7. Ishizaka, K. and Ishizaka, T.: Physicochemical properties of reaginic antibody. I. Association of reaginic activity with an immunoglobulin other than γA or γG globulin. J. Allergy *37:* 169 (1966)
8. Ishizaka, K. and Ishizaka, T.: Physicochemical properties of reaginic antibody. III. Further studies on the reaginic antibody in γA globulin preparation. J. Allergy *38:* 108 (1966).
9. Ishizaka, K. and Ishizaka, T.: Identification of γE antibodies as a carrier of reaginic activity. J. Immunol. *99:* 1187 (1967).
10. Ishizaka, K. and Ishizaka, T.: Reversed type allergic skin reactions by anti-γE globulin antibodies in humans and monkeys. J. Immunol. *100:* 554 (1968).
11. Ishizaka, K. and Ishizaka, T.: Induction of erythema-wheal reactions by soluble antigen-γE-antibody complexes in humans. J. Immunol. *101:* 68 (1968).
12. Ishizaka, K.; Ishizaka, T. and Arbesman, C.E.: Induction of passive cutaneous anaphylaxis in monkeys by human γE antibody. J. Allergy *39:* 254 (1967).

13. ISHIZAKA, K.; ISHIZAKA, T. and HORNBROOK, M.M.: Blocking of Prausnitz-Küstner sensitization with reagin by normal human β_{2a} globulin. J. Allergy 34: 395 (1963).

14. ISHIZAKA, K.; ISHIZAKA, T. and HORNBROOK, M.M.: Physicochemical properties of reaginic antibody. IV. Presence of a unique immunoglobulin as a carrier of reaginic activity. J. Immunol. 97: 75 (1966).

15. ISHIZAKA, K.; ISHIZAKA, T. and HORNBROOK, M.M.: Physicochemical properties of reaginic antibody. V. Correlation of reaginic activity with γE antibody. J. Immunol. 97: 840 (1966).

16. ISHIZAKA, K.; ISHIZAKA, T. and HORNBROOK, M.M.: Allergen-binding activity of γE, γG and γA antibodies in sera from atopic patients: In vitro measurements of reaginic antibody. J. Immunol. 98: 490 (1967).

17. ISHIZAKA, K.; ISHIZAKA, T. and LEE, E.M.: Physicochemical properties of reaginic antibody. II. Characteristic properties of reaginic antibody different from γA isohemagglutinin and γD globulin. J. Allergy 37: 336 (1966).

18. ISHIZAKA, K.; ISHIZAKA, T. and MENZEL, A.E.O.: Physicochemical properties of reaginic antibody. VI. Effect of heat on γE, γG and γA antibodies in the sera of ragweed sensitive patients. J. Immunol. 99: 610 (1967).

19. ISHIZAKA, K.; ISHIZAKA, T. and TERRY, W.D.: Antigenic structure of γE globulin and reaginic antibody. J. Immunol. 99: 849 (1967).

20. JOHANSSON, S.G.O. and BENNICH, H.: Immunological studies of an atypical (myeloma) immunoglobulin. Immunology 13: 381 (1967).

21. LAYTON, L.L.; YAMANAKA, E.; LEE, S. and DENKO, C.W.: Demonstration of human reaginic antibodies to foods, cat dander, an insect and ragweed and grass pollens. J. Allergy 33: 271 (1962).

22. LEDDY, J.P.; FREEMAN, G.L.; LUZ, A. and TODD, R.H.: Inactivation of the skin-sensitizing antibodies of human allergy by thiols. Proc. Soc. exp. Biol., N.Y. 111: 7 (1962).

23. LEVY, D.A. and OSLER, A.G.: Studies on the mechanisms of hypersensitivity phenomena. XIV. Passive sensitization in vitro of human leukocytes to ragweed pollen antigen. J. Immunol. 97: 203 (1966).

24. LICHTENSTEIN, L.M. and OSLER, A.G.: Studies on the mechanisms of hypersensitivity phenomena. IX. Histamine release from human leukocytes by ragweed pollen antigen. J. exp. Med. 120: 507 (1964).

25. PERELMUTTER L.; ROSE, B. and GOODFRIEND, L.: The relationship between the skin-sensitizing antibody and γA protein in the sera of ragweed-allergic individuals. J. Allergy 37: 236 (1966).

26. REID, R.T.; MINDEN, P. and FARR, R.S.: Reaginic activity associated with IgG immunoglobulin. J. exp. Med. 123: 845 (1966).

27. ROCKEY, J.H. and KUNKEL, H.G.: Unusual sedimentation and sulfhydryl sensitivity of certain immunoglobulins and skin-sensitizing antibody. Proc. Soc. exp. Biol., N.Y. 111: 7 (1962).

28. SELA, M. and MOZES, E.: Dependence of the chemical nature of antibodies on the net electrical charge of antigens. Proc. nat. Acad. Sci., Wash. 55: 455 (1966).

29. STANWORTH, D.R.: Reaginic antibodies. Adv. Immunol. 3: 181, (1963).

30. STANWORTH, D.R.; HUMPHREY, J.H.; BENNICH, H. and JOHANSSON, S.G.O.: Specific inhibition of the Prausnitz-Küstner reaction by an atypical human myeloma protein. Lancet 2: 330 (1967).

31. STANWORTH, D.R.; HUMPHREY, J.H.; BENNICH, H. and JOHANSSON, S.G.O.: Inhibition of Prausnitz-Küstner reaction by proteolytic cleavage fragments of a human myeloma protein of immunoglobulin class E. LANCET 2 :17 (1968).

32. TERRY, W.D. and ROBERT, M.S.: Antigenic heterogeneity of human immunoglobulin A protein. Science 153: 1007 (1966).

33. VAERMAN, J.P.; EPSTEIN, W.; FUDENBERG, H. and ISHIZAKA, K.: Direct demonstration of reaginic activity in purified γ_{1a} globulin. Nature 203: 1046 (1964).
34. VAERMAN, J.P. and HEREMANS, J.F.: Subclasses of human immunoglobulin A based on differences in the a polypeptide chains. Science 153: 647 (1966).
35. YAGI, Y.; MAIER, P.; PRESSMAN, D.; ARBESMAN, C.E. and REISMAN, R.E.: The presence of the ragweed-binding antibodies in the β_{2a}, β_{2m} and γ-globulins of sensitive individuals J. Immunol. 91: 83 (1963).

Author's address: KIMISHIGE ISHIZAKA, M.D., Children's Asthma Research Institute and Hospital, Denver, Colo. (USA).

Cellular and Humoral Mechanisms in Anaphylaxis and Allergy, pp. 90–105
(Karger, Basel/New York 1969)

The Homocytotropic Nature of Reaginic Antibodies[1]

L. GOODFRIEND[2], T. HUBSCHER and M. RADERMECKER[3]

Harry Webster Thorp Laboratories, Division of Immunochemistry and Allergy,
McGill University Clinic, Royal Victoria Hospital
Montreal

To the already staggering heterogeneity shown by antibodies, must be added
yet another delineating characteristic: that of *homo- or heterocytotropism*
[3], depending on the ability of a given antibody to sensitize target cells
exclusively within or exclusively outside the species of origin. The particular
class of antibodies implicated in human allergic disease, the so-called
reagins or skin sensitizing antibodies, are considered to be homocytotropic,
i.e., to sensitize target organs and cells of the primate species only [9].
Supportive evidence for this characterization has accrued from studies in
which human allergic serum was employed to passively sensitize tissues and
cells of the non-primate (guinea pig, rabbit) and sub-human primate (monkey)
species [4].

Guinea Pig

FIREMAN *et al.* [10] and CONNELL and SHERMAN [7] were unable to sensitize
guinea pigs for passive cutaneous anaphylaxis (PCA) with sera from *untreated* atopic patients containing positive Prausnitz-Küstner (PK) activity.
These workers did, however, induce PCA in guinea pigs using sera of
treated hay fever patients, sera containing high titers of the non-reaginic,
blocking antibodies. Recently, ARBESMAN *et al.* [1] have shown that serum of
ragweed atopic patients could passively sensitize the isolated guinea pig
ileum to give Schultz-Dale contractions on challenge with ragweed allergen.
However, the *in vitro* anaphylactic reactions were *insensitive* to heating of

[1] Supported by grants from the Medical Research Council, Ottawa, Canada.
[2] Medical Research Associate of the Medical Research Council of Canada.
[3] Research Fellow of the N.F.S.R. (Belgium) and of the M.R.C. (Canada).

the allergic serum at 56° C for as much as 6 h, a classical method of inactivation of human reaginic antibodies.

Rabbit

Close correlations have been reported [30, 31] between the incidence of
hypersensitivity to various drugs, notably penicillin, and the capacity of the
sera of drug sensitive patients to passively sensitize *rabbit basophils* to
degranulation on challenge with the corresponding incitant drugs. However, the immunoglobulin class of the human, drug specific antibody mediating rabbit basophil degranulation, and its correspondence with the reagin
class, have not yet been elucidated. Furthermore, the few studies [5, 11] of
the rabbit basophil degranulation test which have been made for various
pollinoses have given equivocal or contraindicatory results. Evidence from

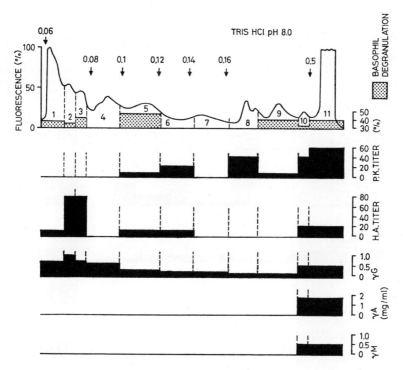

Fig. 1. Antibody activities and immunoglobulin content of DEAE-Sephadex fractions of
serum from treated ragweed allergic patient S. M. [14].

chromatographic studies [14] in this laboratory suggests that the antibodies in human ragweed allergic serum which sensitize rabbit basophils to degranulation are of the *non-reaginic* type.

Figure 1 shows the distribution of the various antibody activities among the DEAE-Sephadex fractions of a treated ragweed allergic serum. *The basophil degranulating activity had no apparent relationship to the reagin content of the fractions.* For example, reagin-rich fractions 6 and 8 were devoid of degranulating activity, while fraction 5, with minimal reagin activity gave maximum degranulation of the basophil cells. It is noteworthy that the most active hemagglutinating fraction 3 had less degranulating activity than the fast γG fraction 5. Indeed, basophil degranulating activity was observed for the DEAE-Sephadex fractions of an *untreated* ragweed allergic serum *containing no detectable hemagglutinating activity* (fig. 2). In this case, too, fast γG-containing fractions 4 and 5 gave maximal degranu-

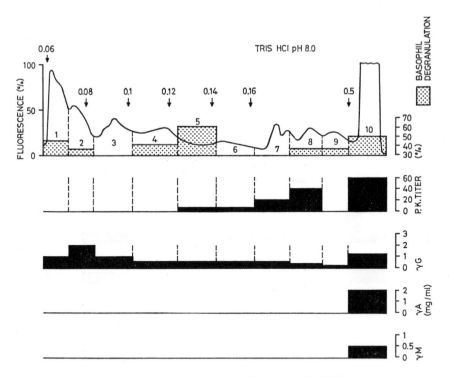

Fig. 2. Rabbit basophil degranulating activities and P-K titers of DEAE-Sephadex fractions of serum from treated ragweed allergic patient J. R. [14].

lating activity although these fractions had no or little reagins, respectively. By Sephadex G-200 gel filtration, the basophil degranulating antibodies were localized essentially to 19S and 7S molecular size components whereas the bulk of the reagins were confined to the ascending portion of the 7S peak [14]. It is probable, therefore, that rabbit basophil degranulating antibodies in ragweed atopic serum do not belong to the reagin class of immunoglobulins (IgE) but to particular, *heterocytotrophic* sub-groups of 7S (likely IgG) and 19S (likely IgM) immunoglobulins. This appears probable also for basophil degranulating antibodies present in human serum sensitive to penicillin G [15]. The role of such non-reaginic antibodies in the full expression of atopic disease remains to be clarified.

Monkey

In contrast to the rodent species, the *sub-human primates*, such as the *monkey*, have been found to be readily sensitized by human reaginic antibodies. STRAUS [31] first demonstrated that human reaginic serum could provoke PCA in the rhesus monkey. Subsequent extensive PCA studies by LAYTON and his associates [19, 20] clearly established *monkey skin* as a target organ for sensitization by human allergic sera of diverse specificity. The antibodies in human allergic serum mediating PCA in monkeys were inactivated by heating at 56°C for 1 h [6, 20]. Intravenous transfer of human allergic serum was found by LAYTON and GREENE [18] and BUCKLEY and METZGAR [6] to sensitize monkeys to severe and fatal systemic anaphylaxis. PATTERSON *et al.* [24, 25] have done extensive studies on the passive transfer of immediate hypersensitivity by intravenous injection of human allergic serum to monkeys. These workers observed *local cutaneous, mucosal and anaphylactic reactions* in monkeys on challenge with appropriate allergen.

Parenthetically, PATTERSON *et al.* [24, 25] observed that monkeys sensitized systemically with human reaginic serum were refractory to PCA with reagins some 2 weeks after the initial sensitization. These workers suggested that the refractory state might be due to the formation of monkey antibodies to the sensitizing serum and its constituent reaginic antibodies. We have observed [26] a similar refractory state following intravenous injection of monkeys with *normal* (non-atopic) human serum (fig. 3), and *even more markedly, with non-immune rabbit serum* (fig. 4). It seems unlikely, therefore, that the refractory state is due specifically to the development of monkey anti-reagin antibodies. Our findings [26] implicate some immunological

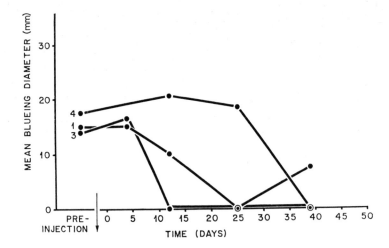

Fig. 3. Effect of i.v. injection of normal human serum (NHS) on reagin-induced PCA in monkeys. PCA tests were done in monkeys 1, 3 and 4 prior to and at various times following i.v. injection of 20 ml NHS/kg [27].

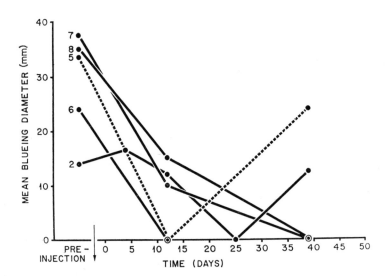

Fig. 4. Effect of i.v. injection of rabbit serum (RS) on reagin-induced PCA in monkeys. PCA tests were done in monkeys 2, 5, 6, 7 and 8 prior to and at various times following i.v. injection of 20 ml RS/kg [27].

mechanism involving the production of monkey antibodies, but the immuno-globulin nature and specificity of these antibodies, and their role in the mechanism of inhibition of PCA with human reagins, require elucidation.

An important contribution to the delineation of human reagins as *primate species specific* was the demonstration by ARBESMAN *et al.* [1] that segments of monkey ileum could be passively sensitized with human reaginic serum *in vitro* to give Schultz-Dale contractions on challenge with appropriate allergen. By diluting the reaginic serum, Schultz-Dale titers could be obtained: *these were found to be closely correlated with P-K titers of reaginic serum as determined in the human.* Furthermore, *unlike the guinea pig ileum reactions, the monkey ileum contractions were abolished by heating the allergic serum at 56°C,* in accord with the heat sensitivity of reaginic antibodies.

These findings stimulated studies in our own laboratory [12, 13, 21] to develop an *in vitro* technique which might be more amenable to the *bio-chemical* investigation of reagin-induced anaphylaxis and we borrowed a leaf from the classical work on *in vitro* anaphylaxis of *chopped guinea pig lung* [2]. In these studies, antigen was added to guinea gip lung suspensions previously sensitized *in vitro* with rabbit antiserum and the amount of histamine diffusing out of the tissue in a fixed time determined by bioassay on the isolated guinea pig ileum preparation. The quantity of histamine released was taken as an index of sensitization. We adopted the same methodological principles for passive sensitization of *suspensions of rhesus monkey lung or skin* by ragweed allergic serum.

Figure 5 shows the anaphylactic reactions obtained with rhesus monkey lung suspensions previously incubated with ragweed-allergic serum and challenged with varying doses of ragweed allergen [21]. In the case of lung suspensions, the dose-response curves were generally of a precipitin-like nature.

As shown in table I, the *in vitro* anaphylactic reactions correlated in a general way with P-K titers but showed no relationship to the tanned cell hemagglutination titers of the allergic sera [12]. Indeed, *non-reaginic, human antisera* to diphtheria toxoid, of high hemagglutination titers, failed completely to sensitize monkey lung fragments.

The *in vitro* anaphylactic reactions were invariably inhibited by pre-heating the sensitizing human allergic serum at 56°C (fig. 6), the inhibition paralleling the inactivation of reaginic antibodies (table II).

The findings of these studies were recently confirmed by MALLEY and HARRIS [28].

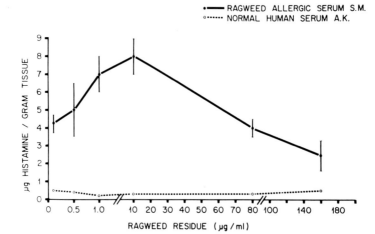

Fig. 5. Effect of allergen concentration on *in vitro* anaphylaxis of monkey lung suspensions [21].

Table I. Comparison of hemagglutination and P-K titers with *in vitro* anaphylaxis of monkey lung fragments

	Hemagglutination titer	P-K titer	Histamine equivalent [μg/g][1]
	Ragweed atopic sera[2]		
V. E.	80	200	0.3
J. P.	160	500	0.8
S. M.	1,280	1,000	1.0
J. L.	80	4,000	1.7
	Human antidiphtheria toxoid sera[3]		
A. K.	1,600	0	0–0.1
J. C.	102,400	0	0–0.1
	Normal serum[2]		
A. K.	0	0	0–0.15

[1] Mean values of duplicate determinations; fragments incubated with serum at 37°C for 1.5 h.

[2] First bleedings: Sept. 1965: fragments challenged with ragweed residue at optimal concentrations: 20 μg/ml (V. E., J. P., S. M.) and 80 μg/ml (J. L.).

[3] Fragments separately challenged with diphtheria toxoid at 10, 20, 40, 80, 160, 640, 1,000, 5,000 and 10,000 μg/ml [12].

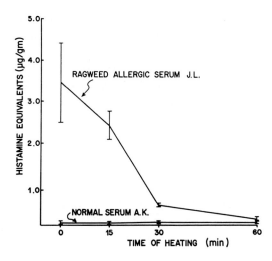

Fig. 6. *In vitro* anaphylaxis of monkey lung fragments: Effect of heating serum at 56°C [12].

Table II. Effect of heating serum at 56°C for 1 h on hemagglutination, P-K titers and *in vitro* anaphylaxis of monkey lung fragments

| | Ragweed atopic sera[2] Hemagglutination titer | | P-K titer | | Histamine equivalent (μg/gm)[1] | |
	unheated	heated	unheated	heated	unheated	heated
V. E.	160	160	250	50	0.4	0.1
J. P.	160	160	500	50	0.9	0.1
S. M.	640	640	1,000	50	2.3	0.1
J. L.	640	640	2,000	200	3.0	0.3
Normal serum						
A. K.	0	0	0	0	0.1	0.1

[1] Mean values of triplicate determinations; fragments incubated with serum at 37°C for 1.5 h.
[2] Second bleeding: Dec. 1965 [12].

In a further study [29], we employed DEAE-Sephadex fractions of ragweed-allergic sera for passive sensitization of monkey lung suspensions and observed close correlations between the *in vitro* anaphylactic reactions and the reagin content of these fractions as determined by P-K test in humans (fig. 7). The lack of correlation with ragweed hemagglutinating antibody was very evident in these studies (fig. 8).

The anaphylactic reactions of monkey skin suspensions contrasted with those of monkey lung suspensions in showing little inhibition of response with high allergen concentrations (fig. 9). The cause of this difference in dose-response relationships is unclear.

The monkey skin suspension reaction was able to discriminate between reagins of different allergen specificity [22]. We have recently [31] isolated a ragweed allergen, Ra 3, differing in allergenic properties from those of Antigen E, isolated by KING and NORMAN [17]. Monkey skin suspensions passively sensitized with human ragweed-allergic serum containing reagins to Antigen E but not to Antigen Ra 3, as determined in the human, gave *in vitro* anaphylactic reactions upon challenge with Antigen E only (fig. 10). On the other hand, skin suspensions reacted equally to Antigens E and Ra 3 when the serum employed for passive sensitization contained equal amounts

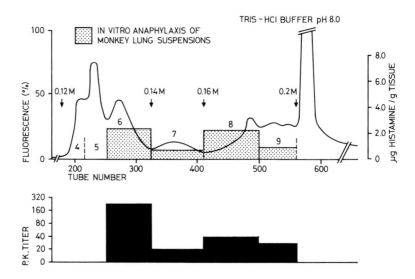

Fig. 7. DEAE-Sephadex chromatography of treated ragweed-allergic serum R.C. [21].

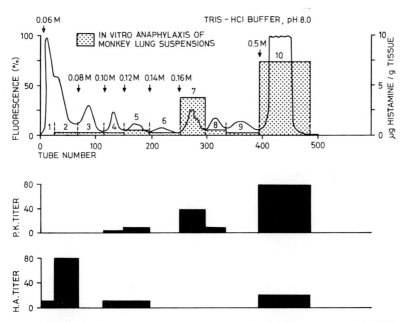

Fig. 8. DEAE-Sephadex chromatography of treated ragweed-allergic serum S.M. [21].

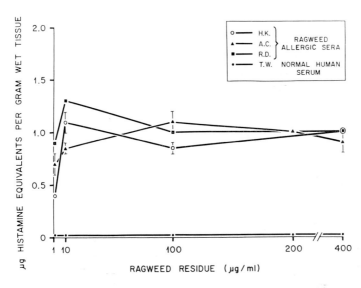

Fig. 9. Effect of allergen concentration on *in vitro* anaphylaxis of monkey skin suspensions [13].

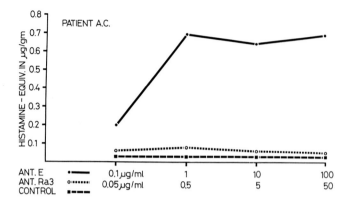

Fig. 10. *In vitro* anaphylaxis of monkey skin suspensions passively sensitized with ragweed allergic serum A.C. and separately challenged with ragweed Antigens E and Ra3 [22].

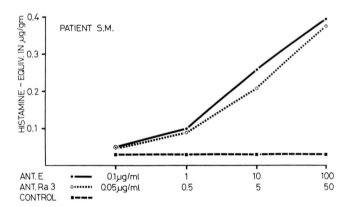

Fig. 11. *In vitro* anaphylaxis of monkey skin suspensions passively sensitized with ragweed allergic serum S.M. and separately challenged with ragweed Antigens E and Ra3 [22].

of reagins to Antigens E and Ra 3 as determined by P-K tests in the human (fig. 11).

As with the lung, the monkey skin suspension responses were abolished by heating allergic serum at 56°C for 1 h (table III). The activity was not restored by incorporating normal human serum as a source of complement.

We have recently attempted [16] to localize the *target cells of human reagins in monkey skin*, utilizing for this purpose the fluorescent 'sandwich'

Table III. Effect of heating allergic serum at 56°C for 1 h on *in vitro* anaphylaxis of monkey skin suspensions

Allergic serum	Histamine equivalents (μg/g) Unheated[1]		Heated[2]		Heated + NHS[3]	
R. D.	1.3,	1.3	0.02,	0.02	0.02,	0.03
A. C.	0.9,	1.0	0.02,	0.02	0.01,	0.02
C. D.	0.4,	0.4	0.02,	0.02	0.02,	0.02
C. P.	0.2,	0.2	0.02,	0.02	0.01,	0.02
NHS	0.01	0.02	0.02,	0.02	–	

[1] Each 200 mg aliquot of monkey skin suspension was sensitized with 0.4 ml of allergic serum.
[2] Allergic serum (0.4 ml) which had been heated at 56°C for 1 h was used to 'sensitize' each skin suspension aliquot.
[3] Heated allergic serum (0.4 ml) and normal human serum D. W. (0.4 ml) as a source of human complement were incorporated in the incubation medium of each aliquot of monkey skin suspension [13].

technique [8]. Monkey skin biopsies were separately incubated with ragweed-allergic or normal human serum and sections overlayered with ragweed Antigen E, followed by a fluorescein-tagged preparation of rabbit immune globulin specific to Antigen E. Sections of monkey skin sensitized with allergic serum showed specific cellular fluorescence, invariably absent from sections treated with normal serum (fig. 12). On counterstaining with toluidine blue, the fluorescent cells were identified as metachromatically staining mast cells (fig. 13). Attempts to localize human IgG, IgA or IgM to the mast cells in monkey skin sections treated with human ragweed-allergic serum and stained either directly or indirectly with fluorescein-tagged specific antisera have been uniformly negative. Our results to date encourage us to believe that the antibodies in human ragweed allergic serum which fix to the mast cells of monkey (and presumably also of the human tissues) belong to the IgE or reagin class of immunoglobulins.

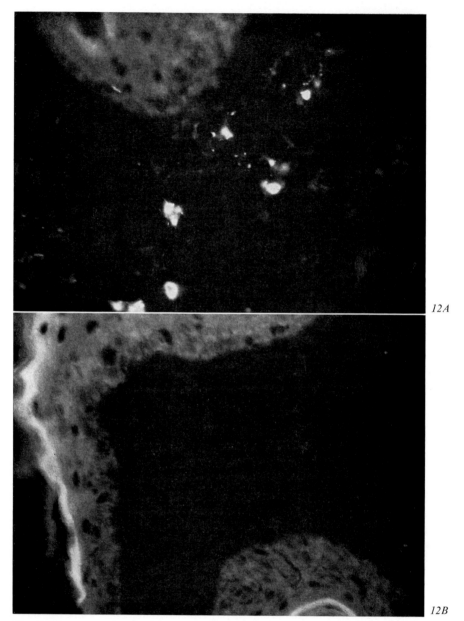

12A

12B

Fig. 12. Fluorescence localization of ragweed-binding antibodies in monkey skin biopsies separately incubated with untreated ragweed-allergic serum J.H. (A) and normal human serum T.W. (B) Sections of the incubated biopsies were exposed to ragweed Antigen E and stained with fluorescein-tagged rabbit anti-Antigen E globulin ($\times$ 400) [16].

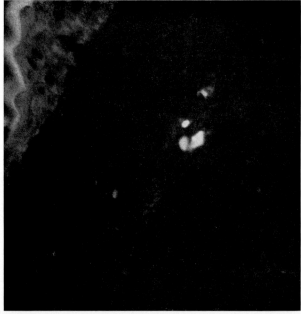

13A

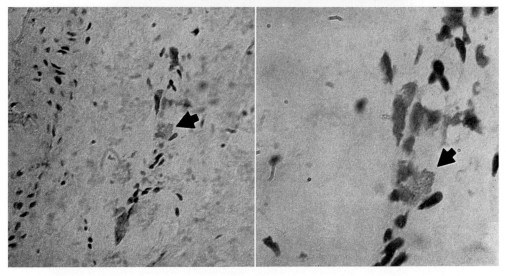

13B   *Fig. 13.* Identification of fluorescent cells in monkey skin sensitized with human ragweed   13C
allergic serum (see text). (A) Isolated area of a section showing a fluorescent cell (×400).
(B) The same area counterstained with toluidine blue (×400). The fluorescence was localized to a metachromatically staining cell (arrow). (C) The same cell at higher magnification
(×700) showed the characteristic morphology of a mast cell [16].

Summary

Anaphylactic antibodies have been delineated into 2 broad categories, hetero- and homo-cytotrophic, depending on their capacity to sensitize target organ cells of foreign species or otherwise. Studies in the literature which relate to the cytotrophic nature of human reaginic antibodies are reviewed, with particular emphasis on those in the authors' laboratory on passive sensitization with reaginic serum of rabbit, monkey and human cells and tissues. The results of such studies favor the conclusion that reagins are exclusively homocytotrophic, sensitizing mast cells of the primate species only.

References

1. ARBESMAN, C. E.; GIRARD, J. P. and ROSE, N. R.: Demonstration of human reagins in the monkey. II. *In vitro* passive sensitization of monkey ileum with sera of untreated atopic patients. J. Allergy *35:* 535 (1964).
2. AUSTEN, K. F. and HUMPHREY, J. H.: *In vitro* studies of the mechanism of anaphylaxis; in Advances in Immunology, F. J. DIXON and J. H. HUMPHREY, eds., p. 1, Vol. 3 (Academic Press, New York/London 1963).
3. BECKER, E. L. and AUSTEN, K. F.: Anaphylaxis; in Immunopathology, H. MULLER-EBERHARD and P. MIESCHER, eds. (Little, Brown, Boston 1966).
4. BLOCH, K. J.: The anaphylactic antibodies of mammals including man. Progr. Allergy, vol. 10, p. 84 (Karger, Basel/New York 1967).
5. BOBITT, J. R.; SCHECHTER, H. and POLLAK, V. E.: A critical evaluation of the indirect basophil degranulation test. Proc. Soc. exp. Biol., N.Y. *117:* 608 (1964).
6. BUCKLEY, R. H. and METZGAR, R. S.: The use of nonhuman primates for studies of reagin. J. Allergy *36:* 382 (1965).
7. CONNELL, J. T. and SHERMAN, W. B.: Relationship of passive cutaneous anaphylaxis to antibodies in the serum of ragweed hay fever patients after injection treatment. J. Immunol. *94:* 498 (1965).
8. COONS, A. H. and KAPLAN, M. H.: Localization of antigen in tissue cells. II. Improvements in a method for detection of antigen by means of fluorescent antibody. J. exp. Med. *91:* 1 (1950).
9. DAVIS, B. D.; DULBECCO, R.; EISEN, H. N.; GINSBERG, H. S. and WOOD, W. B.: Microbiology, Chapt. 17, p. 525 (Harper & Row, New York 1968).
10. FIREMAN, P.; VANNIER, W. E. and GOODMAN, H. C.: The association of skin-sensitizing antibody with the B2A-globulins in sera from ragweed-sensitive patients. J. exp. Med. *117:* 603 (1963).
11. FRIEDLAENDER, S. and FRIEDLAENDER, A. S.: Observation on basophil degranulation as an indicator of antigen-antibody reaction. J. Allergy *35:* 361 (1964).
12. GOODFRIEND, L.; KOVACS, B. A. and ROSE, B.: *In-vitro* sensitization of monkey lung fragments with human ragweed atopic serum. Int. Arch. Allergy *30:* 511 (1966).
13. GOODFRIEND, L. and LUHOVYJ, I.: *In-vitro* detection of reagins in human atopic sera by monkey skin suspension technique. Int. Arch. Allergy *33:* 171 (1968).
14. HUBSCHER, T. and GOODFRIEND, L.: Role of human reaginic and hemagglutinating antibodies in the indirect rabbit basophil degranulation reaction. Int. Arch. Allergy *35:* 298 (1969).
15. HUBSCHER, T. and GOODFRIEND, L.: Unpublished observations.
16. HUBSCHER, T.; GOODFRIEND, L. and WATSON, J. I.: Fluorescent localization of ragweed binding antibodies in monkey skin passively sensitized with human atopic serum. To be submitted for publication in J. Immunol.

17. KING, T. P. and NORMAN, P. S.: Isolation studies of allergens from ragweed pollen. Biochemistry *1:* 709 (1962).
18. LAYTON, L. L. and GREENE, F. C.: Systemic allergic shock induced in monkeys passively sensitized by intravenous injection of human allergic sera. Int. Arch. Allergy *25:* 193 (1964).
19. LAYTON, L. L.; LEE, S. and DEEDS, F.: Diagnosis of human allergy utilizing passive skin sensitization in the monkey *Macaca irus.* Proc. Soc. Exp. Biol., N.Y. *108:* 623 (1961).
20. LAYTON, L. L.; YAMANAKA, E.; GREENE, F. C. and PERLMAN, F.: Atopic reagins to penicillin, pollens and seeds: Thermolability, titer and persistence in the skin of passively sensitized macaque monkeys. Int. Arch. Allergy *23:* 87 (1963).
21. LOENG, A. and GOODFRIEND, L.: In preparation.
22. LUHOVYJ, I.; UNDERDOWN, B. J. and GOODFRIEND, L.: Unpublished observations.
23. MALLEY, A. and HARRIS, R. L., Jr.: Passive sensitization of monkey lung fragments with sera of timothy-sensitive patients. I. Spectrofluorimetric analysis of histamine release. J. Immunol. *100:* 915 (1968).
24. PATTERSON, R.; FINK, J. H.; NISHIMURA, E. T. and PRUZANSKY, J. J.: The passive transfer of immediate type hypersensitivity from man to other primates. J. clin. Invest. *44:* 140 (1965).
25. PATTERSON, R.; MIYAMOTO, T.; REYNOLDS, L. and PRUZANSKY, J. J.: Comparative studies of two models of allergic respiratory disease. Int. Arch. Allergy *32:* 31 (1967).
26. RADERMECKER, M. and GOODFRIEND, L.: Inhibition of reagin-induced PCA in monkeys. Lancet *ii:* 1086 (1968).
27. RADERMECKER, M. and GOODFRIEND, L.: In preparation.
28. REYNOLDS, R. D. and SMITH, R. E.: The indirect basophil degranulation test. Ann. Allergy *25:* 318 (1967).
29. SHELLEY, W. B.: Indirect basophil degranulation test for allergy to penicillin and other drugs. J. amer. med. Ass. *184:* 171 (1963).
30. STRAUS, H. W.: Studies in experimental hypersensitiveness in the rhesus monkey. II. Passive local cutaneous sensitization with human reaginic sera. J. Immunol. *32:* 251 (1937).
31. UNDERDOWN, B. J. and GOODFRIEND, L.: Isolation and characterization of an allergen from short ragweed pollen. In press (Biochemistry).

Authors' address: L. GOODFRIEND, Ph.D., T. HUBSCHER, MSc. and M. RADERMECKER, M.D., Harry Webster Thorp Laboratories, Division of Immunochemistry and Allergy, McGill University Clinic, Royal Victoria Hospital, *Montreal* (Canada).

Cellular and Humoral Mechanisms in Anaphylaxis and Allergy, pp. 106–113
(Karger, Basel/New York 1969)

Is There a Common Receptor for Different Types of Antibody Activating Histamine Release in the Guinea Pig?

Irvin Broder

Departments of Medicine, Pathology and Pharmacology University of Toronto

Anaphylaxis can be activated in the guinea pig either by guinea pig gamma 1, non-complement-fixing antibody or by rabbit gamma 2 complement-fixing antibody [11, 31]. Since these two kinds of antibody differ in electrophoretic mobility and in capacity to fix complement, the question arises of whether they also differ in the tissue receptor occupied during the activation of guinea pig anaphylaxis.

The approach taken in answering this question was based on the premise that the two antibodies could be assumed to act on a common tissue receptor if both were competitively inhibited by a single antagonist [1]. The antagonist selected for study was normal rabbit gamma globulin. It is well known that this reagent interferes with the anaphylactic activity of antibodies [8, 9, 10, 17, 23, 24, 25, 27, 28, 30] but the mechanism of this inhibition has not previously been defined. The following studies in the guinea pig suggest that normal rabbit gamma globulin may inhibit the anaphylactic activity of guinea pig and rabbit antibody by a competitive mechanism.

This work was carried out using the isolated perfused guinea pig lung, in which histamine release was activated by soluble antigen-antibody complexes prepared in excess antigen [13]. Soluble complexes were employed containing either guinea pig gamma 1 antibody (guinea pig complexes) or rabbit gamma 2 antibody (rabbit complexes). This system can be considered to represent anaphylaxis since inhibition occurred in the absence of calcium or glucose and also in the presence of excess sodium chloride. In addition, inhibition was seen at 45° C and in the presence of sulfhydryl reagents, while succinate or maleate produced enhancement [12]. The release of histamine by soluble complexes was accompanied by mast cell degranulation [29]. These characteristics are the same as those defined when anaphylaxis is activated by the addition of antigen to sensitized guinea pig lung tissue [5, 6, 7, 8, 15, 16, 20, 21, 22, 26].

Methods

Antigen and antibodies. Crystalline bovine plasma albumin was used to immunize guinea pigs and rabbits. Immunoelectrophoresis was performed on each antiserum and developed with both antigen and goat antiserum to whole guinea pig or rabbit serum. Each antiserum was also examined for complement-fixing activity. The guinea pig antiserum demonstrated the presence of antibody to bovine plasma albumin, migrating as a gamma 1 globulin; no gamma 2 component was apparent and the serum showed no complement-fixing activity. The rabbit antiserum exhibited antibody migrating as a gamma 2 globulin and fixed 500 C′H50 units of rabbit complement per mg of antibody protein. Soluble antigen-antibody complexes were prepared by precipitating each antiserum with the amount of antigen required for equivalence, washing the equivalence precipitate and then rendering this soluble by the addition of a ninefold excess of antigen.

Fractionation of normal rabbit serum. Normal rabbit serum was fractionated by starch block electrophoresis [14]. The protein content of each fraction was determined by micro-Kjeldahl nitrogen analysis.

Isolated perfused guinea pig lung. Heart-lung preparations were obtained from normal, non-immunized guinea pigs. Each preparation was maintained at 37° C and perfused with Tyrode solution through the pulmonary artery. The Tyrode solution passed through the vascular bed of the lung, escaped from the left atrium and was collected in sequential fractions. Soluble antigen-antibody complexes were injected into the pulmonary artery and led to the appearance of histamine in the effluent perfusion fluid. The histamine was quantitated by biological assay on the guinea pig ileum. A single guinea pig lung responded with appreciable histamine release to 3 or 4 sequential injections of soluble complexes given at intervals of 1½ h. A dose-response relationship could be defined and neither the antigen nor antiserum were active when injected alone. A detailed description of this system has been published previously [13].

Experimental design. The studies to be described consisted of defining dose-response curves, relating amount of soluble complex injected to magnitude of histamine release. The guinea pig lung system exhibited a moderate variability in response to a constant dose of soluble complexes given to separate lungs or given sequentially to a single lung. This variability dictated that multiple observations be made on each treatment and also that a method be established for relating one set of observations to another. These requirements were met by planning each experiment to fit a 3×9 Latin square design. In this design, different treatments were compared in groups of three (triplets) and all three treatments were administered in random order to each of nine lungs. Two approaches were then utilized to enable separate triplets to be related. The first approach was employed in the absence of inhibitor, in constructing the standard dose-response curves. Here, two triplets were used in which one dose was common to each and therefore enabled all 5 doses to be related. The second approach was utilized in constructing dose-response curves under the influence of inhibitor. Here, each triplet consisted of a constant dose of complexes given either alone or when premixed with two different amounts of normal gamma globulin. The assumption was made that the response obtained in the absence of inhibitor fell on the previously defined standard dose-response curve; consequently, the responses obtained within these triplets in the presence of inhibitor could be related to the standard curve.

It was found that within a set of nine observations obtained for a single treatment, occasional values for histamine release were exceedingly high. In order to minimize the heavy weighting which these values would otherwise introduce, the mean for each treatment was calculated from the square root of the nine individual values for histamine release. The mean obtained in this manner was then squared and this value was used in expressing the histamine-releasing activity of one treatment as a percentage of another.

Results

A preliminary study was carried out to define the relative histamine releasing activity of the guinea pig and rabbit complexes. The approach taken was to compare a fixed dose of rabbit complexes with paired doses of guinea pig complexes, using the 3×9 Latin square design. Data were obtained with four doses of the guinea pig complexes, two of which produced smaller responses and two larger responses than the fixed dose of rabbit complexes. It was found by interpolation that a dose of guinea pig complexes containing 5 μg of antibody protein was equal in activity to a 2.5 μg dose of the rabbit complexes.

These equivalent doses of guinea pig and rabbit complexes were used in further preliminary studies to screen the starch block fractions of normal rabbit serum for an inhibitory effect on histamine releasing activity. The influence of each fraction on the two preparations of complexes was individually examined in separate 3×9 experiments. In each experiment, the three treatments consisted of the fixed dose of complexes given alone and given together with 20 and 80 μg protein of the individual starch block fractions. It was found that the fraction containing gamma globulin, but not albumin, alpha globulin or beta globulin, produced an inhibitory effect. The slow and fast migrating gamma globulin fractions were each equally inhibitory and therefore subsequent studies were carried out using the whole gamma globulin fraction. The inhibition produced by gamma globulin was reversible, since no inhibition occurred when the injection of gamma globulin preceded that of the soluble complexes.

The following studies were carried out applying the specific approaches discussed under Experimental Design. Standard dose-response curves were defined for the guinea pig and rabbit complexes (fig. 1 and 2). Each standard curve was utilized in constructing additional dose-response curves obtained with varying doses of soluble complexes in the presence of 20 and 80 μg protein of normal rabbit gamma globulin. It was found that the dose response curve for rabbit complexes was no appreciably shifted in the presence of

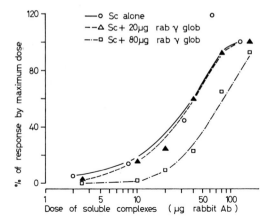

Fig. 1. Dose-response curves for soluble antigen-antibody complexes containing rabbit gamma 2 antibody.

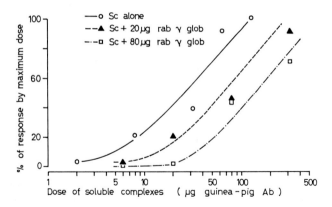

Fig. 2. Dose-response curves for soluble antigen-antibody complexes containing guinea pig gamma 1 antibody.

20 μg of normal rabbit gamma globulin (fig. 1). The same amount of inhibitor increased the requirement of guinea pig complexes by twofold, to achieve a histamine releasing effect equal to that obtained in the absence of inhibitor (fig. 2). In the presence of 80 μg of normal rabbit gamma globulin, there was a twofold shift in the curve for the rabbit complexes and a fourfold shift in that for the guinea pig complexes (fig. 1 and 2). The shift of each curve seen in the presence of inhibitor was parallel to the standard curve.

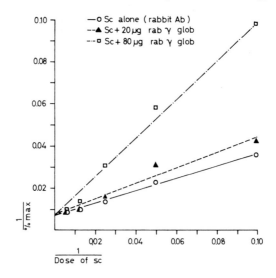

Fig. 3. Lineweaver Burk plot for dose-response curves of soluble antigen-antibody complexes containing rabbit gamma 2 antibody.

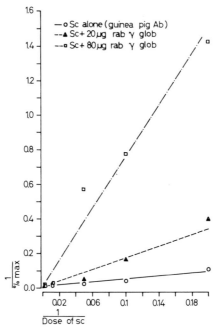

Fig. 4. Lineweaver Burk plot for dose-response curves of soluble antigen-antibody complexes containing guinea pig gamma 1 antibody.

The foregoing data were also examined (fig. 3 and 4) in Lineweaver Burk reciprocal plots [19]. The dose response curves for the rabbit complexes displayed a threshold effect and the plots shown have been corrected for this [18, 4]. No threshold effect was evident in the curves obtained for the guinea pig complexes. The reciprocal plots of the data obtained with the guinea pig and rabbit complexes each defined a straight line relationship. The three lines defined for each soluble complex preparation converged on a common intercept on the vertical ordinate.

Discussion and Summary

The foregoing studies demonstrated that normal rabbit gamma globulin was a more effective antagonist of guinea pig complexes than it was of rabbit complexes (fig. 1 and 2). This may indicate that rabbit antibody has a greater affinity for the anaphylactic histamine releasing site in guinea pig tissue than does guinea pig antibody. Perhaps in keeping with this interpretation was the finding that a dose of rabbit complexes containing 2.5 μg of antibody protein was twofold more active than guinea pig complexes when compared on a weight basis.

The dose response curves for guinea pig and rabbit complexes each underwent a parallel shift in the presence of normal rabbit gamma globulin (fig. 1 and 2). Also, the Lineweaver Burk plots of these data defined straight lines which for each preparation of complexes converged on a common intercept on the vertical ordinate (fig. 3 and 4). Both of these findings can be best explained on the basis that normal rabbit gamma globulin inhibits anaphylactic histamine release by a competitive mechanism [2]. Since the inhibitor displayed competitive kinetics in the presence of both preparations of soluble complexes, this is consistent with the possibility that guinea pig gamma 1, non-complement-fixing antibody acts on the same tissue receptor as rabbit gamma 2, complement-fixing antibody [1]. However, this interpretation must be considered provisional, since similar kinetics could theoretically be encountered under conditions of non-competitive inhibition in a system possessing spare receptors [3]. If this latter mechanism were to be operative here, it would not be valid to conclude that the two kinds of antibody acted upon the same receptor [2]. It will be necessary to define additional curves, using larger amounts of inhibitor, in order to distinguish between the two different mechanisms which could account for the data presented [3].

112   BRODER   Is There a Common Receptor for Different Types

Acknowledgements

This work was supported by the Medical Research Council of Canada. The excellen
technical assistance of Miss CHRISTINE LAWLOR and Miss CAROLYN CROWE is gratefully
acknowledged.

References

1. ARIENS, E. J.; SIMONIS, A. M. and VAN ROSSUM, J. M.: Drug-receptor interaction:
Interaction of one or more drugs with one receptor system; in Molecular Pharmacology, vol. 1, ed. E. J. ARIENS, p. 155 (Academic Press, New York 1964).
2. ARIENS, E. J.; SIMONIS, A. M. and VAN ROSSUM, J. M.: Drug-receptor interaction:
Interaction of one or more drugs with different receptor systems; in Molecular Pharmacology, vol. 1, ed. E. J. ARIENS, pp. 290 and 322 (Academic Press, New York 1964).
3. ARIENS, E. J.; SIMONIS, A. M. and VAN ROSSUM, J. M.: The relation between stimulus
and effect; in Molecular Pharmacology, vol. 1, ed. E. J. ARIENS, p. 408 (Academic
Press, New York 1964).
4. ARIENS, E. J.; VAN ROSSUM, J. M. and KOOPMAN, P. C.: Receptor reserve and threshold
phenomena. 1. Theory and experiments with autonomic drugs tested on isolated
organs. Arch. int. Pharmacodyn. *127:* 459 (1960).
5. AUSTEN, K. F. and BROCKLEHURST, W. E.: Anaphylaxis in chopped guinea pig lung.
1. Effect of peptidase substrates and inhibitors. J. exp. Med. *113:* 521 (1961)
6. AUSTEN, K. F. and BROCKLEHURST, W. E.: Anaphylaxis in chopped guinea pig lung.
2. Enhancement of the anaphylactic release of histamine and slow reacting substance
by certain dibasic aliphatic acids and inhibition by monobasic fatty acids. J. exp. Med.
113: 541 (1961).
7. AUSTEN, K. F. and BROCKLEHURST, W. E.: Anaphylaxis in chopped guinea pig lung.
3. Effect of carbon monoxide, cyanide, salicylaldoxime and ionic strength. J. exp. Med.
114: 29 (1961).
8. BAKER, A. R.; BLOCH, K. J. and AUSTEN, K. F.: *In vitro* passive sensitization of
chopped guinea pig lung by guinea pig 7S antibodies. J. Immunol. *93:* 525 (1964).
9. BINAGHI, R.; LIACOPOULOS, P.; HALPERN, B. N. and LIACOPOULOS-BRIOT, M.: Inter-
ference of non-specific gamma globulins with passive *in vitro* anaphylactic sensitization of isolated guinea pig intestine. Immunology *5:* 204 (1962).
10. BIOZZI, G.; HALPERN, B. N. and BINAGHI, R.: The competitive effect of normal serum
proteins from various animal species on antibody fixation in passive cutaneous
anaphylaxis in the guinea pig. J. Immunol. *82:* 215 (1959).
11. BLOCH, K. J.; KOURILSKY, F. M.; OVARY, Z. and BENACERRAF, B.: Properties of
guinea pig 7S antibodies. III. Identification of antibodies involved in complement
fixation and hemolysis. J. exp. Med. *117:* 965 (1963).
12. BRODER, I.: Unpublished observations.
13. BRODER, I. and SCHILD, H. O.: The action of soluble antigen-antibody complexes in
perfused guinea-pig lung. Immunology *8:* 300 (1965).
14. CAMPBELL, D. H.; GARVEY, D. H.; CREMER, N. E. and SUSSDORF, D. H.: Methods in
Immunology, p. 57 (Benjamin, Inc., New York 1964).
15. CHAKRAVARTY, N.: The mechanism of histamine release in anaphylactic reaction in
guinea pig and rat. Acta physiol. scand. *48:* 146 (1960).
16. DIAMANT, B.: Effect of phlorizin on the *in vitro* release of histamine from lung tissue.
Acta physiol. scand. *56:* 97 (1962).

17. HALPERN, B. N. and FRICK, O. L.: Protection against fatal anaphylactic shock with
γ-globulins in guinea pigs and mice. J. Immunol. *88:* 683 (1962).
18. KIRSCHNER, L. B. and STONE, W. E.: Action of inhibitors at the myoneural junction.
J. gen. Physiol. *34:* 821 (1950–51).
19. LINEWEAVER, H. and BURK, D.: The determination of enzyme dissociation constants.
J. amer. chem. Soc. *56:* 658 (1934).
20. MONGAR, J. L. and SCHILD, H. O.: Inhibition of the anaphylactic reaction. J. Physiol.
135: 301 (1957).
21. MONGAR, J. L. and SCHILD, H. O.: Effect of temperature on the anaphylactic reaction.
J. Physiol. *135:* 320 (1957).
22. MONGAR, J. L. and SCHILD, H. O.: The effect of calcium and pH on the anaphylactic
reaction. J. Physiol. *140:* 272 (1958).
23. MONGAR, J. L. and SCHILD, H. O.: A study of the mechanism of passive sensitization.
J. Physiol. *150:* 546 (1960).
24. MONGAR, J. L. and WINNE, D.: Further studies of the mechanism of passive sensitization. J. Physiol. *182:* 79 (1966).
25. MOTA, I.: The mechanism of anaphylaxis. 1. Production and biological properties of
mast cell sensitizing antibody. Immunology *7:* 681 (1964).
26. MOTA, I. and VUGMAN, I.: Effects of anaphylactic shock and compound 48/80 on the
mast cells of the guinea pig lung. Nature *177:* 427 (1956).
27. OVARY, Z.; BENACERRAF, B. and BLOCH, K. J.: Properties of guinea pig 7S antibodies.
II. Identification of antibodies involved in passive cutaneous and systemic anaphylaxis.
J. exp. Med. *117:* 951 (1963).
28. PROUVOST-DANON, A.; QUEIROZ JAVIERRE, M. and SILVA LIMA, M.: Passive anaphylactic reaction in mouse peritoneal mast cells *in vitro.* Life Sci. *5:* 175 (1966).
29. TAICHMAN, N. and BRODER, I.: Unpublished observations.
30. VUREK, G. G.; PRAGER, D. J. and FEIGEN, G. A.: Antibody concentration and temperature as determinants of *in vitro* sensitization and histamine release in isolated
cardiac tissues. J. Immunol. *99:* 1243 (1967).
31. ZVAIFLER, N. J. and BECKER, E. L.: Rabbit anaphylactic antibody J. exp. Med. *123:*
935 (1966).

Author's address: IRVIN BRODER, M.D., Departments of Medicine, Pathology and
Pharmacology, University of Toronto, *Toronto* (Canada).

Cellular and Humoral Mechanisms in Anaphylaxis and Allergy, pp. 114–118
(Karger, Basel/New York 1969)

Disodium Cromoglycate a Specific Inhibitor
of Certain Reagin (type II) Antibody-Antigen Reactions

A. M. J. N. Blair and A. J. Clarke

Disodium cromoglycate, code number FPL 670, is a new compound which has recently been introduced in the United Kingdom for the treatment of asthma. This compound is a chromone derivative which has the unusual property of specifically inhibiting the liberation of the mediators of tissue reactions in immediate anaphylactic reactions induced by reagin (type II) antibodies, in particular those of man and rat. It is neither a bronchodilator nor has it any corticosteroid activity. Disodium cromoglycate, in concentrations up to 1 mg/ml, did not affect the responses of guinea-pig ileum *in vitro* to histamine, SRS-A, 5-hydroxytryptamine, acetylcholine, nicotine, substance P or bradykinin, neither did it block the effects of prostaglandin E_1 (relaxation) nor prostaglandin $F_2\alpha$ (contraction) on isolated human bronchial muscle.

We would like to mention a few of the actions of disodium cromoglycate on rat reagin reactions. OGILVIE [4] has shown that rats subjected to helminth infections exhibit a self cure phenomenon which is associated with the presence in the blood of reagin antibodies.

We have collected the serum from such rats and injected it intradermally into normal rats and allowed at least a 24 h interval before intravenous challenge with worm antigen and Evans Blue dye. Usually we wait 20 min before killing the animal, reflecting the skin and reading the PCA reaction. Disodium cromoglycate, 0.5 mg/kg i.v., given with antigen substantially inhibited the PCA while 2 mg disodium cromoglycate/kg gave complete inhibition. We have found that the *N. brasiliensis* antibody (serum) shares many properties with the mast cell sensitising or 'early' antibody induced by sensitisation with egg albumen/*B.pertussis* as described by MOTA [3]. Both are labile to heating for 30 min at 56°C and persist in the skin for several

weeks. Their PCA reactions can be completely inhibited by combined treatment with mepyramine (50 mg/kg i.v.) and BOL148 (4 mg/kg i.v.), or 2–8 mg
disodium cromoglycate/kg i.v., or treatment 3 h before challenge with 4 mg
compound 48/80/kg i.p. to disrupt the mast cells. Mast cell disruption (MCD)
was examined by taking a strip of subcutaneous connective tissue (SCCT)
from the axis of the site of the skin reaction, fixed and stained by the method
of BRIGGS [2]. Thus PCA and MCD could be measured for each reaction
site. In preliminary experiments, it was found that maximal MCD and PCA
occurred at 5 min after antigen challenge in sites sensitised with rat reagin.
In contrast, sites sensitised with rabbit hyperimmune anti-serum to egg
albumen showed only slight skin reactions at 5 min, but were maximal at
10 min. At neither 5 nor 10 min was the MCD significantly different from
manipulative controls.

In order to assess the specificity of the action of disodium cromoglycate,
we sensitised rats on one flank with rat reagin (either the *N. brasiliensis* or the
egg albumen/*B. pertussis* induced antibody) and challenged intravenously
24 h later, and on the other flank injected rabbit hyperimmune serum which
was challenged 4 h later. The timing of sensitisation was arranged so that
both antigens could be given together. The sera were diluted so that both
skin reactions were just maximal. The skin reactions and MCD were read at
10 min and various doses of disodium cromoglycate from 0.1 to 8 mg/kg
were given intravenously with the mixture of antigens with Evans blue dye.
The skin reactions to rat reagin and rabbit hyperimmune sera were similar
in diameter, but the MCD varied from 40–80% (dependent on the serum
used) and about 25% respectively. The manipulative control sites which
were sensitised but not challenged showed MCD from 10–20% and were
significantly less than those at the rat reagin sites (P <0.001), but not at the
rabbit hyperimmune sites (P >0.05). Disodium cromoglycate 8 mg/kg was
able to completely inhibit both PCA and MCD induced by rat reagin.
Smaller doses were able to completely inhibit MCD but not the PCA.

We consider that disodium cromoglycate at the lower doses is able to
inhibit MCD without completely preventing the release of the pharmacological mediators of the reaction, but higher doses can prevent both. In contrast
disodium cromoglycate did not inhibit the skin reaction induced with rabbit
hyperimmune serum which was not primarily dependent on MCD for its
manifestation. A further example of the specificity of the action of disodium
cromoglycate in inhibiting MCD induced with rat reagin, was the observation that the skin reaction and MCD caused by the i.d. injection of 5 μg
compound 48/80 was not prevented by 100 mg disodium cromoglycate/kg

i.v. The inhibitory dose of disodium cromoglycate varied according to the rat reagin serum used. In general *N. brasiliensis* serum had higher titres than the egg albumen/*B. pertussis* induced serum.

We have also studied the effect of disodium cromoglycate on the release of spasmogens from portions of actively sensitised rat lung (200 mg) challenged with antigen (500 ng egg albumen/ml) in the presence of isolated guinea-pig ileum. Rats 200–250 g weight were most suitable for sensitisation with an intramuscular injection of 5 mg/kg of filtered egg albumen solution, and an intraperitoneal injection of 20×10^9 organisms of *B. pertussis* [3]. The time course of the sensitisation of rat lung has been followed. Spasmogen release from the lung, as demonstrated by contraction of the guinea-pig ileum, appeared on day 11 or 12 after sensitisation, and persisted through day 20 being much reduced by day 30 when the reagin serum titre was low according to the homologous PCA reaction. Lungs from rats which had received 5 to 9 weeks sensitisation, did not show any spasmogen release on challenge. Antagonist studies with mepyramine (400 ng/ml) and BOL148 (5 μg/ml) indicated that the contraction of the ileum was due in part to release of histamine and 5-hydroxytryptamine from lungs (taken at day 12), the approximate contributions being 65% and 10% respectively.

Analysis of bath fluid suggests that in addition SRS-A was released. Disodium cromoglycate 10 μg/ml given with antigen caused on average a 40% reduction in the height of ileal contraction and 100 μg/ml a 64% reduction (fig. 1). Disodium cromoglycate had no effect on response to spasmogens added to the bath and, therefore, must have inhibited the antigen induced release of these substances.

The first observation of the unusual activity of disodium cromoglycate was made in 1965 by our Clinical Pharmacologist, Dr. ALTOUNYAN [1]. He is an atopic asthmatic sensitive to mixed grass pollen and found that disodium cromoglycate 1 mg inhaled as an aqueous aerosol prevented by 70% the fall in FEV_1, usually induced by inhalation of antigens. At that time we used the guinea pig as a laboratory model of immediate anaphylaxis but were unable to observe any inhibition by disodium cromoglycate of lung shock *in vivo*, of PCA, or of the release of histamine or SRS-A from actively or passively sensitised lung, using the homologous anti-serum to egg albumen. Consequently, we used the rat reagin model since this seems to be more related to the human atopic reaction. PEPYS and his colleagues [5] also found that disodium cromoglycate provided substantial protection against antigen inhalation challenge in 5 patients, who were sensitive to grass pollen or *Dermatophagoides culinae*, which is a major allergen in house dust.

Rat lung shocked in the presence of guinea-pig ileum

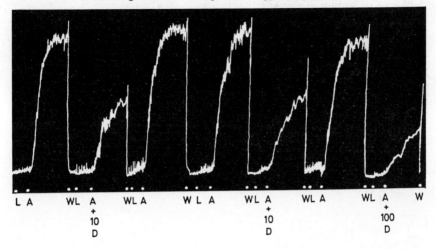

L A   WL A   WL A   W L A   WL A   WL A   WL A   W
+   +   +
10   10   100
D   D   D

Fig. 1. Inhibition by disodium cromoglycate (10 and 100 μg/ml shown as 10D and 100D) of the contraction of guinea-pig ileum in response to spasmogens released from fresh 200 mg portions of rat lung (L) killed 12 days after being sensitised with 5 mg/kg egg albumen i.m. and 20×10^9 *B.pertussis* organisms i.p. and challenged with 500 ng egg albumen/ml (A).

We believe that disodium cromoglycate acts at some critical point in the events after the union of antigen with antibody, which results in an increase in the permeability of cell membranes, particularly those of mast cells. It is possible that the critical pathway, perhaps an enzyme cascade, resulting in mast cell disruption, is common to both the rat and human reagin systems, since both are inhibited by the compound even when different antigen-reagin antibody systems are involved. In summary disodium cromoglycate possesses unusual activity in inhibiting reagin antibody-antigen reactions and should prove useful not only therapeutically but also in the study of allergic mechanisms.

References

1. ALTOUNYAN, R.E.C.: Inhibition of experimental asthma by a new compound disodium cromoglycate, 'Intal'. Acta allerg. *XXII:* 487 (1967).
2. BRIGGS, N.T.: Immunological injury of mast cells in mice actively and passively sensitized to antigens from *Trichinella spiralis*. J. Infect. Dis. *113:* 22–32 (1963).

3. MOTA, I.: The mechanism of anaphylaxis. I. Production and biological properties of 'Mast Cell Sensitizing' antibody. Immunology 7: 681 (1964).
4. OGILVIE, B.M.: Reagin-like antibodies in animals immune to helminth parasites. Nature 204: 91–92 (1964).
5. PEPYS, J.; CHAN, M.; HARGREAVE, F.E. and MCCARTHY, D.S.: Inhibitory effects of disodium cromoglycate on allergen-inhalation tests. Lancet ii: 134–137 (1968).

Author's address: A. M. J. N. BLAIR, Ph.D., Fisons Pharmaceuticals Research Laboratories. Bakewell Road, *Loughborough, Leics.* (England).

Cellular and Humoral Mechanisms in Anaphylaxis and Allergy, pp. 119–121
(Karger, Basel/New York 1969)

Heterogeneity of Homocytotropic Antibodies

G. Strejan and D. H. Campbell

Division of Chemistry and Chemical Engineering, California Institute of Technology,
Pasadena, Calif.

In a study on immediate type hypersensitivity to Ascaris antigens that we started three years ago, we found that guinea pigs immunized with crude extracts emulsified in complete Freund's adjuvant produced both 7S γ_1 and γ_2 precipitating antibodies and that passive cutaneous reactions were induced with serum fractions derived from the entire gamma globulin electrophoretic range. Since the anti-Ascaris immunoglobulins were isolated by preparative electrophoresis, the possibility of γ_1 and γ_2 cross contamination was not ruled out even in the absence of supplementary immunoelectrophoretic arcs [7].

As a subsequent step, several γ_2-containing anti-Ascaris preparations were isolated and purified by exhaustive absorption with a rabbit anti-guinea pig γ_1 serum. The fractions which were found to be free of guinea pig 7S γ_1 globulins – by immunoelectrophoretic criteria – retained the ability to induce passive skin reactions in normal guinea pigs. However, unlike the classical passive cutaneous anaphylactic (PCA) reaction, in which the extravasation of dye appears within a few minutes after the intravenous challenge, the reactions mentioned above appeared not sooner than 30 to 45 min after challenge [8].

The Ascaris extracts are known for their unique ability to induce atopic-type hypersensitivity in a very high percentage of normal, nonatopic individuals following the parenteral introduction of microgram amounts of these extracts. Since the type of immune response depends among others – on the nature of the antigenic determinants injected, the production of a non-γ_1 anti-Ascaris antibody capable of inducing passive cutaneous reactions in the same species might have represented a special situation.

As an alternative, hemocyanin, a highly immunogenic protein was used to produce high-titered precipitating antisera in guinea pigs. The anti-hemocyanin (KLH) antibodies were purified from specific precipitates after dissociation of the immune complexes. The purified anti-KLH antibodies were freed of the 7S γ_1 component by specific absorption with a rabbit anti-guinea pig γ_1 serum. The resulting preparations were found to be free of 7S γ_1 by radio-immunoelectrophoresis. Between 100- and 1,000-fold dilutions of these purified preparations still retained the ability to induce cutaneous reactions in normal guinea pigs, 30 to 45 min after intravenous challenge with KLH [9].

It is interesting to note that the guinea pig 7S γ_2 immunoglobulin was very heterogeneous electrophoretically and was not restricted to the slow γ G zone. Immunoelectrophoretic patterns showed that the γ_2 arc extended into the β_1–α_2 globulin zone; moreover anti-KLH antibodies were found to be associated with this class along the whole range of its electrophoretic mobility.

C^{14}-amino acid incorporation showed different rates of incorporation for three different types of 7S γ G: slow 7S γ_2, fast 7S γ_2 and 7S γ_1 [2].

Guinea pig 7S γ_2 anti-insulin antibodies displaying intermediate to fast electrophoretic mobility were shown to elicit clear PCA reactions in normal guinea pigs [4]. Apart from differences in the rate of synthesis and physico-chemical heterogeneity, the guinea pig 7S γ_2 class might also display differences in biologic properties. On the other hand, however, we must not exclude the possibility that an immunoglobulin type other than 7S γ_2 induced the skin reactions reported.

Regardless of the mechanisms involved (which are probably different for different immunoglobulins) it appears to-day that in a given species, more than one immunoglobulin can display 'homocytotropic' properties. Experimental evidence in this respect was presented also for rabbits [1], for rats [6], for mice [3], and for non-human primates [10].

While very few are contesting to-day, the major role played by IgE in the mechanism of human atopic reactions, there are some indications that it might not be the only one involved [5].

From all the above mentioned evidence it seems that earlier concepts attributing homocytotropic properties exclusively to one immunoglobulin class must be revised.

References

1. HENSON, P. M. and COCHRANE, C. G.: Antigen-antibody complexes and increased vascular permeability (this symposium).

2. Koyama, J. and Miyajima, N.: Heterogeneity of guinea pig 7-S antibodies. I. 7-S Antibodies against ovalbumin produced by various lymphoid tissues. J. Biochem., Tokyo 60: 184 (1966).
3. Mota, I.: Early mouse homocytotropic antibodies. Fed. Proc. 27: 367 (1968).
4. Pondman, K.; van Es, L. and den Harink, I.: Skin-sensitizing antibodies in the guinea pig (this symposium).
5. Reid, R. and Ishizaka, K.: Radioactive tracing of IgE in DEAE fractions containing reagin. J. Allergy 41: 96 (1968).
6. Stechschulte, D.; Austen, F. K. and Bloch, K.: Antibodies involved in antigen-induced release of slow-reacting substance of anaphylaxis (SRS-A), in the guinea pig and rat. J. Exp. Med. 125: 127 (1967).
7. Strejan, G. and Campbell, D. H.: Hypersensitivity to Ascaris antigens. I. Skin-sensitizing activity of serum fractions from guinea pigs sensitized to crude extracts. J. Immunol. 98: 893 (1967).
8. Strejan, G. and Campbell, D. H.: Hypersensitivity to Ascaris antigens. II. Skin-sensitizing properties of 7-S γ_2 antibody from sensitized guinea pigs, as tested in guinea pigs. J. Immunol. 99: 347 (1967).
9. Strejan, G. and Campbell, D. H.: Skin sensitizing properties of guinea pig antibodies to Keyhole Limpet Hemocyanin. J. Immunol. 100: 1245 (1968).
10. Wicher, K.; Girard, J. P.; Reisman, R. E.; Yagi, Y. and Arbesman, C. E.: Demonstration of human reagin in monkey tissues. J. Allergy 41: 63 (1968).

Present address: G. Strejan, Ph.D., Department of Bacteriology and Immunology, University of Western Ontario, London, Ont. (Canada).

Cellular and Humoral Mechanisms in Anaphylaxis and Allergy, pp. 122–128
(Karger, Basel/New York 1969)

The Selective Release of Histamine
from Rat Mast Cells[1]

Alice R. Johnson and Neil C. Moran

Department of Pharmacology, Division of Basic Health Sciences,
Emory University, Atlanta, Ga.

The presence of histamine in cytoplasmic granules of tissue mast cells suggests that the mast cell participates in allergic reactions. Histamine is released from mast cells of sensitized animals by specific antigens [13] or by antibodies directed against antigens fixed by the mast cells [3, 11]. Similarly, histamine is released from mast cells by the polymer amine, compound 48/80 [16], or by physical agents such as heating, freezing and thawing and distilled water [5]. Current evidence suggests that on one hand, the interaction of antigen and antibody or compound 48/80 with the mast cell membrane stimulates release of histamine containing granules by cations in the extracellular medium [15]. On the other hand, physical agents such as distilled water, freezing and thawing or surface active compounds [13] release histamine presumably as a result of lysis of the cells.

When mast cells isolated from rat peritoneal fluid are treated with antigen [14] antibody [8] or 48/80 [16] they undergo morphologic changes such as swelling, vacuolization and degranulation. Although the mast cells do not appear to be completely disrupted by such treatment, it has never been established that the cell membrane remains intact when histamine is released. The percent experiments, in which the release of histamine and several other intracellular substances was measured, test the hypothesis that histamine releasing agents such as antigen, antibody, or 48/80 selectively release histamine containing granules from mast cells without disruption of the cell membrane.

[1] Publication number 898 of the Division of Basic Health Sciences, Emory University. This work was supported by Public Health Service grant 2T1 GM 179 and National Heart Institute grant HE02953.

Materials and Methods

Mast cells were isolated from peritoneal and pleural fluids of male Wistar rats by centrifugation through solutions of FICOLL [9]. The cells of 5–8 animals were pooled for each experiment. Mast cells used for experiments where histamine release was induced by 48/80 or by antibody (rabbit anti-rat gamma globulin)[2] were isolated from normal rats. Sensitized mast cells were isolated from rats sensitized 14–18 days previously by a single subcutaneous injection of horse serum with *H. pertussis* vaccine as an adjuvant.

Mast cells were suspended in 0.2–2.0 ml of buffered medium[3] containing one of the following: 48/80 (10 μg/ml), antigen (2 mg/ml of horse serum), antibody (0.2 mg/ml of anti-rat gamma globulin)[4] or 0.1 % Triton X-100. The samples were incubated for 10 min at 37° in a metabolic shaker. The cells were then separated from the supernatant medium by centrifugation and both cell and supernatant fractions were assayed for histamine, lactic dehydrogenase and ATP.

A perfusion system was used to measure release of ^{42}K from mast cells which had been labeled previously by incubation in buffered medium containing 3–5 μC/ml of $^{42}K_2CO_3$. The cells were washed in isotope-free medium and placed in a funnel lined with filter paper. Buffered solution was fed by gravity into the funnel and consecutive samples of cell-free filtrate were collected. After collection for a control period (15–30 seconds) either 48/80 (final concentration 10 μg/ml) or antigen (final concentration 2 mg/ml) was added to the cells. Collection of cell-free filtrate was continued for 150–300 sec, perfusion was stopped and the residual ^{42}K and histamine were extracted from cells and filter paper with dilute acid.

Histamine was determined by bioassay on atropinized strips of guinea-pig ileum. Lactic dehydrogenase and ATP were determined by standard fluorometric methods. Radioactive potassium was measured in a crystal well counter by a Nuclear Chicago radiation analyzer and scaling unit. Details of these methods have been described [10].

Results

There was no evidence of release of either lactic dehydrogenase or ATP when mast cells were treated with doses of 48/80, antigen or anti-rat gamma globulin (anti-RGG) that released significant amounts of histamine. In contrast, the surface active compound, Triton X-100, caused release of both lactic dehydrogenase and ATP as well as histamine. These data are portrayed in figure 1.

When mast cells labeled with ^{42}K were treated with either antigen or 48/80, the major portion of the label was retained while histamine was

[2] Rabbit anti-rat gamma globulin obtained from Pentex, Inc.

[3] The buffered medium (pH 7.0) contained 150 mM NaCl, 2.7 mM KCl, 0.9 mM CaCl$_2$, 3 mM Na$_2$HPO$_4$, 3.5 mM KH$_2$PO$_4$, 5.6 mM dextrose and 0.1 % human serum albumin.

[4] When anti-rat gamma globulin was used the medium also contained 5 % fresh rabbit serum which had been dialyzed for 6 h at 5° against glucose-free Tyrodes solution.

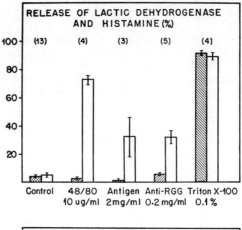

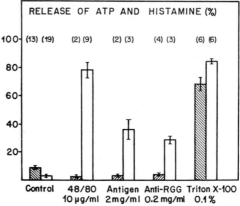

Fig. 1. Comparison of the release of lactic dehydrogenase (LDH) and ATP with the release of histamine from rat mast cells. Ordinates are mean percent release of LDH or ATP (hatched bars) and histamine (open bars) corrected for spontaneous (control) release. Vertical lines indicate standard errors or range where there were two experiments. Number of experiments in parentheses. *Anti-RGG* = anti-rat gamma globulin.

released. Subsequent addition of Triton X-100 to these cells, however, released over 70% of the ^{42}K and an additional store of histamine.

A small portion of ^{42}K (less than 15% of the total label) was released with histamine by 48/80. In four experiments the time course of ^{42}K release coincided with that of histamine release, suggesting that the two substances were released by the same mechanism. The results of a single typical experiment are shown in figure 2.

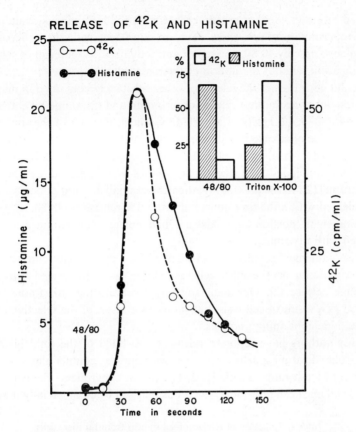

Fig. 2. Comparison of time course of release of ^{42}K and histamine from rat mast cells treated with 48/80 (10 μg/ml). Cell-free filtrate was collected at timed intervals after addition of 48/80 and analyzed for histamine and ^{42}K. The plot of a single experiment shows release of ^{42}K (open circles) and histamine (closed circles) with time. The inset shows percent of total measured histamine (hatched bars) and ^{42}K (open bars) released by 48/80 and by subsequent addition of Triton X-100 to the cells.

Reproduced by permission of the American Physiological Society from Reference 10.

Discussion

The present experiments show that the release of histamine by antigen, antibody or 48/80 is not accompanied by the release of either lactic dehydrogenase or ATP, two intracellular substances which are presumably localized in cellular compartments other than the histamine containing granules. Further, mast cells labeled with ^{42}K retained most of the label when histamine was released by either 48/80 or antigen. Since mast cell histamine is contained in the cytoplasmic granules, these data are consistent with the concept that histamine release by 48/80, antigen or antibody occurs as a result of selective degranulation without disruption of the mast cell membrane.

We did not measure the release of other substances contained in mast cell granules, but concomittant release of serotonin and histamine by antigen [7] and by 48/80 [6, 12] has been reported by others. Because of the similarities in time course of release and dose-response relationships between serotonin and histamine when rat mast cells were treated with 48/80, MORAN and associates concluded that these two amines were released by the same mechanism [12]. In the present investigation, a small amount of potassium-42 was released within the time course of histamine release by 48/80, suggesting that this small portion of potassium had entered the granules and was released with histamine.

The complement requiring reaction of anti-rat gamma globulin with fixed gamma globulin on the mast cell membrane has been termed 'cytotoxic' histamine release [2]. Our data suggest, however, that histamine is not released as a result of cell lysis, but rather as a result of the selective release of histamine containing granules.

Other authors have reported release of 70–80% of the total histamine when isolated rat mast cells are treated with anti-rat gamma globulin in the presence of fresh rabbit serum [1, 2, 11]. In our experiments the percentage of the total mast cell histamine which was released by commercially prepared

Table I. Summary of release of substances from rat mast cells

Substance	Intra-cellular location	Estimated molecular weight	Releasing Agent[1]			
			48/80	Antigen	Anti-RGG	Other
LDH	cytoplasm	126,000	–	–	–	+
ATP	cytoplasm mitochondria	518	–	–	–	+
Serotonin[2]	granules	192	+	+	0	+
Histamine	granules	115	+	+	+[3]	+
Potassium	cytoplasm	39–42	–	–	0	+
	granules		+	+	0	+

[1] Symbol + means released and – means not released. Symbol 0 means not determined. 'Other agents' refers to surface active compounds such as Triton X-100 or n-decylamine.
[2] References 6, 7, 12.
[3] References 1, 2, 11.

anti-rat gamma globulin was comparable to that released by antigen reacting with sensitized mast cells. In either system histamine release rarely exceeded 50% and was usually between 20% and 40%. In contrast, 48/80, in a dose of 10 μg/ml, consistently released over 70% of the total mast cell histamine. The reason for these differences is not readily apparent, but the two antigen-antibody reactions may be limited by the number of reactive sites on the mast cells.

Release of granules from isolated rat mast cells by 48/80 [16] and antigen [14] has been observed with the light microscope. Although mast cells treated with anti-RGG exhibited changes such as swelling and vacuolization, HUMPHREY and associates [8] did not observe release of granules from the cells. In a study of fine structure of rat mast cells BLOOM and HAEGERMARK [4] found numerous 'altered' granules in mast cells that had been treated with 48/80. Electron photomicrographs of these cells suggest that there is fusion of perigranular membranes with each other and with the cell membrane which effectively excludes the granules from the intracellular compartment. According to the model of UVNAS [15] histamine is displaced from the granules by exchanging with cations in the extracellular medium. Thus, if the granules are externalized by a rearrangement of intracellular membranes the release of histamine may occur without obvious extrusion of the granules from the cell. The selective release of amines from mast cells is compatible with such a mechanism.

The release of substances from rat mast cells is summarized in table I. The selective release of amines by 48/80, antigen, or antibody is emphasized by the fact that substances ranging in size from potassium ions to a protein are retained while amines are released. In contrast, agents that lyse the cells release all of the intracellular constituents as well as histamine. Assuming that the release of histamine indicates that the mast cell granules or their contents are released, these data support the hypothesis that 48/80, antigen or antibody cause selective release of histamine containing granules without disrupting the mast cell membrane.

References

1. AUSTEN, K. F. and BECKER, E. L.: Mechanisms of immunologic injury of rat peritoneal mast cells. II. Complement requirement and phosphonate ester inhibition of release of histamine by rabbit anti-rat gamma globulin. J. exp. Med. 124: 397 (1966).
2. AUSTEN, K. F.; BLOCH, K. J.; BAKER, A. R. and ARNASON, B. G.: Immunological histamine release from rat mast cells in vitro: Effect of age of cell donor. Proc. Soc. exp. Biol., N.Y. 120: 542 (1965).

3. AUSTEN, K. F. and HUMPHREY, J. H.: Release of histamine from rat peritoneal mast cells by antibody against rat gamma globulin. J. Physiol. *158:* 36 P. (1961).

4. BLOOM, G. D. and HAEGERMARK, O.: A study of morphological changes and histamine release induced by compound 48/80 in rat peritoneal mast cells. Exp. Cell Res. *40:* 637 (1965).

5. BRAY, R. E. and VAN ARSDALE, P. P.: *In vitro* histamine release from rat mast cells by chemical and physical agents. Proc. Soc. exp. Biol., N.Y. *106:* 255 (1961).

6. GARCIA AROCHA, H.: Release of histamine and 5-hydroxytryptamine from cells of the peritoneal fluid of rats. Canad. J. Biochem. *39:* 395 (1961).

7. GARCIA AROCHA, H.: Liberation of 5-hydroxytryptamine and histamine in the anaphylactic reaction of the rat. Canad. J. Biochem. *39:* 403 (1961).

8. HUMPHREY, J. H.; AUSTEN, K. F. and RAPP, H. J.: *In vitro* studies of reversed anaphylaxis with rat cells. Immunology *6:* 226 (1963).

9. JOHNSON, A. R. and MORAN, N. C.: Comparison of several methods for the isolation of rat peritoneal mast cells. Proc. Soc. exp. Biol., N.Y. *123:* 886 (1966).

10. JOHNSON, A. R. and MORAN, N. C.: The selective release of histamine from rat mast cells by compound 48/80 and antigen. Amer. J. Physiol. (In press 1968).

11. KELLER, R.: Effect of antibodies against rat gamma globulin or rat albumin on isolated peritoneal mast cells. Nature *193:* 282 (1962).

12. MORAN, N. C.; UVNAS, B. and WESTERHOLM, B.: Release of 5-hydroxytryptamine and histamine from rat mast cells. Acta physiol. scand. *56:* 24 (1962).

13. MOTA, I.: Effect of antigen and octylamine on mast cells and histamine content of sensitized guinea pig tissues. J. Physiol. *147:* 425 (1959).

14. MOTA, I. and DIAS DA SILVA, W.: Antigen-induced damage to isolated sensitized mast cells. Nature *186:* 245 (1960).

15. UVNAS, B.: Release processes in mast cells and their activation by injury. Ann. N.Y. Acad. Sci. *116:* 880 (1964).

16. UVNAS, B. and THON, I.: Evidence for enzymatic histamine release from isolated rat mast cells. Exp. Cell Res. *23:* 45 (1961).

Authors' address: ALICE R. JOHNSON and NEIL C. MORAN, M.D., Department of Pharmacology, Division of Basic Health Sciences, Emory University, *Atlanta, Ga. 30322* (USA).

Cellular and Humoral Mechanisms in Anaphylaxis and Allergy, pp. 129–143
(Karger, Basel/New York 1969)

Antigen-Antibody Complexes, Platelets and Increased Vascular Permeability[1]

Peter M. Henson[2] and Charles G. Cochrane[3]

Department of Experimental Pathology
Scripps Clinic and Research Foundation
La Jolla, Calif.

Acute experimental serum sickness of rabbits is a useful model of tissue injury produced by immune complexes in which a number of the etiological processes have been determined. Rabbits are given a large single intravenous injection of an antigen such as bovine serum albumin. During immune elimination of this antigen immune complexes circulate in the blood stream. The induction of lesions follows the deposition of the complexes in blood vessel walls of the heart, arteries and veins of several organs and the glomerulus. It has been shown [4, 12] that this deposition involves an increase in vascular permeability and can be prevented if the rabbits are depleted of their platelets or treated with antagonists of vasoactive amines. The production of the necrotizing cardiovascular lesion is also dependent upon the presence of neutrophils.

Since, in serum sickness, there appears to be an increase in vascular permeability when the immune complexes circulate, studies have been performed on the types of antibody produced by rabbits to BSA which can induce such permeability increase. Passive cutaneous anaphylaxis was used to demonstrate the ability of the antibody to cause vascular permeability increase upon reaction with its antigen in the skin.

In experiments recently described, it was found [8] that two types of rabbit antibody would persist in the rabbit skin for 48 to 72 h and produce a blueing reaction upon subsequent intravenous injection of antigen and

[1] This is Publication No. 305 from the Department of Experimental Pathology, Scripps Clinic and Research Foundation. The work was supported by United States Health Service Grant AI-07007 and National Multiple Sclerosis Society Grant 459.

[2] Dr. Henson is supported by U.S.P.H.S. Training Grant 5 TI GM 683.

[3] Dr. Cochrane is an Established Investigator of the Helen Hay Whitney Foundation.

Evan's blue dye. One of these antibodies resembled that described by ZVAIFLER and BECKER [16], and this has been called homocytotropic antibody. Its activity could be inhibited by treating the rabbits with antihistamine, but not by depleting them of C3, platelets or neutrophils.

The other antibody was a γ_2, heat-stable antibody which did require the presence of complement, platelets and neutrophils for its activity. This second type of PCA reaction has been called the complement-dependent PCA reaction (C-dependent PCA). It can be differentiated from the Arthus reaction by the small amount of antibody (2.5 μg N) required, its inhibition with antihistamine and platelet depletion, and the increasing reactivity over a 24–72 h sensitization period. The inhibitory effect of antihistamine requires a sensitization period of more than 24 h before the antigen injection. Shorter sensitization periods with these small doses of antibody result in greater neutrophil infiltration and a mild Arthus reaction.

It may be seen, therefore, that the lesions of serum sickness and the C-dependent PCA reaction have certain features in common. These are summarized in table I. There is a requirement for platelets and an inhibitory action of antagonists of vasoactive amines in both systems. For this reason, the release of histamine from platelets by antigen-antibody reactions *in vitro* was studied. It was hoped therby to elucidate the source and mechanism of release of the mediators of the increased vascular permeability.

Four mechanisms have been found by which the reaction of rabbit antibody with antigens unrelated to the platelet may cause rabbit platelets to

Table I. Inhibition of lesions of serum sickness and passive cutaneous anaphylaxis[1]

Treatment of rabbits	Serum sickness		PCA reaction	
	Arteritis	Glomerulo-nephritis	C-dependent Ab	Homocytotropic Ab
Untreated	+	+	+	+
Antagonists of vasoactive amines	−[2]	−[2]	−	−
Depletion of: neutrophils	−	+	−	+
platelets	−[2]	−[2]	−	±
Depletion of C3	−[3]	+	−	+

[1] − = inhibited; ± = partially inhibited; + = not affected.
[2] Shown to prevent deposition of circulating complexes in vessels.
[3] Intimal changes noted (see text), but neutrophil accumulation and destruction of arterial wall absent.

release their histamine *in vitro*. *One* of these has been shown with a soluble antigen and a *second* with particulate antigens. The *third* requires neutrophil interaction and the *fourth* is apparently associated with homocytotropic antibody. Some of the properties of these mechanisms will be described. Preliminary indications as to which of the processes may be involved in the production of vascular permeability increase in the *in vivo* conditions will then be presented.

1. Soluble Antigen

Many workers have shown that soluble antigen reacting with rabbit antibody in the presence of plasma and rabbit platelets results in the release of platelet histamine into the supernatant [1, 2, 3, 6, 7, 10, 15]. Recent studies in our laboratory [9] have extended this work and clarified the role of complement in the system. Some of these results are indicated in table II. In the presence of normal plasma and with conditions of antibody excess, clumping of platelets was observed microscopically and release of platelet histamine occurred. Both clumping and release were inhibited if the plasma was heat-inactivated or depleted of C3. C6-deficient plasma, on the other hand, was effective in inducing clumping, but not in producing histamine release. Since normal releasing activity could be produced if C6 was restored to C6-deficient plasma, this releasing system apparently requires activation of the

Table II. Plasma factors involved in histamine release from platelets using *soluble* antigen

	Plasma	Platelet clumping[2]	% histamine release[3]
	None	–	0
	Normal plasma	+	75
Antigen (BSA)[1] + Antibody + Platelets	Heated plasma (56°C 30 min)	–	0
	C3-depleted plasma (cobra factor)	–	0
	C6-deficient plasma	+	0
	C6-deficient plasma + C6 preparation	+	80

[1] Antibody (12 μg N) + BSA (0.05 μg N) + 2.5 × 10^8 platelets.
[2] Platelet clumping was observed microscopically.
[3] Released histamine was assayed after 30 min at 37°C. The figure represents the percent of the total histamine which was released.

complement system through C6. The clumping may represent immune adherence to fixed C3, which is followed by an as yet undefined release process involving later-acting complement components.

2. Particulate Antigens

In a study of the effect of platelet immune adherence on histamine release, particulate antigens such as zymosan and erythrocytes were used, since they could be readily washed free of excess plasma components [9]. Results obtained with this system are summarized in table III. Once again, heat-inactivated or C3-depleted plasma was ineffective. With this type of antigen, however, the adherence of platelets to zymosan which had been treated with C6-deficient plasma did result in histamine release. This was confirmed with the erythrocyte as antigen, where a requirement for C3 for both adherence and histamine release was demonstrated. C6, on the other hand, did not play a part in this release process. Preliminary experiments have suggested that during immune adherence a release mechanism in the platelet is activated by its reaction with the C3 or the antigen surface.

3. Neutrophil-mediated Histamine Release from Platelets

The increased vascular permeability of the complement-dependent PCA reaction required the presence of neutrophils as well as of platelets. Conse-

Table III. Plasma factors involved in histamine release from platelets using particulate antigens

	Adherence of platelets	% histamine release[2]
Zymosan treated with[1]		
Normal plasma	+	62
Heated plasma (56°C 30 min)	−	0
C3-depleted plasma (cobra factor)	−	0
C6-deficient plasma	+	60
EAC1, 4, 2	−	0
EAC1, 4, 2 + rabbit C3 preparation	+	25

[1] EAC and ZC were washed before addition of washed platelets.
[2] Released histamine was assayed after 30 min at 37°C. The figure represents the percent of the total histamine which was released.

quently the *in vitro* platelet histamine release reactions were examined to see if the presence of normal neutrophils could affect the release.

Neutrophils were obtained from the rabbit peritoneum following glycogen stimulation [5]. After washing, they were added to the platelet histamine releasing system described above and in table IV. Peripheral blood leukocytes obtained following dextran sedimentation of erythrocytes were also employed. The immune reactants and platelets were allowed to react together for 10 min at 37°C before addition of the neutrophils, as this was found to give optimal neutrophil effects. The results are given as the percentage of total histamine released after subtraction of the control, background values which varied from 9 to 20%.

Representative results are expressed in table IV. Both soluble and particulate antigen releasing systems were augmented by the presence of neutrophils. This was most marked with the washed zymosan previously treated with plasma, where 50% (600 ng) of the histamine was released under the influence of the neutrophils. Leukocytes from the peripheral circulation were also effective. As noted in table IV, BSA-anti-BSA complexes, with C6-deficient plasma, which did not release histamine from platelets alone, could be caused to release platelet histamine if neutrophils were also present. This neutrophil-dependent reaction therefore represents a third mechanism for immunological histamine release from platelets.

The mechanism of neutrophil action has not yet been clarified. Preliminary evidence suggests that substances damaging to platelets are not released from the neutrophils. Consequently either phagocytosis of the

Table IV. Augmentation of platelet histamine release by neutrophils

Histamine releasing system	% histamine release		% release due to neutrophils
	Platelets alone	Platelets plus neutrophils[1]	
Ag.Ab[2] + normal plasma	33	57	24
Ab.Ab + C6-deficient plasma	0	36	36
Z[3] + normal plasma	45	82	37
Z + normal plasma (washed)	46	96	50

[1] Platelets (2.5×10^8) were allowed to react with the releasing system for 10 min before addition of the neutrophils (1×10^6).

[2] Antibody (5 µg N) + BSA (0.05 µg N) + 0.25 ml plasma.

[3] Zymosan (2.5×10^8 particles) + 0.25 ml plasma.

immune complex and adherent platelets, or mutual immune adherence of platelets and neutrophils resulting in surface activation of the platelets could be the operative mechanism.

4. Homocytotropic Antibody and Platelet Histamine Release: A Complement-Independent Mechanism

Recent evidence from a number of sources [13, 14, 9] has indicated that under certain circumstances platelets from actively immunized rabbits will release their histamine upon contact with antigen in the absence of plasma. This reaction also requires the participation of blood leukocytes. In a system involving *Schistosoma mansoni* as antigen, SCHOENBECHLER and BARBARO [13] showed that the leukocyte involved was the small lymphocyte. There appears to be some correlation between the production of homocytotropic antibody by the rabbit and release of histamine from washed blood cells.

The involvement of platelets and the correlation with homocytotropic antibody production using BSA as the antigen is shown in a representative experiment in table V. Homocytotropic antibody was produced as described

Table V. Histamine release from platelets of rabbits producing homocytotropic antibody

Rabbits from which cells taken	Washed cells[3]	Histamine release in the presence of 5 μg antigen	
		ng	%[4]
	Whole blood cells	5,400	66
Rabbit producing	Platelets	60	2
homocytotropic antibody[1]	Platelet-poor		
	buffy-coat cells	700	57
	Buffy-coat cells + platelets	2,450	53
Rabbit producing	Whole blood cells	0	0
C-dependent PCA antibody[2]	Platelets	0	0

[1] Serum from these animals gave PCA reactions in normal and C3-depleted rabbits. The results described are for one rabbit. Cells from 11 out of 12 of such rabbits that were examined exhibited this histamine release.

[2] Serum from these animals gave PCA reactions in normal rabbits only. Fourteen rabbits were tested but in no case was histamine released from washed cells.

[3] For preparation of cells, see text.

[4] Figure represents percent of total histamine released.

previously [8] and was characterized by its ability to give a PCA reaction in both normal and C3-depleted rabbits. C-dependent PCA antibody was characterized by its inability to produce a PCA reaction in rabbits depleted of C3 with cobra venom factor. Blood cells from animals producing these types of antibody were washed and examined for histamine release. Washed cells from 1 ml of whole blood were employed. Washed platelets were obtained as described previously, and 5×10^8 were used for testing. Platelet-poor buffy-coat cells were obtained by washing the buffy-coat from 5 ml of blood by repeated centrifugation at 170 × g for 10 min. Upon addition of 5 μg BSA N and incubation at 37°C for 30 min the released histamine was assayed on the atropinized guinea-pig ileum. The percentage release obtained without antigen was subtracted to give the specific histamine release due to antigen.

Eleven out of twelve rabbits producing homocytotropic antibody exhibited histamine release from washed blood cells (table V). Some release was found with the platelet-poor buffy-coat cells, but this was much greater if platelets were present, showing that release from platelets had occurred. No release from washed platelets themselves was observed. The histamine release from washed blood cells was not seen if the rabbits were producing C-dependent PCA antibody.

The Occurrence of the Histamine Release Mechanisms in the in vivo Reactions

The C-dependent PCA reaction and experimental serum sickness were examined in order to try and determine which of the histamine-releasing mechanisms might be involved in the increased permeability observed in the reactions.

1. The complement-dependent PCA reaction. The C-dependent reaction was inhibited in rabbits depleted of C3 [8], and hence complement appeared to be involved. In contrast, when the reaction was performed on C6-deficient rabbits, no inhibition was observed and identical antibody titers were obtained on both normal and C6-deficient animals (table VI). As noted above, neutrophils are also required for the reaction [8] (table I). These findings suggest that the histamine releasing mechanism which is operative here is that in which neutrophils augment the effect of soluble antigen in combination with antibody. Alternatively, the surface effect, as exhibited by particulate antigens, may be involved when antigen-antibody complexes react with platelets in the skin. This mechanism of release is also augmented by the presence of neutrophils.

Table VI. Titers of PCA antibody tested in rabbits depleted of C3 or deficient in C6

| Rabbits | Number of rabbits | Titer of Ab giving PCA reaction[1] | |
		C-dependent PCA antibody	Homocytotropic antibody
Normal	10	32	8
C6-deficient	2	32	8
C3-depleted (CoF)	6	0	8

[1] The rabbits were given intradermal injections of antibody dilutions, and after 48 h, challenged with antigen and Evan's blue dye. The lesions were examined after 30 min. The titers represent the reciprocal of the highest dilution of antiserum giving more than 50 mm[2] of blueing.

2. Serum sickness. C3 depletion offers an experimental means of differentiating between some of these releasing mechanisms. Consequently an experiment was performed to examine the effect of C3 depletion on the deposition of circulating complexes and the production of lesions of serum sickness.

Acute serum sickness was produced by methods described previously [11]. C3 depletion was effected by administration of cobra venom factor [8] starting on the fifth day after the injection of antigen (500 units of cobra factor/kg as a divided dose) and continuing as daily injections of 200 units/kg until the animals were sacrificed. This procedure reduced the hemolytic complement levels to an average of 26% on the sixth day. Less than 10% of the hemolytic complement was present at the time of maximal lesions, and daily tests for C3 by a sensitive agar diffusion test revealed no precipitin line with the sera from CoF-treated rabbits. Moreover, plasma from these rabbits were incapable of inducing histamine release from platelets with zymosan or with an antigen-antibody reaction.

Table VII summarizes the results of the experiment. Both groups of rabbits (normal and C3-depleted) exhibited roughly equal amounts of proteinuria during the time of immune elimination of the antigen. Examination of histological sections of the kidneys revealed glomerular lesions of equal severity in both groups (fig. 1).

Fig. 1. Glomerular lesions in acute serum sickness. A. Rabbit depleted of C3. B. Rabbit with normal C3. Note strong endothelial proliferation in both circumstances. × 450.

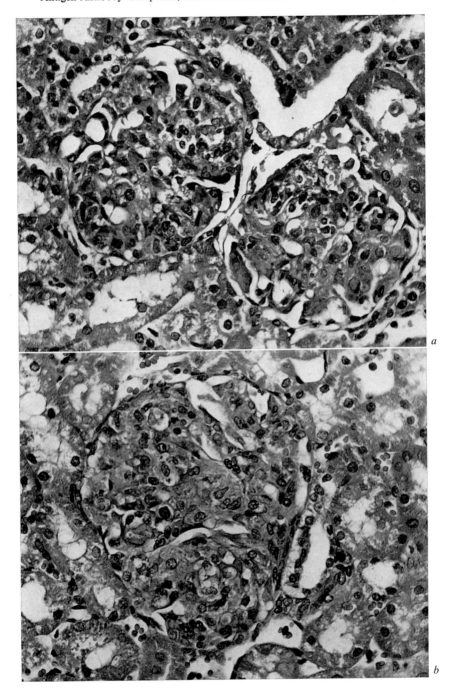

a

b

Table VII. The production of acute serum sickness in C3-depleted and normal rabbits

	Number of animals showing lesions	
	Untreated	C3-depleted (CoF)
Cardiovascular lesions[1]		
Intimal changes	5/5	5/6[3]
Neutrophil infiltration	5/5	0/6
Glomerular lesions	5/5	6/7
Proteinuria	5/5 (450)[2]	6/7 (440)

[1] Characteristic lesions are shown in the figures and described in the text.
[2] Average mg protein in urine for the 24 h immediately preceding the point when 99%
of the injected antigen was eliminated.
[3] One of these rabbits failed to give a good immune response.

On the other hand, a clear difference between the two groups was observed when the cardiovascular lesions were examined. In the group depleted of C3, intimal changes consisted of lifting of the endothelial cell layer leaving a space between these cells and the internal elastic lamina. An accumulation of mononuclear cells and/or proliferation of endothelial cells was also apparent (fig. 2). This type of lesion has been described as the earliest reaction in serum sickness arteritis and is evidence of complex deposition [12]. As might be expected, neutrophil accumulation and necrosis were not observed in these C3-depleted rabbits. In contrast, the animals with normal C3 exhibited massive neutrophil accumulation and medial necrosis (fig.2).

Thus the deposition of complexes and early cardiovascular lesions of serum sickness, along with the glomerular damage, appear to occur in the absence of complement. This finding precludes the involvement of anaphylatoxins in the initiation of the early serum sickness lesions. These are the lesions which were inhibited by antagonists of vasoactive amines and by platelet depletion [12]. The mechanism of histamine release from platelets associated with homocytotropic antibody therefore seemed the most likely mechanism to be involved in the initiation of these lesions.

To investigate this possibility, rabbits stimulated to produce serum sickness were examined to see if they produced homocytotropic antibody. Before elimination of the antigen occurs, the circulating antigen would be expected

Fig. 2. Arterial lesions (coronary artery) in acute serum sickness. A. Rabbit depleted of C3. Note lifting of endothelium and absence of neutrophils. B. Rabbit with normal C3. Note endothelial proliferation, neutrophil accumulation and breaks in the internal elastic lamina. The vessel lumen is toward the top. × 300.

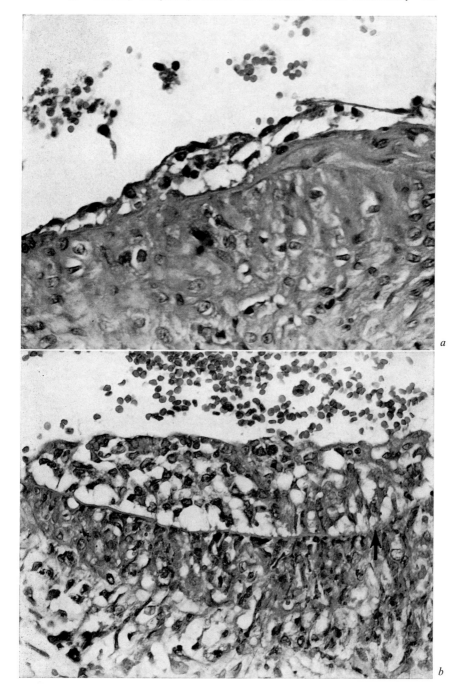

a

b

to prevent any detection of this reaction *in vitro*. Consequently the rabbits were examined after complete immune elimination for the ability of added antigen to release histamine from washed blood cells. Blood was taken into EDTA (0.01 M) as anticoagulant and the cells were washed four times. Cells from 1 ml blood were reacted with 5 μg BSA N for 30 min at 37°C. Control tubes contained cells without antigen. Plasma were also examined for PCA reactivity but were all negative, suggesting that even if homocytotropic antibody was being produced it was not present free in the plasma in large enough quantities to give the passive cutaneous reaction. Fifteen rabbits were used in this experiment. Of these animals, only nine rabbits exhibited immune elimination of antigen. The production of proteinuria was taken as an indication of tissue damage.

Five of the nine rabbits which showed immune elimination of antigen exhibited proteinuria (table VIII). After the elimination, cells from all five animals showed the complement-independent histamine release in the presence of antigen. This reaction, which suggests the presence of antibody on the washed cells, has been associated with the homocytotropic variety of antibody. Four rabbits showed immune elimination without proteinuria. Only one of these had cells that, after washing, released histamine with antigen, and these were found somewhat later, after elimination. Since it has

Table VIII. Correlation of complement-independent histamine release from blood cells and glomerular damage in serum sickness

| Rabbit no. | Proteinuria (mg total) | % histamine release from washed blood cells[1] | |
		Before Ag elim.[2]	After Ag elim.[3]
1	1,622	0	30
2	1,095	0	57
7	870	0	50
12	914	0	59
14	300	0	56
3	0	0	0
6	0	0	0
8	0	0	0
11	0	0	15

[1] The percentage of total histamine in washed cells from 1 ml blood which was released by 5 μg BSA N.

[2] Tested two days after injection of serum sickness-inducing antigen.

[3] Cells from rabbits 1 and 2 were tested 3 days after immune elimination of antigen. The other animals were tested one day after elimination.

been shown that parameters other than the vascular permeability also influence the production of lesions (e.g., size and quantity of immune complexes), the finding of the complement-independent histamine release mechanism in one rabbit which did not exhibit proteinuria probably does not discount this hypothesis.

These results were felt to show very good correlation between the development of glomerular lesions and the presence of cell bound antibody (possibly homocytotropic antibody) after antigen elimination. It may be inferred that this antibody is produced before antigen elimination but cannot be detected because of the continued presence of antigen. The initiation of immune complex localization appears, therefore, to result from platelet histamine release by a mechanism which does not require complement and may be associated with homocytotropic antibody. There is also a possibility, however, that this is an entirely cell-mediated immunological reaction. Initiation of release from platelets by the mechanisms described above may be followed by ADP-dependent platelet aggregation and subsequent release of more histamine and serotonin.

Once complex deposition has occurred, neutrophil accumulation in the arteries fails to occur in the absence of C3. These findings are in keeping with previous results from this laboratory on the requirement for complement for neutrophil accumulation in other lesions. Neutrophils will adhere to immune complexes with fixed C3 on them and, moreover, are attracted to sites of immune reaction by chemotactic agents resulting from complement activation. Either or both of these processes may therefore be involved in the neutrophil accumulation. Previous work has clearly shown that it is the reaction of these neutrophils which results in breakdown of the internal elastic lamina and in the subsequent production of typical arteritis lesions [4, 11].

Summary

The production of serum sickness arteritis and of complement-dependent passive cutaneous anaphylaxis (PCA) in rabbits have been shown to require the participation of platelets and neutrophils. Since increased vascular permeability appears to play an important role in inducing the lesions and since the permeability increase can be inhibited by antihistamine, the immunologic release of histamine from platelets has been studied.

Two mechanisms by which antigen-antibody complexes release histamine from rabbit platelets are described, both requiring complement. One of these involves particulate antigens and requires complement fixation as far as the C3 component. The other results from the action of soluble antigens and requires complement activation through C6. Both appear to result from the adherence of the platelet to the antigen-antibody-complement complex.

The presence of neutrophils during the reaction of immune complexes with platelets augments the release of histamine from the latter and is therefore a third mechanism of inducing histamine release. Still another mechanism, not requiring complement, involves homocytotropic antibody together with platelets and leukocytes

Preliminary indications have been obtained as to which of these mechanisms is involved in the production of the *in vivo* lesions. The complement-dependent PCA reaction was inhibited in rabbits depleted of C3 with cobra venom factor but not in C6-deficient animals. The lesions might therefore result from the mechanism described for particulate antigens and/or the neutrophil augmentation process. In serum sickness, on the other hand, the glomerular and early arteritic lesions were not inhibited in rabbits depleted of C3. The histamine-releasing mechanism associated with homocytotropic antibody was observed in animals which had undergone serum sickness, suggesting that this process might be involved in the deposition of circulating immune complexes and the initiation of the serum sickness lesions.

References

1. Barbaro, J. F.: The release of histamine from rabbit platelets by means of antigen-antibody precipitates. I. The participation of the immune complex in histamine release. J. Immunol. *86:* 369–376 (1961).
2. Barbaro, J. F.: The release of histamine from rabbit platelets by means of antigen-antibody precipitates. II. The role of plasma in the release of histamine. J. Immunol. *86:* 377–381 (1961).
3. Bryant, R. and Des Prez, R.: Mechanisms of immunologically-induced rabbit platelet injury. Clin. Res. *16:* 318 (1968).
4. Cochrane, C. G. and Aikin, B. S.: Polymorphonuclear leukocytes in immunologic reactions. The destruction of vascular basement membrane *in vivo* and *in vitro*. J. exp. Med *124:* 733–752 (1966).
5. Cohn, Z. A. and Hirsch, J. G.: The isolation and properties of the specific cytoplasmic granules of rabbit polymorphonuclear leukocytes. J. exp. Med. *112:* 983–1004 (1960)
6. Gocke, D. J.: *In vitro* damage of rabbit platelets by an unrelated antigen-antibody reaction. II. Studies of the plasma requirement. J. Immunol. *94:* 247–252 (1965).
7. Gocke, D. J. and Osler, A. G.: *In vitro* damage of rabbit platelets by an unrelated antigen-antibody reaction. I. General characteristics of the reaction. J. Immunol. *94:* 236–246 (1965).
8. Henson, P. M. and Cochrane, C. G.: Immunological induction of increased vascular permeability. I. A rabbit PCA reaction requiring complement, platelets and neutrophils. J. exp. Med. *129:* 153–165 (1969).
9. Henson, P. M. and Cochrane, C. G.: Immunological induction of increased vascular permeability. II. Two mechanisms of histamine release from rabbit platelets involving complement. J. exp. Med. *129:* 161–184 (1969).
10. Humphrey, J. H. and Jaques, R.: The release of histamine and 5-hydroxy-tryptamine (serotonin) from platelets by antigen-antibody reactions (*in vitro*). J. Physiol. *128:* 9–27 (1955)
11. Kniker, W. T. and Cochrane, C. G.: Pathogenic factors in vascular lesions of experimental serum sickness. J. exp. Med. *122:* 83–98 (1965).
12. Kniker, W. T. and Cochrane, C. G.: The localization of circulating immune complexes in experimental serum sickness. The role of vasocative amines and hydrodynamic forces. J. exp. Med. *127:* 119–136 (1968).

13. Schoenbechler, M. J. and Barbaro, J. F.: The requirement for sensitized lympho-cytes in one form of antigen-induced histamine release from rabbit platelets. Proc. nat. Acad. Sci., Wash. *60:* 1247–1251 (1968).
14. Siraganian, R. P. and Oliveira, B.: The allergic response of rabbit platelets and leukocytes. Fed. Proc. *27:* 315 (1968).
15. Spielvogel, A. R.: An ultrastructural study of the mechanisms of platelet-endotoxin interaction. J. exp. Med. *126:* 235–250 (1967).
16. Zvaifler N. J. and Becker, E. L.: Rabbit anaphylactic antibody. J. exp. Med. *123:* 935–950 (1966).

Authors' address: Peter M. Henson, Ph.D. and Charles G. Cochrane, M.D., Department of Experimental Pathology, Scripps Clinic and Research Foundation, *La Jolla, Calif.* (USA).

Cellular and Humoral Mechanisms in Anaphylaxis and Allergy, pp. 144–150
(Karger, Basel/New York 1969)

The Allergic Responses of Human Leukocytes and Rabbit Platelets[1]

ABRAHAM G. OSLER and REUBEN P. SIRAGANIAN

Department of Medical Immunology
The Public Health Research Institute of the City of New York, Inc.
New York, N.Y.

It is now generally accepted that allergic reactions of the immediate type follow different pathways in the sequence which begins with an immune event and terminates in the release of vasoactive compounds. The diversity of these mechanisms has been traced to the nature and species of the mediating immunoglobulin, the requirement for serum cofactors, the utilization of soluble intermediates, the type of target cell, its species of origin and its reservoir of permeability-enhancing factors. In this report, we shall summarize studies exemplifying some of these differences as they emerged from experiments dealing with the *in vitro* responses of human leukocytes and rabbit platelets. In addition, a new allergic reaction mechanism will be documented, one which involves the sequential participation of both leukocytes and platelets.

The studies with human leukocytes, carried out with Drs. DAVID A. LEVY and LAWRENCE M. LICHTENSTEIN, typify the classic reaginic type of allergic response [1]. Here we are concerned with reaginic immunoglobulins of the IgE class whose outstanding property from an immunopathologic viewpoint is cytophilia, the ability to bind firmly and enduringly to homologous and autologous host cells.

The cytophilic property of human reagins for human cells can be readily demonstrated under *in vitro* conditions. In experiments with Dr. LEVY, it has been found that peripheral leukocytes from non-ragweed sensitive

[1] Support for this investigation has been available, in part, from the National Science Foundation, Grant No. GB-1120; The American Cancer Society, Inc., Grant. No. T-257; The National Institute of Allergy and Infectious Diseases of the United States Public Health Service, Grant. No. AI-03151; and from the Office of The Surgeon General, Department of the Army, under the auspices of the Commission on Immunization of the Armed Forces Epidemiological Board, Contract No. DA-49-193-MD-2468.

individuals can be passively sensitized by incubation with reagin-containing human serum. Even after several cycles of centrifugation and resuspension in a serum-free buffer, these cells release histamine after interaction with specific antigen. Since the lymphocytic and monocytic cells contain little if any histamine, these experiments establish that reaginic immunoglobulins are cytophilic for polymorphonuclear leukocytes. Although cytophilia has thus been demonstrated, its *in vitro* manifestation is relatively inefficient in that only 20 % of donors provide cells which can be sensitized passively. In addition, cells sensitized under *in vitro* conditions are far less reactive (about 1000-fold) in terms of their antigen requirements, than leukocytes furnished by ragweed sensitive donors.

An important feature of *in vitro* sensitization experiments is that they provide a useful approach to the study of cell-antibody interaction. For example, positively charged cations like calcium inhibit the fixation process of reagin to human cells. In contrast, polyanionic compounds like EDTA and heparin enhance the cellular response. The mechanism of these events is as yet undefined, but two possibilities may be mentioned. Calcium may interfere through the imposition of a positive charge on the cell membrane fixation site, thereby preventing interaction with positively charged residues on the immunoglobulin. Alternatively, calcium may stabilize the membrane in a more rigid condition which prevents the reaginic immunoglobulin from being fixed or assuming the conformational state required for the sequence of cell fixation, antigen binding and histamine release. The importance of conformational changes in the immunoglobulin as a pre requisite for histamine release will be mentioned again with respect to the platelets.

It had been established by earlier studies with animal tissues, and later with human leukocytes, that the extent of antibody fixation varies directly with time, temperature and the concentration of antibody in the fluid phase. These findings have been utilized in the design of an *in vitro* assay for human reagins. This assay procedure can now be used to monitor reagin levels as a function of natural immunization, specific desensitization therapy, etc., as described by OSLER *et al.* [1].

Reagin-sensitized leukocytes derived from ragweed sensitive individuals have been used in several laboratories for studies of the immunologically mediated histamine release mechanism. Here, we wish to mention only those characteristics of the cellular response which can be contrasted with the rabbit platelets. These can be briefly summarized as follows:

1. Minute amounts of antigen suffice to initiate the release mechanism. Threshold levels may be less than 10^{-6} μg of protein, with maximal reactions

frequently occurring at about 10^{-3} µg. Since histamine release from cell suspensions is diminished by excessive amounts of antigen, these findings imply that 10^7 highly sensitive human leukocytes may carry a reagin burden in the nanogram range. This value ignores the reagin content of the blood lymphocytes and monocytes whose lack of histamine excludes any recognition of their participation in these events.

2. The histamine release process requires metabolically-active cells maintained at physiologic temperatures.

3. Normal human leukocytes as well as heated and fresh human sera contain one or more dialyzable components which participate in the release process. These components have not yet been characterized.

4. The histamine release reaction can be completed in a medium lacking complement components in the fluid phase. The cells carry components of the complement system, but their involvement in this allergic response has not yet been demonstrated.

5. Histamine release requires the participation of two divalent cations, calcium and magnesium. We do not yet know the sequential nature of the metal-requiring steps, although there is suggestive evidence that magnesium involvement precedes that of calcium.

6. Several reaction steps in the overall sequence have been identified, but the reaction products have not yet been isolated.

7. The experimental evidence suggests, but does not establish, that the integrity of the leukocyte membrane is not violated during the release process. This allergic response may therefore represent only a heightened secretory reaction of the cells which is mediated by a reagin-antigen complex of appropriate conformation. Dr. Alice Johnson's report to this symposium leads to similar conclusions for the allergic release of histamine from rat mast cells.

8. Drs. SIRAGANIAN and OLIVEIRA in our laboratory recently reported that peripheral leukocytes from immunized rabbits carry reagin-like antibodies [2, 3], a finding which has now been extended by SCHOENBECHLER and BARBARO [4].

The data in table I clearly show that leukocytes from immunized rabbits react with the immunizing antigen and release histamine into the fluid phase of reaction mixtures. The reaction mechanism resembles that of human leukocytes in that exogenous serum is not required to mediate this response. As also shown by the data in table I, the *in vitro* reaction system involving leukocytes and antigen is more sensitive than the homologous PCA in rabbits in the sense that most of the animals can be expected to furnish reactive leukocytes.

Table I. The release of histamine from washed leukocyte suspensions of immunized rabbits

Days after injection	No. of rabbits	No. of rabbits whose sera yielded positive PCA reactions	No. of rabbits whose WBC released histamine with antigen	Average histamine release when positive % (S. E.)	% of rabbits positive	
					PCA	WBC
3–7	12	1	3	16.3 (0.9)	8	25
8–9	14	6	12	53.6 (9.4)	43	86
10–14	15	5	13	49.2 (8.0)	33	87
18–28	14	8	11	56.8 (5.1)	57	79
36–52	11	5	7	38.0 (6.7)	46	64

Rabbits were immunized on day 0 with 10 mg of either human serum albumin or egg albumin in complete Freund's adjuvant.

Isolated washed leukocytes from these animals were tested for histamine release with 3 different levels of the immunizing antigen i.e. 1.0, 0.1 and 0.01 μg of N/ml. Specificity of the reaction was tested by addition of the non-immunizing protein.

Sera from the bleeding used for WBC isolation was also used for PCA tests, either undiluted or at a 1 → 5 dilution.

Positive histamine release = > 10% release.

The response of rabbit platelets results from a completely different reaction sequence [5, 6]:

1. Rabbit platelets are incapable of fixing homologous, or even autologous reaginic immunoglobulins. Rabbit platelets also fail to bind 7S immunoglobulins in hyperimmune serum. As mentioned above, leukocytes furnished by an immunized rabbit carry cytophilic, reagin-like immunoglobulins. It is therefore clear that the manifestation of cytophilia or cell binding results from unique properties of both the immunoglobulin and the cell under study.

2. In the case of rabbit platelets, the release mechanism is initiated by an immune event in the fluid phase of the reaction medium.

3. In contrast to the antigen requirements of human leukocytes, rabbit platelets respond only to microgram quantities of antigen and antibody.

4. The most efficient complexes for initiating a platelet response are those formed in the region of antibody excess. It can therefore be stated that non-

cytophilic immunoglobulins also bind to cells after they have assumed an appropriate steric configuration, one that is imposed by antibody excess ratios.

5. Pepsin digested immunoglobulins which can still be precipitated by antigen, do not activate the release process.

6. The last two statements suggest that the allergic response of rabbit platelets requires a specific conformation of the Fc portion of rabbit immunoglobulins. It may be further proposed that the conformation achieved by the Fc fragment at antibody excess ratios exposes a site on the immunoglobulin which interacts with the platelet membrane.

7. The interaction between the platelets and the immune complexes as judged by the release of histamine requires the presence of fresh rabbit plasma.

8. Magnesium fulfills the divalent cation requirement for the platelet response. In the presence of optimal magnesium levels (ca. 3×10^{-4} M), calcium prolongs the lag phase and diminishes both the rate and extent of the reaction.

9. This allergic response is cytotoxic for the platelet and is signaled by three successive events; the enhanced efflux of intracellular potassium or rubidium, histamine and finally, macromolecular substances.

Rabbit platelets also discharge their store of vasoactive compounds when an allergic response occurs on other cells in their presence. Thus, platelets from non-immunized animals lose their intracellular rubidium and histamine when they are placed in a reaction medium containing sensitized leukocytes and specific antigen.

Documentation of this novel reaction emerges from the data in table II. In each experiment, the total histamine of 10^6 leukocytes is far less (usually about 5-fold) than that which can be released from the cells in the presence of platelets from non-immunized animals. Since the platelets are inactive in the absence of sensitized leukocytes, it is clear that the response of the leukocytes triggers the release of histamine from platelets in the immediate environment. This response can take place in the absence of plasma.

It has recently been suggested that lymphocytes provide the initial cellular response in the sequence which destroys the platelets although the participation of other cells could not be dismissed. Sequential reactions of this type may also take place during the course of an Arthus reaction in actively immunized rabbits. They further suggest that reactions occurring on the surface of cells which do not carry vasoactive agents can be monitored by this means. These cells, the lymphocytes and/or the poly-

Table II. Interaction of rabbit leukocytes and platelets in the allergic release of histamine

Rabbit number	Reaction mixture	Total number of cells/tube leukocytes × 10⁶	Platelets × 10⁶	Total histamine per tube (μg)	Histamine released on addition of antigen 1.0 μg of antigen N/ml	0.1 μg of antigen N/ml
684	Leukocyte preparation	0.8		0.06	0.05	0.06
	Leukocyte preparation + normal platelets	0.8	182.4	0.47	0.36	0.33
685	Leukocyte preparation	1.1		0.18	0.11	0.07
	Leukocyte preparation + normal platelets	1.1	181.7	0.59	0.42	0.30
690	Leukocyte preparation	2.5		0.17	0.095	0.08
	Leukocyte preparation + normal platelets	2.5	182.2	0.57	0.32	0.27

Experiment 021268.
Leukocytes were obtained from rabbits injected 21 days previously in the foot pads with 10 mg of egg albumin in complete Freund's adjuvant. Reaction mixtures contained Tyrode buffer, rabbit serum albumin 1 mg/ml, Ca^{2+} 6 × 10⁻⁴ and Mg^{2+} 1.0 × 10⁻³ M. Antigen used was ovalbumin 1.0 and 0.1 μg of N/ml.
Platelets were obtained from an unimmunized animal and isolated as described previously.

morphonuclear leukocytes react with the immunizing antigen and release intracellular products as a consequence of this immune event which are cytotoxic to platelets [7].

References

1. OSLER, A. G.; LICHTENSTEIN, L. M. and LEVY, D. A.: *In vitro* studies of human reaginic allergy. Adv. Immunol. *8:* 183 (1968).
2. SIRAGANIAN, R. P.; SECCHI, A. G. and OSLER, A. G.: Biochemistry of the acute allergic reactions, edited by K. Frank Austen and E. L. Becker, Blackwell Scientific Publications, Oxford, p. 229 (1968).
3. SIRAGANIAN, R. P. and OLIVEIRA, B.: The allergic response of rabbit platelets and leukocytes. Fed. Proc. *27:* 315 (1968).
4. SCHOENBECHLER, M. J. and BARBARO, J. F.: The requirement for sensitized lymphocytes in one form of antigen-induced histamine release from rabbit platelets. Proc. Nat. Acad. Sci. *60:* 1247 (1968).
5. GOCKE, D. L. and OSLER, A. G.: *In vitro* damage of rabbit platelets by an unrelated antigen-antibody reaction. J. Immunol. *94:* 236 (1965).
6. SIRAGANIAN, R. P.; SECCHI, A. G. and OSLER, A. G.: The allergic response of rabbit platelets. I. Membrane permeability changes. J. Immunol. *101:* 1130 (1968) – II. Dependence on magnesium. J. Immunol. *101:* 1140 (1968) – III. Its cytotoxic nature. J. Immunol. *101:* 1148 (1968).
7. SIRAGANIAN, R. P. and OSLER, A. G.: Platelet lysis and histamine release resulting from antigen interaction with sensitized rabbit leukocytes. J. Immunol. (submitted for publication).

Authors' address: ABRAHAM G. OSLER, Ph.D. and REUBEN P. SIRAGANIAN, Ph.D. and M.D., Dept of Medical Immunology, The Public Health Research Institute of the City of New York, Inc., *New York, N.Y.* (USA).

Cellular and Humoral Mechanisms in Anaphylaxis and Allergy, pp. 151–163
Karger, Basel–New York (1969)

The Platelet in Intravascular Immunological Reactions

J. F. Mustard, G. Evans, M. A. Packham and E. E. Nishizawa

Department of Pathology, Faculty of Medicine, McMaster University
Hamilton, Ont.
and the Department of Biochemistry, Faculty of Medicine, University of Toronto,
Toronto, Ont.

Platelets in circulating blood take part in the response of the organism to several types of injury. Not only are they involved in hemostasis [24] and thrombosis [42], but they are also concerned in inflammatory and immunological processes [51]. This review will describe the reactions of platelets to antigen-antibody complexes, endotoxin and organ transplantation.

In vitro Studies

It is possible to study some of these reactions *in vitro* using platelet-rich plasma, or suspensions of washed platelets.

Circulating platelets are disc-shaped and contain a number of organelles including granules and mitochondria [23]. The granules are believed to be of at least two types: storage granules similar to those in the adrenal gland, and lysosomes. When platelets are exposed to antigen-antibody complexes, a number of events may occur. The platelets may phagocytose the complexes [35, 45] incorporating them into vacuoles within their cytoplasm. During this process, some of the platelet granules disappear. This reaction is similar to phagocytosis by leucocytes in which degranulation also occurs. Other responses of platelets to exposure to antigen-antibody complexes include swelling, the development of breaks in the outer membranes, and loss of cytoplasmic constituents. Among the contents which are discharged from the platelets are nucleotides [adenosine diphosphate (ADP) and adenosine triphosphate (ATP)], adrenaline, serotonin, histamine, a material (other than serotonin and histamine) which increases vessel permeability, and probably some lysosomal enzymes. Depending on the strength of the stimulus, this discharge of platelet constituents may involve as many as three mechanisms [16, 45, 51]: 1. a discharge of serotonin and nucleotides which resembles that from the adrenal gland, 2. a degranulation and release of permeability factors which may resemble that of leucocytes [43, 51], and 3. an extensive loss of platelet constituents similar to that which occurs when cells are lysed. This last reaction takes place when the platelets have been exposed to a strong stimulus, and if such platelets are examined by electron microscopy they are seen to have lost their organelles and to have retained very little electron-dense material [45].

The ADP released from the platelets induces the formation of platelet aggregates or platelet thrombi [51]. In addition, the serotonin and adrenaline which are released can themselves cause platelet aggregation, and have been shown to potentiate the action of ADP [5]. The serotonin, histamine, permeability factors and lysosomal enzymes which escape from the platelets may alter the endothelial lining of the blood vessels.

The interaction between platelets and antigen-antibody complexes is not specific; for example, human and pig platelets will react with an antigen-antibody complex prepared from rabbit antibovine serum albumin and bovine serum albumin. Furthermore, it is likely that the reaction of platelets with antigen-antibody complexes involves the gamma-globulin in these complexes because pig and human platelets will react with surfaces coated with gamma-globulin from guinea pigs, rabbits, pigs and humans [40].

Rabbit platelets differ from those of the other species studied in that suspensions of washed rabbit platelets do not interact with either antigen-antibody complexes or gamma-globulin coated surfaces unless an additional factor from serum is present [18, 40]. It has been found that with particulate antigens, complement fixation as far as the C'-3-component is required, whereas with soluble antigens, complement activation through C'-6 is necessary [17]. It is possible that complement is also involved in the inter-action of antigen-antibody complexes with human or pig platelets, which themselves contain complement-like activity [47, 51].

When a suspension of washed rabbit platelets is exposed to bacterial endotoxin, platelet aggregation does not occur unless serum is added. In these studies it has been found that only serum from old rabbits, or from rabbit presensitized with endotoxin, is active [39]. This could mean that antibodies to endotoxin may be involved in the reaction of endotoxin with platelets. However, DES PREZ described the factor from plasma as heat-labile and found that it had a close relationship to properdin [9].

Although it is possible that endotoxin may induce platelet aggregation by releasing platelet ADP, this had not yet been established.

The endothelial lining of vessels may be damaged during immunological processes, either by antibody acting directly on the endothelium, or by material released from leucocytes and platelets by antigen-antibody complexes. If the injury to the endothelium is such that the subendothelial tissues are exposed, platelets will interact with the collagen or the basement membrane. Collagen causes the same changes in platelets as are produced by the stimuli already discussed, and induces platelet aggregation at the site of endothelial injury. The reaction of platelets with collagen has been studied extensively both *in vitro* and *in vivo* in investigations of hemostasis and thrombosis [23, 24, 42, 51, 56].

The release of platelet constituents by collagen does not require a plasma cofactor in any of the species studied, including the rabbit, and in this way differs from release induced by antigen-antibody complexes or gamma-globulin coated surfaces, which require a plasma cofactor with rabbit platelets [39].

In all species examined, the release of serotonin and nucleotides from platelets is dependent on the presence of divalent cations in the medium in which the platelets are suspended and calcium ions appear to be required [13, 22, 40]. There is evidence that when platelets are exposed to stimuli which cause the release of platelet constituents, the amount of ATP [15] in the platelet falls and there is a burst of lactate production [4, 54]. This indicates that the release reaction may be energy dependent.

The release of platelet constituents by the various stimuli can be inhibited by prostaglandin (PGE$_1$) and colchicine [28]. PGE$_1$ has been found to either inhibit or activate contractile protein [3], and colchicine is known to disorganize the microtubular system in the platelets [2]. This evidence could be interpreted to mean that the platelet contractile protein is involved in the release of platelet constituents.

The platelet aggregates produced by ADP are not stable and in both *in vitro* and *in vivo* experiments it has been shown that these aggregates break up within a few minutes [6, 46]. However, under conditions in which blood coagulation occurs, the formation of fibrin around the platelet aggregates stabilizes them [38]. The fibrin is found to be closely associated with the platelets [23, 26] and little or no fibrin is found remote from the platelet aggregates. There are at least three relationships between platelet aggregation and blood coagulation which may be responsible for this proximity of fibrin to the platelets: 1. A number of coagulation factors are associated with the platelet membrane. These include fibrinogen, factor V, factor VIII, factor XII and factor XIII [5]; 2. When platelet aggregates form under the

influence of adenosine diphosphate, the platelet phospholipoid which acceler-
ates blood coagulation is made available [14, 41]; and 3. Thrombin, which is
generated in the vicinity of the platelet aggregates, not only causes fibrin
formation but also induces the platelets to release their constituents, including ADP [15]. This leads to further platelet aggregation. One of the unsolved
problems is the mechanism by which blood coagulation is initiated or
accelerated *in vivo*. Collagen [48] and antigen-antibody complexes [34] have
been shown to activate factor XII which is considered to initiate coagulation. However, the significance of factor XII *in vivo* can be questioned
because the hemostatic process is normal in subjects with factor XII deficiency [38]. Since it is known that partially altered fibrinogen (which has
lost the A-peptide by the action of thrombin) is present in the plasma of
normal individuals [55] it may be that some coagulation is taking place
continually. Platelet aggregates may accelerate this process.

The release of platelet constituents produced by the stimuli discussed can
be inhibited by a number of compounds. Some of these are listed in table I
[11, 28, 49, 50, 52, 57]. The mechanism by which these compounds inhibit
platelet aggregation appears to be by suppressing the release of platelet
constituents including the ADP which induces aggregation [11, 51, 52].
Studies with suspensions of washed platelets have shown that the presence
of increasing concentrations of these inhibitors reduces the amount of ADP
appearing in the suspending fluid and the extent of platelet aggregation is
decreased proportionately [11, 51, 52].

Table I. The effect of anti-inflammatory and related compounds on platelet aggregation

| Compound | Stimulus for platelet aggregation[1] | | | |
	ADP[2]	collagen	thrombin	Ag-Ab[3]
Sulfinpyrazone	−	+	+	+
Phenylbutazone	−	+	+	+
Indomethacin	−	+		
Phenacetin		−		
Acetalsalicylic acid	−	+	+	+
Sodium salicylate	−	+	+	+
Mefanamic acid		+		
Meclofenamic acid		+		

[1] − no effect   + inhibits platelet aggregation.
[2] Primary phase of ADP-induced aggregation.
[3] Ag-Ab − Antigen-Antibody complexes.

Stimuli which cause platelet aggregation induce the release of material from pig, human or rabbit platelets which increases the permeability of small vessels [43, 51]. The activity of this material has been measured by intradermal injection into rabbits or guinea pigs given Evans blue and I^{131}-labelled serum albumin intravenously. The radioactivity and colour which accumulate at the injection sites reflect the permeability of the vessels in the skin to serum albumin. The increased permeability observed cannot be attributed solely to serotonin and histamine because serotonin does not increase vessel permeability in rabbits and the amount of histamine in the material released from the platelets is insufficient to cause the increased permeability observed [51]. Pig and human platelets, from which the material can be prepared, contain very little histamine [30, 31], and active material can be prepared from pig platelets which have been depleted of serotonin by the administration of reserpine to the animal prior to isolation of the platelets [44, 51]. However, treatment of rabbits with antihistamine drugs (mepyramine maleate or triprolidine hydrochloride) decreases their response to the intradermal injection of the material released from the platelets [51]. This may indicate that the increased vessel permeability is due to the release of the rabbit's own histamine at the injection site.

If phenylbutazone, sulfinpyrazone or acetylsalicylic acid is present during the exposure of platelets to stimuli which ordinarily cause the release of platelet constituents, the suspending fluid is less active in causing increased vessel permeability [51]. However, these drugs do not affect the activity of the permeability factor after it is released.

The factor (or factors) which increase vessel permeability pass through a dialysis sac and are heat stable. Fractionation of this material on the basis of molecular size by passage through Diaflo filters [44] has indicated that there may be a number of components in it which affect the permeability of small vessels (table II). Some activity was found in a fraction containing substances of molecular weight greater than 10,000, but less than 20,000; some in a fraction comprised of compounds with molecular weights between 1,000 and 10,000; and some activity apparently resided in molecules smaller than 1,000 in weight. Some of the activity in this low molecular weight fraction may be due to histamine.

Material released from pig or human platelets under the influence of aggregating stimuli can also be shown to cause the contraction of smooth muscle, e.g. guinea-pig ileum and rat uterus [44, 51]. The characteristics of this material are the same as those which have been studied in connection with the permeability factors and this activity also cannot be attributed

Table II. Effect of fractions of permeability factor from pig platelets on the accumulation of I[131]-labelled serum albumin at injection sites in the skin of rabbits and guinea pigs[1]

Material injected	Radioactivity at injection site (cpm)			
	Exp. 1[2]	Exp. 2[2]	Exp. 3[3]	Exp. 4[3]
Unfiltered	1,779	3,306	2,320	4,016
UM-1 filtrate	1,221	1,931	1,333	2,836
Retained material		1,517		2,026
UM-2 filtrate	693	1,416	560	2,280
Retained material		1,451		760
UM-3 filtrate	1,823	1,915	979	950
Retained material		683		850
Tyrode's solution	978	718	373	560

[1] The preparation of this permeability factor has been described (51). UM-1 Diaflo filters retain molecules greater than 10,000 in molecular weight. UM-2 and UM-3 filters retain molecules greater than 1,000 and the UM-3 filter is charged. The material retained was washed twice on the filter with Tyrode's solution and then reconstituted to the original volume with Tyrode's solution.
[2] Rabbits.
[3] Guinea pigs.

solely to histamine and serotonin [51] because inhibitors of the action of these compounds do not abolish the effect of the material from platelets [44].

The relationship of the material released from the platelets to that released from other cells remains to be determined. However, it does not appear to be anaphylatoxin, which has been found to originate from complement [29], since the platelet material contracts both guinea-pig ileum and rat uterus [44]. While there may be kinins present, the activity cannot be due entirely to these because some activity is found in a high molecular weight fraction. The activity does not appear to be similar to that of slow reacting substances [58] because the platelet material does not cause delayed contraction of the isolated guinea-pig ileum. It could be related to the material which has been described as originating from the lysosomes of granulocytes [25, 61].

In vivo Studies

Shock and death frequently occur in anaphylaxis induced either by the intravenous infusion of antigen-antibody complexes or the infusion of antigen into a presensitized animal [1, 32]. In association with the acute shock, the platelet count falls and blood coagulation is accelerated [59, 60]. Both thrombi and antigen-antibody precipitates have been found obstructing the pulmonary vessels. Many investigators consider that the shock is due to obstruction of these vessels by the antigen-antibody precipitates rather than by the platelet-fibrin thrombi [1]. In addition, the vasoactive compounds released during anaphylaxis could contribute to peripheral vasodilatation which can produce shock.

To examine the possible relationship between platelet aggregation and shock associated with the intravenous infusion of antigen-antibody complexes in rabbits, we investigated the effects of inhibiting platelet aggregation with compounds such as sulfinpyrazone. Administration of sulfinpyrazone in doses which inhibited antigen-antibody induced aggregation, prevented the acute shock and death which occurred upon the infusion of these complexes into untreated rabbits (table III) [39]. If the shock were due solely to the immune precipitates blocking pulmonary blood flow, shock would have occurred even though platelet aggregation was inhibited. This evidence suggests, therefore, that platelet aggregation may be involved in the acute shock seen with the intravenous infusion of antigen-antibody complexes in rabbits. However, it must be pointed out that drugs such as the pyrazole compounds and the salicylates also inhibit other cellular systems [12], and can antagonize vasoactive agents such as histamine, catechola-

Table III. The effect of intravenous antigen-antibody complexes on platelet count and arterial and venous blood pressure in rabbits

Rabbits	Mean platelet count No/cu. mm		Mean blood pressure mm Hg Arterial		Venous	
	Pre	Post	Pre	Post	Pre	Post
Untreated (5)	358,000	53,000	84.8	50.0	3.3	7.6
Treated[1] (6)	321,000	136,000	84.2	77.7	3.7	3.8
P values[2]		$P < 0.01$		$P < 0.02$	$P < 0.05$	

[1] Sulfinpyrazone (150 mg/kg) was infused intravenously 20 min before rabbit bovine serum albumin-anti bovine serum albumin complexes (10 ml at a concentration of 0.1 mg antibody nitrogen/ml) were administered. Platelet counts and blood pressures were measured 5 min later.

[2] The P values represent the differences between the mean values post infusion for the untreated and treated animals.

mines, bradykinin, serotonin and slow reacting substances [20]. The effects of these drugs on the leucocytes and vascular tissues may also be important in the protection given these animals.

The main changes which occur immediately after intravenous infusion of endotoxin are a fall in the platelet count and shock, due to failure of cardiac output [7, 21]. A decline in venous return associated with hepatic pooling of the blood has been proposed as a mechanism to explain the shock [62]. In rabbits given intravenous endotoxin, arterial pressure falls and pulmonary arterial pressure rises, which may indicate increased pulmonary resistance to blood flow. Although the vasoactive compounds released from the platelets might be a factor in producing shock, it is also possible that the initial shock is in part due to the obstruction of the pulmonary circulation by the platelet aggregates as is the case with the antigen-antibody complex reaction described above. Examination of lung tissue immediately following the intravenous infusion of endotoxin has shown platelet aggregates plugging the pulmonary microcirculation [10]. If the rabbits were treated with pyrazole compounds, sodium salicylate, or acetylsalicylic acid prior to the endotoxin infusion, the fall in platelet count and arterial pressure did not occur. Furthermore, none of the animals treated with the compounds died during the two days following the infusion, whereas all the untreated animals died within four hours [10]. These studies provide evidence that inhibition of endotoxin-induced platelet aggregation is associated with the prevention of the acute shock effect seen with this material.

To investigate further the role of platelet aggregates in these reactions we examined the effect of producing platelet aggregates by the infusion of adenosine diphosphate (ADP). When intravenous ADP is given to animals such as pigs or rabbits there is a marked fall in the arterial pressure and a rise in venous pressure similar to that produced by the antigen-antibody complexes or endotoxin [26, 39, 46]. ADP does not cause leucocyte or red cell aggregation and causes only a slight release of platelet constituents [33, 43], in contrast to the effects of antigen-antibody complexes or endotoxin on platelets. It can be assumed, therefore, that the primary effects of ADP are due to vasodilatation and platelet aggregation. The effects on platelet aggregation and blood pressure cannot be prevented by pretreating these animals with acetylsalicylic acid, sulfinpyrazone or related compounds [39]. This is hardly surprising, since these compounds do not inhibit ADP-induced platelet aggregation [11, 52]. However, if the animals' platelets are made insensitive to ADP or the animals are made thrombocytopenic (by pretreatment with P^{32}), ADP infusion does not produce the acute shock effect. The degree of shock produced in these experiments in which platelet aggregation does not occur is moderate and similar to that produced by the adenine compounds which do not cause platelet aggregation [26]. Although this evidence is not conclusive, it does appear to indicate that the acute shock seen with compounds which can cause platelet aggregation could be the result, initially, of the platelet aggregates blocking the circulation in small vessels such as those in the lung.

The generalized Shwartzman reaction is usually induced in animals by two intravenous injections of bacterial endotoxin separated by 24 h. The distinguishing characteristic of the reaction which occurs after the second injection is the formation of renal glomerular capillary fibrin thrombi which cause renal cortical necrosis [32]. Several lines of evidence indicate that these fibrin deposits form in the glomerular capillaries as a result of the trapping in the glomeruli of microscopic fibrin aggregates formed elsewhere in the circulation [8]. The mechanism by which endotoxin initiates blood coagulation and leads to intravascular fibrin formation is still not clearly understood. Although there are many possibilities, one mechanism could be that the endotoxin-induced platelet aggregates either initiate or accelerate the coagulation process, because when endotoxin is infused intravenously, much of it becomes associated with the platelets and the platelet count falls [19, 21]. Therefore, inhibition of endotoxin-induced platelet aggregation might prevent the coagulation changes and therefore protect the animals from the changes associated with the formation of fibrin deposits in the glomeruli. We examined the effect of pretreating rabbits with compounds which inhibit endotoxin-induced platelet aggregation. It was found that when rabbits were given compounds such as the pyrazole or salicylate compounds in doses which would inhibit endotoxin-induced platelet aggregation, none of the animals developed the generalized Shwartzman reaction [10]. In these studies, the treatment had to be initiated before the first infusion of endotoxin and maintained throughout the study. Although this evidence suggests that endotoxin-induced platelet aggregation may be involved in producing the changes giving rise to the renal lesions characteristic of the generalized Shwartzman reaction, it is, of course, possible that these compounds may also be interfering with other mechanisms which take part in the development of this reaction.

Immunological reactions are important in the rejection episodes seen with kidney transplants. There is evidence from the studies by PORTER et al. [53] and MOWBRAY [36], that during the rejection episodes which occur 7–50 days after the transplantation, the formation of platelet aggregates in the renal arteries and capillaries leads to renal dysfunction. They have found that in biopsies taken from kidneys at the time of a rejection episode, there are platelet aggregates in the lumen of the glomerular capillaries and small arteries. In patients given platelets labelled with chromium-51 prior to such rejection episodes, the radioactivity accumulated in the transplanted kidney at the time of the rejection episode but not in the recipient's own kidney. When therapy was increased, in this case increasing doses of immuran and prednisone, the radioactivity left the transplanted kidney, the platelet count rose, the radioactive platelets returned to the circulation and kidney function was restored. Both 6-mercaptopurine (the metabolic product of immuran) and cortisone in appropriate doses inhibit the response of platelets to surface stimuli in *in vitro* studies [36]. More recently MOWBRAY [37] found that the intravenous administration of phenylbutazone during such an episode will also reverse the process in terms of restoring the platelet count and renal function.

The mechanism by which the platelet aggregates are initiated is not clear but it could be related to the vessel injury induced by an immunological reaction. The stimulus for this may be gamma-globulin, which is known to line the vessels of the transplanted kidney at this stage, or disruption of the endothelium exposing the basement membrane and/or collagen fibres. The results of this study are interesting in that they provide evidence that extensive platelet thrombi which are formed as a result of vessel injury can be made unstable by inhibiting the response of platelets to surface stimuli. It appears that in thrombus formation there is an equilibrium between the factors producing thrombi and the factors involved in their dissolution. If the balance is changed in favour of those factors which disrupt thrombi, the platelet mass breaks up. This dissolution of platelet thrombi by agents which interfere with the response of platelets to surface stimuli appears to be possible for several hours until fibrin formation around the platelet aggregates is extensive.

References

1. AUSTEN, K. F.: Anaphylaxis: Systemic, local cutaneous and *in vitro;* in The Inflammatory Process. B. W. ZWEIFACH, L. GRANT, R. T. McCLUSKEY, eds, p. 587 (Academic Press, N.Y. 1965).
2. BEHNKE, O. and FORER, A.: Evidence for four classes of microtubules in individual cells. J. Cell. Sci. *2:* 169 (1967).
3. BERGSTRÖM, S.; CARLSON, L. A. and WEEKS, J. R.: The prostaglandins: A family of biologically active lipids. Pharmacol. Rev. *20:* 1 (1968).

4. Bettex-Galland, M. and Lüscher, E. F.: Studies on the metabolism of human blood platelets in relation to clot retraction. Thromb. Diath. haemorrh. *4:* 178 (1960).
5. Born, G. V. R.: The platelet membrane and its functions. XII. Cong. Int. Soc. Hemat. N. Y., 1968, p. 95.
6. Born, G. V. R. and Cross, M. J.: The aggregation of blood platelets. J. Physiol. *168:* 178 (1963).
7. Brockman, S. K.; Thomas, C. S. and Vasko, J. S.: The effect of Escherichia coli endotoxin on the circulation. Surg. Gynec. Obstet. *125:* 763 (1967).
8. Cohen, M. H. and Lee, L.: Effect of ureteral blockade on localization of circulating fibrin aggregates in the kidney. Fed. Proc. *23:* 446 (1964).
9. Des Prez, R. M.: The effects of bacterial endotoxin on rabbit platelets. V. Heat labile plasma factor requirements of endotoxin-induced platelet injury. J. Immunol. *99:* 966 (1967).
10. Evans, G. and Mustard, J. F.: Inhibition of the platelet-surface reaction in endotoxin shock and the generalized Shwartzman reaction. J. clin. Invest. *47:* 31a (1968).
11. Evans, G.; Packham, M. A.; Murphy, E. A. and Mustard, J. F.: The effect of acetylsalicylic acid on platelet function. J. exp. Med. *128:* 877 (1968).
12. Forbes, I. J. and Smith, J. L.: Effects of anti-inflammatory drugs on lymphocytes. Lancet *2:* 334 (1967).
13. Grette, K.: Studies on the mechanisms of thrombin catalysed hemostatic reactions in blood platelets. Acta. physiol. scand. Suppl. *56:* 195 (1962).
14. Hardisty, R. M. and Hutton, R. A.: Platelet aggregation and the availability of platelet factor 3. Brit. J. Haemat. *12:* 764 (1966).
15. Haslam, R. J.: Mechanisms of blood platelet aggregation; in Physiology of Hemostasis and Thrombosis. S. A. Johnson, W. H. Seegers, eds, p. 88 (Thomas, Springfield 1967).
16. Haslam, R. J.: Biochemical aspects of platelet function. XII. Cong. Int. Soc. Hemat. N.Y., 1968, p. 198.
17. Henson, P. M. and Cochrane, C. G.: Antigen-antibody complexes and increased vascular permeability; in 3rd Int. Symp. on Cellular and Humoral Mechanisms in Anaphylaxis and Allergy, 1968.
18. Henson, P. and Cochrane, C.: Complement-dependent release of histamine from rabbit platelets by antigen-antibody reactions. Fed. Proc. *27:* 479 (1968).
19. Herion, J. C.; Herring, W. B.; Palmer, J. H. and Walker, R. I.: Cr[51]-labeled endotoxin distribution in granulocytopenic animals. Amer. J. Physiol. *206:* 947 (1964).
20. Hinshaw, L. B.; Solomon, L. A.; Erdös, E. G.; Reins, D. A. and Gunter, B. J.: Effects of acetylsalicylic acid on the canine response to endotoxin. J. Pharmacol. exp. Ther. *157:* 665 (1967).
21. Horowitz, H. I.; Des Prez, R. M. and Hook, E. W.: Effects of bacterial endotoxin on rabbit platelets. II. Enhancement of platelet factor 3 activity *in vitro* and *in vivo*. J. exp. Med. *116:* 619 (1962).
22. Hovig, T.: The effect of calcium and magnesium on rabbit blood platelet aggregation *in vitro*. Thromb. Diath. haemorrh. *12:* 179 (1964).
23. Hovig, T.: The ultrastructure of blood platelets in normal and abnormal states. Ser. haemat. I, *2:* 3 (1968).
24. Hovig, T.; Rowsell, H. C.; Dodds, W. J.; Jørgensen, L. and Mustard, J. F.: Experimental hemostasis in normal dogs and dogs with congenital disorders of blood coagulation. Blood *30:* 636 (1967).
25. Janoff, A.; Schaeffer, S.; Scherer, J. and Bean, M.: Mediators of inflammation in leukocyte lysosomes. II. Mechanism of action of lysosomal cationic protein upon vascular permeability in the rat. J. exp. Med. *122:* 841 (1965).

26. JØRGENSEN, L.; ROWSELL, H. C.; HOVIG, T.; GLYNN, M. F. and MUSTARD, J. F.: Adenosine diphosphate-induced platelet aggregation and myocardial infarction in swine. Lab. Invest. *17:* 616 (1967).

27. JØRGENSEN, L.; ROWSELL, H. C.; HOVIG, T. and MUSTARD, J. F.: Resolution and organization of platelet-rich mural thrombi in carotid arteries of swine. Amer. J. Path. *51:* 681 (1967).

28. KINLOUGH, R. L. and MUSTARD, J. F.: Unpublished observations.

29. LEPOW, I. H.; DIAS DA SILVA, W. and PATRICK, R. A.: Biologically active cleavage products of components of complement; in 3rd Int. Symp. on Cellular and Humoral Mechanisms in Anaphylaxis and Allergy, 1968.

30. MARCUS, A. J. and ZUCKER, M. B.: The physiology of blood platelets (Grune and Stratton, Inc., N.Y. 1965).

31. MARKWARDT, F.: Studies on the release of biogenic amines from blood platelets; in Biochemistry of Blood Platelets. E. KOWALSKI, S. NIEWIAROWSKI, eds., p. 105 (Academic Press, N.Y. 1967).

32. McKAY, D. G.: Disseminated intravascular coagulation (Hoeber Med. Divn., Harper and Row, N.Y. 1965).

33. MILLS, D. C. B.; ROBB, I. A. and ROBERTS, G. C. K.: The release of nucleotides, 5-hydroxytryptamine and enzymes from human blood platelets during aggregation. J. Physiol. *195:* 715 (1968).

34. MOVAT, H. Z.: Activation of the kinin system by antigen-antibody complexes; in Int. Symp. on Vasoactive Polypeptides: Bradykinin and Related Kinins. M. ROCHA E SILVA and H. A. ROTHSCHILD, eds., p. 177 (Pergamon Press, Oxford, 1967).

35. MOVAT, H. Z.; MUSTARD, J. F.; TAICHMAN, N. S. and URIUHARA, T.: Platelet aggregation and release of ADP, serotonin and histamine associated with phagocytosis of antigen-antibody complexes. Proc. Soc. exp. Biol. N.Y. *120:* 232 (1965).

36. MOWBRAY, J. F.: Methods of suppression of immune responses. Proc. 9th Int. Cong. of Internal Medicine. Excerpta med. Int. Cong. Ser. *137:* 106 (1966).

37. MOWBRAY, J. F.: Personal communication.

38. MUSTARD, J. F.: Hemostasis and thrombosis. Seminars Hemat. *5:* 91 (1968).

39. MUSTARD, J. F.; EVANS, G. and LEWIS, A. F.: Unpublished observations.

40. MUSTARD, J. F.; EVANS, G. and PACKHAM, M. A.: Unpublished observations.

41. MUSTARD, J. F.; HEGARDT, B.; ROWSELL, H. C. and MACMILLAN, R. L.: Effect of adenosine nucleotides on platelet aggregation and clotting time. J. Lab. clin. Med. *64:* 548 (1964).

42. MUSTARD, J. F.; JØRGENSEN, L., HOVIG, T.; GLYNN, M. F. and ROWSELL, H. C.: Role of platelets in thrombosis; in Pathogenesis and Treatment of Thromboembolic Diseases. Thromb. Diath. haemorrh. Suppl. *21:* 131 (1966).

43. MUSTARD, J. F.; MOVAT, H. Z.; MACMORINE, D. R. L. and SENYI, A.: Release of permeability factors from the blood platelet. Proc. Soc. exp. Biol. N.Y. *119:* 988 (1965).

44. MUSTARD, J. F. and PACKHAM, M. A.: Unpublished observations.

45. MUSTARD, J. F. and PACKHAM, M. A.: Platelet phagocytosis. Ser. Haemat. 1, *2:* 168 (1968).

46. MUSTARD, J. F.; ROWSELL, H. C.; LOTZ, F.; HEGARDT, B. and MURPHY, E. A.: The effect of adenine nucleotides on thrombus formation, platelet count, and blood coagulation. Exp. molec. Path. *5:* 43 (1966).

47. NAGAKI, K.; FUJIKAWA, K. and INAI, S.: Studies on the fourth component of complement. II. The fourth component of complement in guinea-pig and human platelets. Biken J. *8:* 129 (1965).

48. NIEWIAROWSKI, ST.; BANKOWSKI, E. and ROGOWICKA, I.: Studies on the adsorption and activation of the Hageman factor (factor XII) by collagen and elastin. Thromb. Diath. haemorrh. *14:* 387 (1965).

49. NISHIZAWA, E. E.; BUCHANAN, M. and MUSTARD, J. F.: The effect of phosphatidyl-serine on platelet function and hemostasis. Blood (abstract) *28:* 1013 (1966).

50. O'BRIEN, J. R.: Effect of anti-inflammatory agents on platelets. Lancet *1:* 894 (1968).

51. PACKHAM, M. A.; NISHIZAWA, E. E. and MUSTARD, J. F.: Response of platelets to tissue injury. Biochem. Pharmacol. Suppl. 171 (1968).

52. PACKHAM, M. A.; WARRIOR, E. S.; GLYNN, M. F.; SENYI, A. S. and MUSTARD, J. F.: Alteration of the response of platelets to surface stimuli by pyrazole compounds. J. exp. Med. *126:* 171 (1967).

53. PORTER, K. A.; DOSSETOR, J. B.; MARCHIORO, T. L.; PEART, W. S.; RENDALL, J. M.; STARZL, T. E. and TERASAKI, P. I.: Human renal transplants. I. Glomerular changes. Lab. Invest. *16:* 153 (1967).

54. PUSZKIN, E. and JERUSHALMY, Z.: Effect of connective tissue and collagen on platelet lactate production: Possible role of acid mucopolysaccharides. Proc. Soc. exp. Biol. N.Y. *129:* 346 (1968).

55. SHAINOFF, J. R. and PAGE, I. H.: Significance of cryoprofibrin in fibrinogen-fibrin conversion. J. exp. Med. *116:* 687 (1962).

56. SPAET, T. H. and ZUCKER, M. B.: Mechanism of platelet plug formation and role of adenosine diphosphate. Amer. J. Physiol. *206:* 1267 (1964).

57. THOMAS, D. P.: The role of platelet catecholamines in the aggregation of platelets by collagen and thrombin. Exp. Biol. Med. *3:* 129 (1968).

58. VOGT, W.: Slow reacting substances; in 3rd Int. Symp. on Cellular and Humoral Mechanisms in Anaphylaxis and Allergy, 1968.

59. WALTER, J. B. and FRANK, J. A.: The relationship of hyaline emboli to other manifestations of anaphylaxis. Brit. J. exp. Path. *42:* 609 (1961).

60. WALTER, J. B.; FRANK, J. A. and IRWIN, J. W.: Hyaline emboli in the microcirculation of rabbits during anaphylaxis. Brit. J. exp. Path. *42:* 603 (1961).

61. WASI, S.; MURRAY, R. K.; MACMORINE, D. R. L. and MOVAT, H. Z.: The role of PMN-leucocyte lysosomes in tissue injury, inflammation and hypersensitivity. II. Studies on the proteolytic activity of PMN-leucocyte lysosomes of the rabbit. Brit. J. exp. Path. *47:* 411 (1966).

62. WEIL, M. H.; MACLEAN, L. D.; VISSCHER, M. B. and SPINK, W. W.: Studies on the circulatory changes in the dog produced by endotoxin from gram-negative microorganisms. J. clin. Invest. *35:* 1191 (1956).

Authors' address: J. F. MUSTARD, M.D., G. EVANS, M.D., M. A. PACKHAM, Ph.D., E. E. NISHIZAWA, Ph.D. Dept. of Pathology, McMaster University, *Hamilton, Ont.* (Canada).

Cellular and Humoral Mechanisms in Anaphylaxis and Allergy, pp. 164–175
(Karger, Basel/New York 1969)

Chemical Mediators Released by PMN-leukocytes During Phagocytosis of Ag-Ab Complexes[1]

Henry Z. Movat[2], David R. L. Macmorine, Yuko Takeuchi and
Clement E. Burrowes

Division of Experimental Pathology, Department of Pathology
University of Toronto, Toronto

The lysosomes of polymorphonuclear (PMN)-leukocytes have been implicated as mediators of tissue injury and enhanced vascular permeability in many experimental models of immediate hypersensitivity. Included in this list are: the Arthus reaction [17, 4, 2, 19], certain forms of cutaneous anaphylaxis [18, 8], systemic aggregate anaphylaxis [14] and some of the manifestations of serum sickness [7]. In some of the above immune reactions the initiating event leading to lysosomal release is phagocytosis of antigen-antibody complexes.

In vivo Studies Implicating PMN-leukocytes as Mediators of Tissue Injury

Cutaneous anaphylaxis elicited with heterologous (rabbit) antibody in guinea pigs is mediated primarily by histamine. However, there is a PMN-leukocyte component in this type of PCA-reaction. When guinea pigs are rendered neutropenic with a rabbit anti-leukocyte serum or with nitrogen mustard there is partial yet significant inhibition of the reaction. Ultrastructurally one can see micro-precipitates of antigen and antibody, some in digestive vacuoles or phagosomes of degranulating PMN-leukocytes [18].

The findings with PCA in the rat are more clear-cut. When rats are rendered neutropenic with an anti-leukocyte serum there is almost complete suppression of the bluing response induced with homologous or heterologous complement (C)-fixing antibody, while antihistamine and a serotonin antagonist have no suppressive effect [8]. In contrast PCA induced with

[1] Supported by the J. P. Bickell Foundation and the Medical Research Council of Canada.

[2] Dr. Movat is a research associate of the MRC.

homologous anaphylactic (reaginic, homocytotropic) antibody is completely suppressed by the amine antagonists, but neutropenia has no effect on the reaction (fig. 1). PCA induced with anaphylactic antibody is associated with mast cell degranulation [11, 13] and a negligible infiltration of poly-morphs, whereas the reaction induced with the complement-fixing, electro-phoretically slow antibody is accompanied by a considerable accumulation of PMN-leukocytes (fig. 2), which show phagocytosis and degranulation, similar to the PCA of the guinea pig and to systemic aggregate anaphylaxis (see below).

The mechanisms underlying the PCA induced with the C-fixing antibody can be visualized as follows: When antigen and antibody interact, the micro-precipitates fix C and this is followed by generation of the chemotactic complex C 5, 6, 7 [20]. The chemotactic agent attracts PMN-leukocytes which phagocytose the immune aggregates. In this process the membrane of the granules (lysosomes) of the PMN-leukocytes fuse with those of the vacuoles containing the ingested aggregates and the granule contents are emptied in the vacuole, now referred to as 'digestive vacuole'. The phago-cytosing cells gradually use up their glycogen and undergo regressive changes. While these changes can be observed ultrastructurally, it is un-certain whether extracellular enzyme release is due to the cell becoming 'leaky' or a consequence of overt cell death. Some of the *in vitro* data give us an idea which components of the lysosome may contribute to enhanced vascular permeability (see below).

In *systemic aggregate anaphylaxis* the principal change consists of accu-mulation of immune aggregates in the pulmonary vessels [9]. These initial changes are soon followed by accumulation of PMN-leukocytes and platelets, which phagocytose the immune precipitates. They form digestive vacuoles, consisting of the precipitates and fragments of lysosomes (fig. 3). When animals (rabbits, swine) are rendered neutropenic they have less hypotension, show less tendency to develop protracted shock and do not develop the hemorrhagic pulmonary lesions encountered in animals with normal white cell counts. In animals with normal white cell counts there is a rise in certain hydrolytic enzymes known to be present in PMN-leukocyte lysosomes [14]

In vitro Studies on the Release of Phlogistic Agents from Phagocytosing
PMN-leukocytes

The *in vitro* model was designed in an attempt to imitate the *in vivo* happenings observed ultrastructurally and at the same time obtain ma-

PCA IN THE RAT

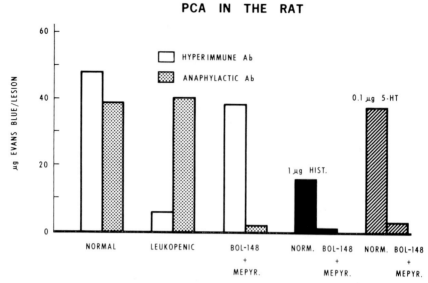

Fig. 1. Passive cutaneous anaphylaxis in the rat elicited with homologous hyperimmune, complement-fixing antibody and with anaphylactic (reaginic, homocytotropic) antibody. The cutaneous lesion induced with the complement-fixing hyperimmune antibody is suppressible by rendering the rats neutropenic.

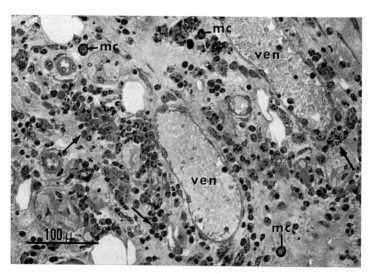

Fig. 2. Accumulation of numerous PMN-leukocytes (arrows) in a one-hour old PCA reaction induced with complement-fixing hyperimmune antibody. Note that the mast cells (mc) appear intact and that the venules (ven) are dilated and filled with blood.

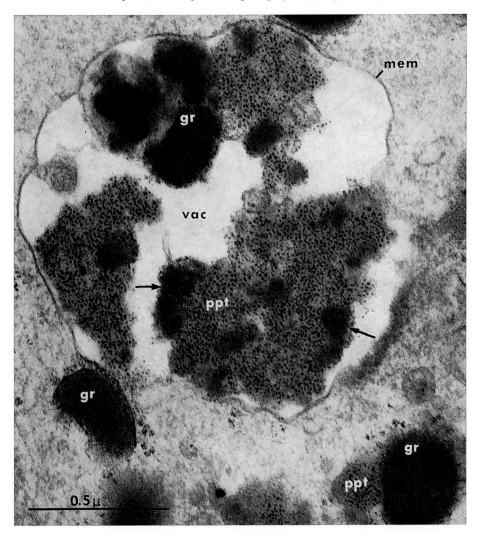

Fig. 3. Electron micrograph of part of a PMN-leukocyte from a pulmonary vessel during systemic aggregate anaphylaxis. A phago-lysosome or digestive vacuole (vac) is shown. It contains phagocytosed ferritin-anti-ferritin precipitates (ppt) and fragments of granules (gr). The limiting double membrane of the digestive vacuole is designated 'men'. Between the arrows a fusion of granule fragments and immune precipitates is seen.

terial released by the phagocytosing cells for biological and physico-chemical analysis.

PMN-leukocytes were obtained from the peritoneal cavity of rabbits, rats or guinea pigs that have been injected intraperitoneally 16–18 h before with 0.1% glycogen in physiological saline. The cells were incubated with precipitates of bovine serum albumin-anti bovine serum albumin, the procedure being essentially the same as described earlier [12], except that the washed immune precipitates were incubated with fresh guinea-pig serum (as a source of complement).

After incubation and centrifugation the cell pellet was prepared for and examined by electron microscopy. The supernatant (ambient fluid in which the cells phagocytosed the immune precipitates referred to as 'Pf/Phag', ref. 1) was examined for its biological and physico-chemical properties.

(a) Evidence for release of lysosomal material: 1. The pellet consisted mainly of PMN-leukocytes in the process of phagocytosing immune aggregates and degranulating, identical to the changes observed ultrastructurally *in vivo* (see fig. 3). 2. When S^{35}-sulfate or H^3-arginine labeled PMN-leukocytes were used (experiments carried out in collaboration with Dr. J. F. Mustard), radioactive material was released into the ambient fluid (parallel studies showed that the radioactivity resides mainly in the 8,000 g or granule fraction) (table I). 3. By acrylamide electrophoresis (EC-Apparatus Corp.) more or less the same pattern was obtained when Pf/Phag was compared with lysed PMN-leukocyte granules (fig. 4). 4. By immunodiffusion a reaction of identity between several components of Pf/Phag and lysed granules could be demonstrated.

Table I. Release of S^{35}-sulfate and H^3-arginine from phagocytosing PMN-leukocytes

Incubation for 1 hour	Release CPM/ml[1]	
	S^{35}-sulfate	H^3-arginine
PMNL + Ag-Ab-C′ (37° C)	1215.00	552.00
PMNL + Tyrode (37° C)	267.00	253.70
PMNL + Tyrode (4° C)	57.00	52.00

PMN-leukocytes were labeled *in vivo* by injecting i.v. 100 μc of S^{35}-sulfate or 20 μc H^3-arginine per rabbit. The S^{35}-sulfate injected rabbits were used 4 days and H^3-arginine injected animals 6 days after the injection. Cells collected from the peritoneal cavity were incubated with or without antigen-antibody precipitates as described in the text. The radioactivity of the ambient fluid in which phagocytosis of the immune precipitates occurred was tested in a liquid scintilation counter after centrifugation of the cells.

[1] Counts per minute per ml of ambient fluid.

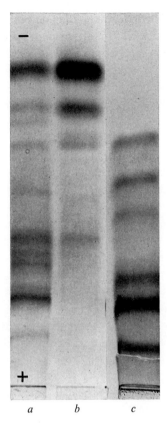

Fig. 4. Acrylamide gel electrophoresis at pH3 (Tris-citric acid buffer) of rabbit Pf/Phag (a), of lysed rabbit PMN-leukocyte granules (b) and of rat Pf/Phag (c). Migration was upwards (catode).

(b) Biological and physicochemical properties of Pf/Phag. When injected intradermally into animals, Pf/Phag enhanced vascular permeability. The vascular permeability induced with Pf/Phag obtained from rabbit leukocytes was almost completely suppressible in the rat with a combination of mepyramine (5 mg/kg) and BOL-148 (2 mg/kg), but only partly suppressible when only one antagonist was used. The bluing effect of rabbit-Pf/Phag was partly suppressible with antihistamine in the guinea pig, while in rabbits the antihistamine had little suppressive effect. Pf/Phag obtained from PMN-leukocytes of rats and guinea pigs induced bluing in the homologous animal, the amine antagonists having little suppressive effect. The bluing in guinea pigs and rats developed rapidly and the animals were killed 30 min after the

intradermal injections. In rabbits the bluing developed slowly and therefore these animals were sacrificed 1½ h after the intradermal injections.

Pf/Phag from all three species induced contraction of several smooth muscle preparations. Contraction was rapid, but relaxation was slow, often with repeated contractions during the wash. The rapidity of the contraction and the height of the contraction was reduced when antihistamine was added to the guinea-pig ileum and BOL-148 to the rat uterus. In the presence of the amine antagonists, both contraction and relaxation was slow. The active material was designated 'SRS/Phag' (slow reacting substance released during phagocytosis). Its properties are shown in table II.

Sucrose density gradient ultracentrifugation (2.5–10% sucrose, 20 h at 134,000 g) showed that the vascular permeability of rabbit Pf/Phag resided in low molecular weight fractions, sedimenting like cytochrome-c or slower.

Further information was obtained from gel filtration on Sephadex G-50 (5 × 90 cm column equilibrated with Tyrode solution). Peak I (eluting with the void volume) contained the hydrolytic enzymes and some bluing activity when tested in the rabbit. Peaks II–IV contained the cationic proteins (bands 1–4) shown in figure 4. Of these, peak II (band 4 by acrylamide gel electrophoresis) with an elution volume slightly greater than cytochrome-c (M.W. 12,300) was most active when tested in the rabbit. Antihistamine did not suppress the bluing in the rabbit. This same moderately cationic protein obtained from rabbit leukocytes caused little bluing in the rat. However, the three most cationic bands (eluting in peaks III and IV) induced marked bluing in the rat. This could be partly suppressed by either mepyramine or BOL-148 and was almost completely inhibited when both amine antagonists were used. Some of these findings are in keeping with those of RANADIVE and COCHRANE [15].

Peak IV obtained by gel filtration contained a blurred band (band 3). Its elution volume was approximately that of Vitamine B_{12} (M.W. 1,360).

Table II. Properties of SRS-Phag

---

1. Contracts guinea-pig ileum (in the presence of mepyramine), rat uterus (in the presence of BOL-148) and rabbit jejunum
2. Heat resistant-boiling 20 min
3. Passes UM-3 (Amicon) membrane (MW < 500)
4. Extractable with diethyl ether
5. Resistant to chymotrypsin and carboxypeptidase-B
6. Inactivated by IBr and phenylisocyanate[1]

---

[1] AMBACHE, N.; REYNOLDS, M. and WHITING, J. M. C.: J. Physiol. *166:* 251 (1963).

This peak contained the SRS/Phag-activity. The smooth muscle contracting activity could be separated from the vascular permeability enhancing activity by membrane partition chromatography. Using the UM-3 (Amicon) membrane (cut off M.W. ∾500), the bluing activity was retained in the concentrate, whereas the SRS/Phag-activity passed into the filtrate.

When crude Pf/Phag and peaks I–IV obtained by gel filtration were further tested, it was found that the crude material and peaks III and IV (bands 1–3) caused disruption of rat peritoneal mast cells and release of both histamine and serotonin (assayed on the guinea-pig ileum and rat uterus respectively; suppressible by the appropriate antagonists). However, neither crude Pf/Phag nor the fractions released histamine from chopped guinea-pig lung preparations[2].

Peak I, eluting with the void volume, was further chromatographed on DEAE-Sephadex. It yielded a fraction which contained both acid protease

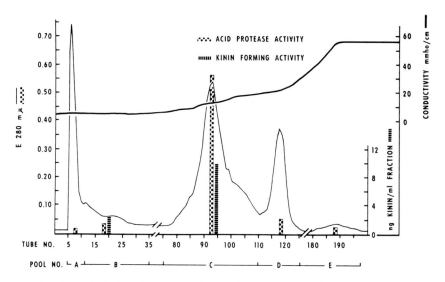

Fig. 5. DEAE-Sephadex chromatography (1 × 25 cm column) of peak I (void volume, see text) obtained by chromatographing rabbit Pf/Phag first on a Sephadex G-50 (5 × 90 cm column). Elution was with a linear gradient consisting of 0.1 M Tris-HCl (pH 8.0) and this buffer plus 0.5 M NaCl. To test kinin-forming activity fresh rabbit serum containing 1 mg/ml of hexadimethrine bromide (to prevent activation of Hageman factor) was incubated with 1 ml of pools A–E, concentrated to the volume of the sample applied to the column. After incubation for 18 h at pH5 (see ref. 3) the heat denatured incubation product was tested on the rat uterus. Note that the kinin-forming activity parallels the acid protease activity.

[2] These findings will be described in detail in another publication.

(measured as described in ref. 21) and kinin forming [3] (assayed on the estrus rat uterus) activities (fig. 5).

In more recent studies rat Pf/Phag (fig. 4c) was chromatographed. Here again the bluing activity was in low molecular size fractions (fig. 6) eluting between protamine sulfate (M.W. $\sim$6,000) and vitamine B_{12} (M.W. 1,360). As with rabbit Pf/Phag, when tested in the homologous animal (rat), the increased vascular permeability could not be suppressed by amine antagonists. The active material in guinea pig Pf/Phag was separated by Sephadex G-50 chromatography into an active fraction eluting with the void volume (giving rise to immediate bluing) and into a low molecular size fraction (causing a delayed bluing response). Antihistamine caused slight inhibition with all fractions.

The findings reported here indicate that the cationic proteins of a given pecies when tested in the same species, induce enhanced vessel permeability, not as generally believed [6, 16], by release of vasoactive amines, but by another, as yet unidentified, mechanism. Many cationic substances

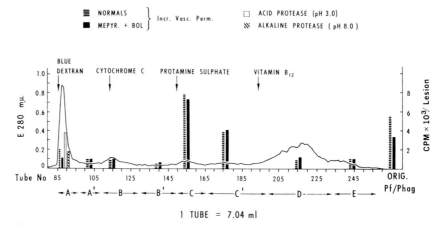

Fig. 6. Gel filtration on Sephadex G-50 of 20 ml rat Pf/Phag on a 5 × 90 cm (K 50/100 Pharmacia) column equilibrated with Tyrode solution (pH 7.4). The bluing activity of the original Pf/Phag is shown on the right. Note that phlogistic fractions eluted between protamine sulfate (M.W. $\sim$ 6,000) and vitamine B_{12} (M.W. 1,360). Amine antagonists did not suppress the bluing response.

CPM = counts per minute. It expresses increase in vascular permeability. I^{125}-labeled human serum albumin was injected intravenously together with Evans blue. The radioactivity of the punched out skin lesions was measured in a γ-scaler, as described by Movat and DiLorenzo, Lab. Invest. *19:* 187 (1968).

release histamine from rat mast cells [6]. The fact that intensly cationic (basic) fractions of rabbit leukocyte lysosomes disrupt rat mast cells and release vasoactive amines does not seem to have any biologic significance, since the phenomenon is unlikely to occur *in vivo*.

Summary and Conclusions

PMN-leukocyte lysosomes are probably mediators of tissue injury and inflammation; their release triggered by the formation of Ag-Ab-C complexes. This includes certain forms of local and systemic anaphylaxis and other reactions of immediate hypersensitivity.

Evidence was presented that *in vitro* PMN-leukocytes undergo ultra-structural changes (phagocytosis and degranulation) identical to changes observed *in vivo*. Evidence was also presented that these phagocytosing cells release lysosomal materials.

The phlogistic agents released *in vitro* by the phagocytosing leukocytes of a certain species when tested in the same species induce the vascular alterations of inflammation by a mechanism other than release of vasoactive amines. The enhanced vessel permeability induced in the rat with leukocyte lysosomes of the rabbit (which is mediated by released amines from the mast cells) has no *in vivo* significance. The vasoactive substances of the leukocyte lysosomes are mainly cationic proteins of low (approx. 1,300–12,000) molecular weight. The acid proteases released by the phagocytosing cells can generate kinin from plasma. This may also contribute to the induction of the vascular phenomena of acute inflammation.

The material released by the phagocytosing cells contains also a slow reacting substance. This can be separated from the permeability agents. Therefore, this substance plays probably no role in acute inflammatory reactions, but may contribute to smooth muscle contraction in conditions such as systemic aggregate anaphylaxis.

References

1. Burke, J. S.; Uriuhara, T.; Macmorine, D. R. L. and Movat, H. Z.: A permeability factor released from phagocytosing PMN-leukocytes and its inhibition by protease inhibitors. Life Sci. *3:* 1505 (1964).

2. Cochrane, C. G.; Weigle, W. O. and Dixon, F. J.: The role of polymorphonuclear leukocytes in the initiation and cessation of Arthus vasculitis. J. exp. Med. *110:* 481 (1959).

3. Greenbaum, L. and Kim, K. S.: The kinin-forming and kininase activities of rabbit polymorphonuclear leukocytes. Brit. J. Pharmacol. *29:* 238 (1967).

4. Humphrey, J. H.: The mechanism of the Arthus reaction. I. The role of polymorphonuclear leukocytes and other factors in reversed passive Arthus reactions in rabbits. Brit. J. exp. Path. *36:* 268 (1965).

5. Janoff, A.; Schaefer, S.; Scherer, J. and Bean, M. A.: Mediators of inflammation in leukocyte lysosomes. II. Mechanism of action of lysosomal cationic protein upon vascular permeability in the rat. J. exp. Med. *122:* 841 (1965).

6. Keller, R.; Mueller-Eckhardt, C.; Kayser, F.-H. and Keller, H. V.: Interrelations between different types of cells. I. A comparative study of the biological properties of a cationic polypeptides from lysosomes of polymorphonuclear leukocytes and other cationic compounds. Int. Arch. Allergy *33:* 239 (1968).

7. Kniker, W. T. and Cochrane, C. G.: Pathogenetic factors in vascular lesions of experimental serum sickness. J. exp. Med. *122:* 1 (1965).

8. Lovett, C. A. and Movat, H. Z.: The role of PMN-leukocyte lysosomes in tissue injury, inflammation and hypersensitivity. III. Passive cutaneous anaphylaxis induced in the rat with homologous and heterologous hyperimmune antibody. Proc. Soc. exp. Biol. *122:* 991 (1966).

9. McKinnon, G. E.; Andrews, E. C.; Heptinstall, R. H. and Germuth, F. G.: An immunologic study on the occurrence of intravascular antigen-antibody precipitation and its role in anaphylaxis in the rabbit. Bull. Johns Hopkin Hosp. *101:* 258 (1957).

10. Mota, T.: The mechanism of anaphylaxis. I. Production and biological properties of 'mast cell sensitizing' antibody. Immunology *7:* 681 (1964).

11. Mota, T.: Release of histamine from mast cells; in Hb. of Exp. Pharmacol., Vol. XVIII/1, p. 569 (Springer, Berlin 1966).

12. Movat, H. Z.; Uriuhara, T.; Macmorine, D. R. L. and Burke, J. S.: A permeability factor released from leukocytes after phagocytosis of immune complexes and its possible role in the Arthus reaction. Life Sci. *3:* 1025 (1964).

13. Movat, H. Z.; Lovett, C. A. and Taichman, N. S.: Demonstration of antigen on the surface of sensitized rat mast cells. Nature, Lond. *212:* 851 (1966).

14. Movat, H. Z.; Uriuhara, T.; Taichman, N. S.; Rowsell, H. C. and Mustard, J. F.: The role of PMN-leucocyte lysosomes in tissue injury, inflammation and hypersensitivity. VI. The participation of the PMN-leucocyte and the blood platelet in systemic aggregate anaphylaxis. Immunology *14:* 637 (1968).

15. Ranadive, N. S. and Cochrane, C. G.: Fractionation and purification of cationic proteins of PMN-leukocytes. Fed. Proc. *26:* 574 (Abstract) (1967).

16. Seegers, W. and Janoff, A.: Mediators of inflammation in leukocyte lysosomes. VI. Partial purification and characterization of a mast-cell rupturing component. J. exp. Med. *124:* 833 (1966).

17. Stetson, C. A., Jr.: Similarities in the mechanisms determining the Arthus and Shwartzman phenomenon. J. exp. Med. *94:* 347 (1951).

18. Taichman, N. S. and Movat, H. Z.: Do polymorphonuclear leukocytes play a role in passive cutaneous anaphylaxis of the guinea pig? Int. Arch. Allergy *30:* 97 (1966).

19. Uriuhara, T. and Movat, H. Z.: The role of PMN-leukocyte lysosomes in tissue injury, inflammation and hypersensitivity. I. The vascular changes and the role of PMN-leukocytes in the reversed passive Arthus reaction. Exp. Molec. Path. *5:* 539 (1966).

20. WARD, P. A.; COCHRANE, C. G. and MÜLLER-EBERHARD, H. J.: The role of serum complement in chemotaxis of leukocytes *in vitro*. J. exp. Med. *122:* 327 (1965).
21. WASI, S.; MURRAY, R. K.; MACMORINE, D. R. L. and MOVAT, H. Z.: The role of PMN-leukocytes in tissue injury, inflammation and hypersensitivity. II. Studies on the proteolytic activity of PMN-leukocyte lysosomes of the rabbit. Brit. J. exp. Path. *47:* 411 (1966).

Recent experiments (with K. Udaka) indicate that anionic phlogistic substances reside in the fractions eluting with the void volume in Sephadex G-50.

Author's address: Dr. HENRY Z. MOVAT, Division of Experimental Pathology, Medical Sciences Building, University of Toronto, *Toronto, Ontario* (Canada).

Cellular and Humoral Mechanisms in Anaphylaxis and Allergy, pp. 176–186
(Karger, Basel/New York 1969)

Characteristics of Leukocytic Histamine Release by Antigen and by Anti-immunoglobulin and Anti-cellular Antibodies[1]

L. M. LICHTENSTEIN[2]

Division of Allergy and Infectious Diseases, Department of Medicine, The John Hopkin's University School of Medicine, Baltimore, Md.

Although exciting new work on the kinins, SRS, and anaphylatoxin is beginning to challenge its preeminent position, the case for histamine as a major mediator of allergic and anaphylactic reactions remains the strongest. Several quite different systems have been developed to study the mechanism of immunologic histamine release *in vitro;* this report deals with some of our experiences with the technique which utilizes isolated human peripheral blood leukocytes [9]. Most of this work was carried out with ragweed antigen E, a protein with a M.W. of 38,000, which can release histamine from the cells of ragweed sensitive donors in picogram concentrations [5]. When this or other appropriate antigens are added to a suspension of cells prepared from a sensitive donor there is a lag period of from one to several minutes before histamine release begins; the release process itself requires 10–40 min, depending on the antigen concentration. The reaction goes to completion with washed cells in buffer, although at sub-optimal antigen concentrations serum can enhance histamine release somewhat. We have shown that the C′ system is not involved in this enhancement [10].

The histamine is localized in the whole granulocytic series, perhaps about half in the basophils and the rest in the eosinophils and neutrophils. This is based on the data of GRAHAM [2], and the more recent studies of STYLER and REMINGTON [17] who showed that high dose corticosteroids decreased the eosinophil and basophil count to essentially zero while dropping the total blood histamine about 50%. The remaining basophil-eosinophil poor granulocyte

[1] Part of the work in this report is a result of collaboration with several investigators including Drs. K. ISHIZAKA; S. MARGOLIS; D. LEVY; H. BRAIN; J. RUSSO and M. RHYNE.
[2] Teaching and Research Scholar of the American College of Physicians Supported by grants No. AI 08270 and AI 07290.

preparations release histamine in essentially the same fashion as the usual preparations. Morphologically, there is little or no change to be seen in leukocyte preparations which have released their histamine. Experiments carried out with radioactive potassium have shown that all of the histamine can be released from the leukocytes by antigen without causing the cells to manifest a detectable loss of intracellular potassium [11].

All of these experiments demonstrate that this type of histamine release, that is, histamine release induced by the interaction of antigen and cell bound reaginic or IgE antibody, is not a cytotoxic process. The cells release their preformed histamine in an active multi-step process which is similar in many respects to the manner in which a pancreatic islet cell secretes insulin in response to the stimulus of hyperglycemia.

The important questions at the present time concern the mechanism of this allergic histamine release. We know that the process requires a metabolizing cell. Histamine release can be stopped immediately with the use of inhibitors of the glycolytic pathways – such as 2-deoxyglucose or fluoride. On the other hand, a variety of inhibitors of oxidative metabolism do not block the reaction [6]. In the first figure we see that cells which are releasing histamine do not increase either their utilization of oxygen or the rate of oxidative metabolism of glucose, the latter judged by the production of labelled CO_2 from C^{14} glucose. This is in contrast to the events which occur when the same cells are involved in phagocytosis, which might be viewed as the reverse of a secretory process, in which the leukocytes increase both O_2 utilization and CO_2 production as compared to controls. The requirement for oxidative metabolism in anaphylactic reactions has been in question for many years [15]. In this system, however, histamine release appears to be independent of oxidative pathways.

Another approach in attempting to understand the mechanism of histamine release is the use of various inhibitors of other metabolic processes. A wide variety of enzymatic inhibitors have been shown to block histamine release in the several *in vitro* systems [12]. It is often difficult to interpret these data, however, since one cannot sort out those inhibitors which poison the cell from those involved more intimately in the histamine release process. In the last few years BECKER and AUSTEN [1] have studied DFP and a series of phosphonate compounds whose action appears more specific in that the inhibition occurs only if the antigen is added in the presence of inhibitor. Recently, Dr. S. MARGOLIS and I have studied two groups of compounds which have the same type of activity: the methylxanthines and catecholamines [7]. The next figure shows dose-response curves

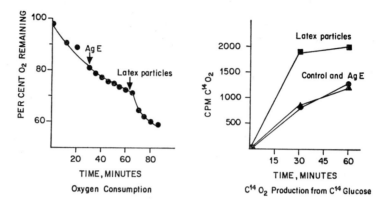

Fig. 1. A comparison of oxygen uptake and the oxidative metabolism of glucose in cells phagocytosing latex particles or releasing histamine after challenge with antigen E.

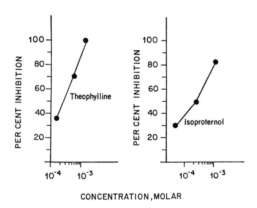

Fig. 2. Dose-response curves showing the inhibition of antigen E induced histamine release by theophylline and isoproterenol.

for inhibition by theophylline, the most active of the methylxanthines, and for isoproterenol, the most active of the catecholamines. Actually, in showing this activity of the catecholamines we are confirming the observation of Dr. SCHILD who, more than 30 years ago, showed that epinepherine inhibits histamine release from guinea-pig lung [14]. As shown in the figure 3 with theophylline, both of these compounds will stop histamine release virtually instantaneously if added after the reaction has already started.

One aspect of these compounds which makes them of interest is that they inhibit only if present when antigen is added. That is, if the cells are preincubated with the inhibitor and this is then washed away before antigen is added, there is no inhibition. Table I shows the type of experiment which demonstrates this: preincubation of the cells with 4×10^{-3} M theophylline, a very high concentration shown here to give virtually complete inhibition, did not cause any significant decrease in histamine release compared to the buffer preincubated control. Similar experiments have been carried out with isoproterenol. Thus, both compounds not only inhibit at pharma-

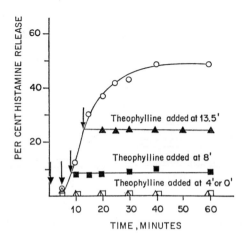

Fig. 3. The effect of theophylline on the rate of histamine release. Theophylline, 2.5×10^{-3} M, was added to samples taken from the control population of cells (open circles) at the times indicated (arrows).

Table I. The effect of the preincubation of cells with theophylline. The cells were mixed with either buffer or 4×10^{-3} M theophylline for 15′ at 37° following which the cells were washed and exposed to antigen E

Concentration of Theophylline [MOLAR] during		
Preincubation	Experiment	% Histamine release
None	None	67
None	4×10^{-3}	0
4×10^{-3}	None	61
4×10^{-3}	4×10^{-3}	1

cologic levels but act only on cells which have been 'activated' by antigen, suggesting that they interact with a system intimately related to the histamine release process.

The next step, of course, was to ascertain on what system these inhibitors were operating. There were ample indications in the pharmacologic literature that the scheme shown on figure 4 tied the two compounds together [13]. That is, the catecholamines are known to stimulate the adenylcyclase which generates cyclic 3′5′ AMP from ATP while an action of the methylxanthines is to inhibit the action of a phosphodiesterase which destroys cyclic AMP. The pertinency of this scheme was further attested to by our observation that isoproterenol and theophylline operated synergistically in inhibiting histamine release. A direct demonstration of the validity of this hypothesis is shown in figure 5 which illustrates the inhibition of histamine release by the dibutryrl derivative of cyclic AMP.

The action of these inhibitors in the direct *in vitro* allergic or anaphylactic reaction prompted us to consider their role in leukocytic histamine release

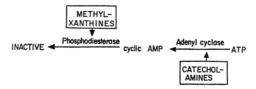

Fig. 4. A diagram of the action of the methylxanthines and catecholamines on the cyclic AMP system.

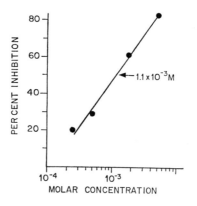

Fig. 5. Dose-response curve showing the inhibition of histamine release by dibutryrl cyclic AMP.

mediated by other modalities. In the so-called 'reversed' anaphylactic reaction histamine release is induced by antibodies against immunoglobulins which are presumably present on the surface of the cells. This reaction was first studied in our hands in Dr. OSLER's laboratory using antisera against crude HGG preparations containing mostly anti-IgG antibodies. We found that histamine could be released with nanogram concentrations of such antisera. The reaction did not require serum and in preliminary experiments, since confirmed by SIRAGANIAN and OSLER [16], there was no loss of cellular potassium during histamine release.

Using this type of antiserum Dr. HAYDEN BRAIN and I carried out dose response curves on the leukocytes of a number of allergic and normal individuals. The results are shown in figure 6. There is a difference between the response of allergic and normal individuals, in that the leukocytes of the former are considerably more sensitive than those of the latter. Thus, as shown in figure 6, at a concentration of 0.04 μg of antibody N per ml the average release for normal donors is less than $1/_3$ that for allergics. Moreover, at this level less than $\frac{1}{4}$ of the normals released a significant amount of histamine whereas more than $\frac{3}{4}$ of the allergics responded. There

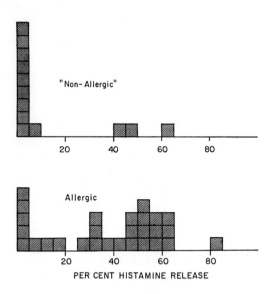

Fig. 6. A comparison between the maximal histamine release induced by rabbit anti-HGG from leukocytes of allergic and non-allergic donors. Each square represents the results with the cells of a single donor suspended in a serum free medium.

is considerable overlap, but this may be partially of a function of the difficulty in defining a patient who is truly non-allergic. Recently, with the Ishizakas' demonstration that reaginic antibody is IgE [3] and JOHANNSON's observations that allergic individuals have higher IgE levels than normals [4], it seemed useful to reexamine this system. Dr. ISHIZAKA was kind enough to absorb out the anti-L chain activity from the serum used for these studies and, as shown in figure 7, we found that this removed more than 99% of the histamine releasing activity. It seems, therefore, that the release we had been observing was not due to anti-IgG activity but rather to antibody reacting with the L chains of cell fixed IgE. In collaboration with Dr. ISHIZAKA we explored this directly using his antisera to IgE and IgG. The results are shown on table II. In previous experiments we had found little histamine release to be mediated by antisera directed against IgA or IgM. The table shows that it is possible to get some histamine release with an anti-IgG serum but that it always takes an antiserum concentration 100 or more times greater than is necessary for histamine release with the anti-IgE serum. It is difficult to rule out the possibility that the release apparently mediated by the anti-IgG serum is due to a one part in several hundred contamination by anti-L chain or anti-IgE antibodies. In any event, it appears clear that the reversed anaphylactic reaction, as carried out in the leukocyte system, is mediated primarily by anti-IgE antibodies.

Figure 8 shows the inhibition of this anti-IgE mediated histamine release by theophylline, comparing the dose response curve with that of the activity of theophylline in antigen E mediated histamine release. The inhibition curves are essentially identical. Thus, there are many similarities between the reversed and direct anaphylactic reactions as studied *in vitro:* Both occur with washed cells in the absence of serum factors; in neither is the cell injured as judged by morphological criteria or by the more sensitive indication of cellular potassium loss. Both are inhibited by the methyl-xanthines, which presumably indicates a role for the cyclic-AMP system. It would appear reasonable to suggest that both reactions result from an 'activation' of cell bound IgE antibody and proceed similarly from this common event.

In accord with this basic similarity between the two types of histamine release is the data shown on figure 9. Here we are plotting the maximal histamine release from the leukocytes of a series of ragweed allergic children run simultaneously with ragweed antigen E and ISHIZAKA's anti-IgE. I might remind you that we have previously shown a significant correlation between the sensitivity of a patient's cells to antigen E and the degree of allergic

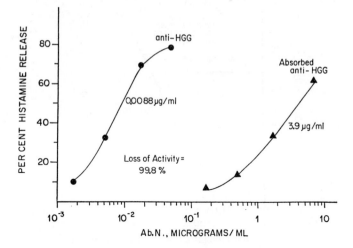

Fig. 7. The effect of the absorption of rabbit anti-HGG with isolated human L chains on the ability of the anti-serum to release histamine from human leukocytes. The numbers refer to the concentration of the native and absorbed antiserum required for 50% hist-amine release.

Table II. Histamine release from human leukocytes by a-IgE and a-IgG

Patient	a-IgE[1]	a-IgG[2]	Minimum Ratio: a-IgE a-IgG
AD	0.013	36%	160
DE	0.0038	25%	260
CO	0.0093	17%	215
MO	0.0037	22%	260
FE	0.038	5%	210
WA	0.0054	34%	185
WE	max. 44%	0%	–
DO	0.0023	22%	430
LY	0.013	18%	230
PA	0.010	25%	100

[1] μg/ml Ab. N. required for 50% histamine release.

[2] Histamine release at 0.6 μg Ab. N./ml anti-IgG antisera. The second column lists the concentration (μg ab. N./ml) of anti-IgE required for 50% histamine release. The third column lists the percent histamine release at 0.6 μg anti-IgG ab. N./ml, the highest concentration tested. The last column expresses the minimum ratio for 50% histamine release by anti-IgE and anti-IgG (extrapolated).

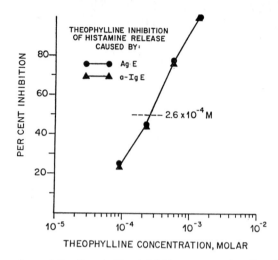

Fig. 8. A comparison of the theophylline inhibition curves of antigen E and anti-IgE induced histamine release.

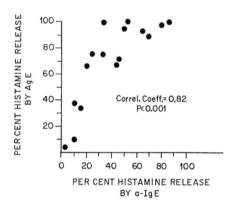

Fig. 9. A plot of the maximal leukocytic histamine release caused by antigen E against that caused by anti-IgE: The cell donors were ragweed allergic children. Spearman Rank Correlation Coefficient = 0.82 p<.001.

symptomatology he suffers during the ragweed season [8]. With the present data we show a high degree of correlation between the sensitivity of a given leukocyte suspension to antigen E and to anti-IgE. This further supports the suggestion that the direct and reversed anaphylactic reactions are twin functions of cell bound IgE. It is also compatible with the hypothesis that in a highly ragweed allergic individual a significant portion of the total IgE is present as antibody directed against ragweed antigens, an idea generated from the observation of increased levels of IgE in allergic individuals.

Finally, I would like to turn ta a very brief consideration of the type of leukocyte histamine release mediated by antibodies directed against constituents of the cell wall. As we have described elsewhere, this system is of a cytotoxic nature [11]. Fresh serum is required and the reaction leads to frank cell destruction. As demonstrated in figure 10 the methylxanthine inhibitors are relatively ineffective in the cytotoxic system. At high antiserum concentrations there is little or no inhibition of histamine release by theophylline. At lower antiserum concentrations the methylxanthines inhibit partially. This moderate inhibition is of some interest, but has not been fully studied.

In summary, I have presented data demonstrating that the methylxanthines and catecholamines, both of which increase the intracellular level of cyclic AMP, inhibit antigenically induced histamine release *in vitro*. Dibutryrl cyclic AMP added extracellularly can also block the reaction. Inasmuch as these inhibitors are active only in the presence of antigen it suggests that the cyclic AMP system is an intimate part of the *in vitro* allergic response. The cyclic AMP system is also active in the histamine release induced by antibody against cell bound immunoglobulins. In this 'reversed anaphylactic' reaction it appears that the mediating antibodies are directed against cell bound IgE. We have pointed out that with the data now available the direct and reversed anaphylactic reactions seem mechanistically very similar. The cells of allergic individuals are more sensitive to anti-IgE than the cells of normal donors; moreover, there is a high degree of correlation

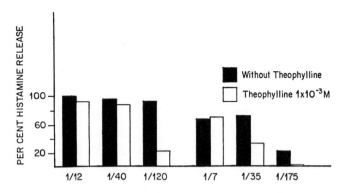

Fig. 10. The action of the theophylline on histamine release mediated by a rabbit antiserum to human leukocytes. The results of two separate experiments are shown.

between the sensitivity of a given donor's cells to antigen E and anti-IgE. Thus, cell sensitivity to anti-IgE may perhaps be useful as a non-specific indicator of an allergic potential.

References

1. BECKER, E. L. and AUSTEN, K. F.: A comparison of the specificity of inhibition by phosphonate esters of the first component of complement and the antigen-induced release of histamine from guinea-pig lung. J. exp. Med. *120:* 491 (1964).
2. GRAHAM, H. T.; LOWRY, O. H.; WHEELWRIGHT, F.; LENZ, M. A. and PARISH, H. H.: Distribution of histamine among leukocytes and platelets. Blood *10:* 467 (1955).
3. ISHIZAKA, K. and ISHIZAKA, T.: Identification of μE antibodies as a carrier of reaginic activity. J. Immunol. *99:* 1187 (1967).
4. JOHANSSON, S. G. O.: Raised levels of a new immunoglobulin class (IgND) in asthma. Lancet *ii:* 951 (1967).
5. KING, T. P. and NORMAN, P. S.: Isolation studies of allergens from ragweed pollen. Biochemistry *1:* 709 (1962).
6. LICHTENSTEIN, L. M.: Mechanism of allergic histamine release from human leukocytes; in International Symposium on The Biochemistry of Acute Allergic Reactions, edited by E. BECKER and K. F. AUSTEN (Blackwell, London 1968).
7. LICHTENSTEIN, L. M. and MARGOLIS, S.: The inhibition of *in vitro* histamine release by the methylxanthines and catecholamines. Science *161:* 902 (1968).
8. LICHTENSTEIN, L. M.; NORMAN, P. S.; OSLER, A. G. and WINKENWERDER, W. L.: *In vitro* studies of human ragweed allergy: Changes in cellular and humoral activity associated with specific desensitization. J. clin. Invest. *45:* 1126 (1966).
9. LICHTENSTEIN, L. M. and OSLER, A. G.: Studies on the mechanisms of hypersensitivity phenomena. IX. Histamine release from human leukocytes by ragweed pollen antigen. J. exp. Med. *120:* 507 (1964).
10. LICHTENSTEIN, L. M. and OSLER, A. G.: Studies on the mechanisms of hypersensitivity phenomena. XI. The effect of normal human serum on the release of histamine from human leukocytes by ragweed pollen antigen. J. Immunol. *96:* 159 (1966).
11. LICHTENSTEIN, L. M. and OSLER, A. G.: Comparative studies of histamine release and potassium efflux from human leukocytes. Proc. Soc. exp. Biol., N.Y. *121:* 808 (1966).
12. MONGAR, J. L. and SCHILD, O. H.: Cellular mechanisms in anaphylaxis. Physiol. Rev. *42:* 226 (1962).
13. ROBISON, G. A.; BUTCHER, R. W. and SUTHERLAND, E. W.: Cyclic AMP. Ann. Rev. Biochem. *37:* 149 (1968).
14. SCHILD, H. O.: Histamine release and anaphylactic shock in isolated lungs of guinea pigs. Quart. J. exp. Phys. *26:* 165 (1937).
15. SCHILD, H. O.: Mechanism of anaphylactic histamine release; in International Symposium on The Biochemistry of Acute Allergic Reactions, ed. by C. BECKER and K. F. AUSTEN (Blackwell, London 1968).
16. SIRAGANIAN, R. P. and OSLER, A. G.: Personal communication.
17. STYLER, H. R. and REMINGTON, J. S.: Glucocorticoid effects on *in vitro* histamine release and total blood histamine content. J. Allergy *41:* 110 (1968).

Author's address: L. M. LICHTENSTEIN, M.D., Division of Allergy and Infectious Diseases, Dept. of Medicine, The Johns Hopkin's University School of Medicine, *Baltimore, Md.* (USA).

Cellular and Humoral Mechanisms in Anaphylaxis and Allergy, pp. 187–195
(Karger, Basel/New York 1969)

Slow Reacting Substances

W. Vogt

Department for Biochemical Pharmacology, Max-Planck-Institute for Experimental
Medicine, Göttingen

Slow reacting substances (SRSs) were detected and the term coined when
FELDBERG and KELLAWAY [13] investigated the mechanism of tissue injury
induced by toxins, drugs and anaphylaxis. They perfused isolated organs with
one of these challengers and found that not only histamine was released,
but in addition another smooth muscle contracting compound. Whereas histamine produced a quickly proceeding contraction of the guine-apig ileum, the
perfusates of the organs showed a delayed component in their effect on the
isolated guinea-pig ileum. Nowadays the pure action of SRS can be demonstrated and assayed in that organ after chemical separation from
histamine or by the use of antihistaminics.

SRS has been found in perfusates of lungs, liver, skin, paws, later also in
mast cell suspensions, and in supernatants of chopped tissue. The organs
were derived from guinea pigs, cats, dogs, rats, monkeys, and even human
lung has been used successfully. SRS appears besides histamine, after
exposure of the tissues to bee venom, snake venoms, phospholipase A,
compound 48/80, antigen if acting on sensitized tissue, or simply heat. Thus
the number of liberators and sources is big, and the question arises whether
the same principle is released and the same mechanism of liberation is at work
in all conditions. FELDBERG and KELLAWAY were already aware of this problem. They used the term SRS only as non-specific description of what in fact
might be different substances. Indeed, a strict definition has never been given,
and the term could be used and has been used also to designate compounds like
bradykinin, which name actually means the same as 'slow reacting', in Latin.

Which substances can then be called 'SRS', and what is common to
them? I think a reasonable limitation and definition is to call SRS all those
substances which slowly contract the guinea-pig ileum and are released from

tissues or cells – as opposed to body fluids like plasma – by any injury or potentially injurious stimulation.

The SRSs have more in common than their origin and action: they are not just released from stores by the nocious stimulus, but formed *de novo*. This does not exclude that some SRS may be present also in non-challenged organs, but much more is obtained after the challenge. In order to investigate SRS one has therefore to prepare it from extracts or perfusates of *treated* tissues.

The investigation into chemical properties of SRSs revealed a further common feature. All SRSs of which the respective properties are known, are acids and show more or less marked lipid-solubility. Quantitatively, however, there are differences in this latter respect.

So far, three types of SRS have been investigated more thoroughly. These are SRS-C, the substance released by cobra and bee venoms, SRS-A, the slow reacting substance appearing in anaphylaxis, and a SRS, which has not been supplied with a suffix, which is released by histamine liberators like compound 48/80. This latter SRS is regarded as identical with SRS-A [2]. SRS-A and -C appear to be different, chemically. They both are not necessarily single substances but each may represent a group of related compounds.

SRS-C. When the lung of a guinea pig is perfused with cobra venom the blood vessels contract, the perfusion flow decreases unless the pressure is raised considerably, and the bronchi also contract increasing the resistance to ventilation of the lungs. The walls of the lung vessels become leaky and much fluid drains into the tissue and from the lung surface. These symptoms can be explained by released histamine, but as SRS also appears and has smooth muscle contracting actions FELDBERG and KELLAWAY [13] concluded that SRS contributes. It was known at that time that cobra venom like practically all other snake and insect venoms contains phospholipase A and that lysolecithin is a pharmacologically active product of this enzyme. In fact, FELDBERG, HOLDEN and KELLAWAY [12] were able to generate SRS activity by incubating egg yolk which is rich in lecithin with cobra venom. However, the smooth muscle contracting principle formed was different from lysolecithin. I have later used egg yolk and egg lecithin as a first convenient source of an SRS. After incubation with cobra venom the smooth muscle contracting activity was followed through several fractionation procedures and it was found to be associated with the fraction of unsaturated fatty acids [24].

The SRS which is released from perfused guinea-pig lung after envenomation also showed the behaviour of unsaturated fatty acids, in liquid-

liquid distribution, in chromatography and in some chemical reactions. It seemed reasonable to conclude that these acids derived from phosphatides which were cleaved by the action of the phospholipase A contained in the venoms injected. Indeed, SRS activity was also obtained from purified lecithin on incubation with purified phospholipase A [24].

Now, SRS-C is not just any unsaturated fatty acid known to occur in phosphatides. Neither oleic, nor the poly-unsaturated acids linoleic, linolenic or arachidonic acid have a smooth muscle contracting effect on the guinea-pig ileum. But we know two groups of derivatives of such acids which have smooth muscle effects and which were actually found in perfusates of envenomed lungs. The one group comprises unspecific autoxidation products of unsaturated fatty acids, notably hydroperoxides, but also secondary products which contain hydroxy- or keto-groups. It is not certain whether these oxidized derivatives actually form in the tissue. They may be generated from the liberated unsaturated fatty acids after escape from the tissue, during the handling of the perfusates. Then they would be merely artifacts. Moreover, usually only a small part of the total SRS activity can be ascribed to the autoxidation products, it may amount to 50% of the action on the guinea-pig ileum, but if tested in other organs it is much less. Thus the unspecific autoxidation products are probably of minor if any biological significance.

The other group of acids which is responsible for SRS-C activity are prostaglandins. This is also a kind of oxidation product of unsaturated fatty acids which are constituents of phosphatides. However, prostaglandins are formed by specific enzyme systems [5, 23], in a series of reactions by which tris- or more highly unsaturated C 20 acids are converted to a corresponding PGE or PGF compound. The two classes E and F differ by one group in the 5 membered ring which is characteristic of all prostaglandins. It is hydroxyl in the F series but carbonyl in the E series. Depending on the number of double bonds of the parent acids one obtains PGEs or Fs 1, 2 or 3.

In guinea-pig lung predominantly $PGF_2\alpha$ has been found [1]. The major fraction of prostaglandin activity in SRS-C from guinea-pig lung has also been identified as a PGF compound [25]. Guinea-pig lung tissue contains only traces of preformed PG and in perfusates obtained without venom injection one does not find any activity except when many perfusates are combined and concentrated. However, after envenomation or injection of phospholipase A there is a marked increase of PG in the perfusate. We found even more to be released than we could extract from non-challenged lungs. This indicates that the PG is not liberated from a store, but is formed. This

formation of prostaglandin after injection of phospholipase A is not restricted to guinea-pig lung, it has been observed also in frog intestine and in rat
stomach tissue [4, 18].

As the tissue phosphatides do not contain preformed prostaglandins as
acid constituents, it follows that the formation of SRS is a two-step process.
In the first step unsaturated fatty acids which are suitable precursors of PG
are released by the venom phospholipase and thus substrate is provided. Then
the precursors are converted to the corresponding PGs, by the specific
enzyme system. This system is not present in cobra or bee venom, it is
confined to the tissue. The first step seems to be the rate limiting.

From this mechanism of formation of SRS-C it would follow that
whatever venom acts on a tissue it would always trigger the same process –
liberation of PG precursors – by its content of phospholipase A. And,
provided the converting enzyme system is present PG should be formed.
Thus all slow reacting substances which have been described after envenomation of tissues will most likely contain PG. This does not exclude that
other biologically active substances can be formed by venoms, in addition.
An example is the formation of bradykinin by bothrops venom. But this
is not an SRS according to the definition given before.

SRS-A. The discussion of this compound will be confined to its possible
nature and mechanism of formation, and the relation to SRS-C. Kellaway
and Trethewie [16] first found a slow reacting substance after injection of
antigen into sensitized perfused guinea-pig lungs. Its action and some
properties appeared to be the same as those of SRS-C, at first sight. But, in
fact, there are differences, and we are much less certain about the nature,
origin and mechanism of formation of SRS-A than of SRS-C. It is even
doubtful whether there exists only one SRS-A and whether different investigators have been dealing with the same material. Common to all investigations
and preparations is that SRS-A has been found after immunological
challenge of tissues and that it is assayed on the isolated guinea-pig ileum
where it produces the same kind of contraction as SRS-C. It is also well
established that SRS-A is formed, not only released from stores.

Three groups have studied the chemistry of SRS-A and have prepared
purified samples: Brocklehurst, then in Mill Hill, Uvnäs and his colleagues
in Stockholm and W. G. Smith in Durham. Brocklehurst obtained SRS-A
from perfusates of sensitized guinea-pig lung, after injection of antigen. A
similar or the same SRS was released from pieces of human asthmatic lung,
after challenge with the specific allergen. The purified preparation was an
acid according to its behaviour in electrophoresis and solvent partition. It

was a small, dialyzable compound which was firmly bound by plasma proteins. It was not a peptide, and it was moderately soluble in some organic solvents, reasonably stable to heat and labile to oxidation [7, 8].

CHAKRAVARTY [9, 10] in Uvnäs' laboratory used preferably chopped lung and incubated it with the antigen to obtain SRS-A. His preparation, also acidic, was much more lipid-soluble than that of BROCKLEHURST. In this respect it could well be a fatty acid, perhaps a prostaglandin, but BROCKLE-HURST's compound could not. Thus the two preparations of SRS-A appear to be different. The slow reacting substance obtained by CHAKRAVARTY after treatment of perfused cat paws with compound 48/80 had the same chemical properties as that generated by the anaphylactic reaction in chopped guinea-pig lung and was considered to be identical.

The chemical nature and properties became even more complicated when ÄNGGARD et al. [2] found that at least two unknown smooth muscle contracting substances emerged from organs after challenge with the specific antigen or compound 48/80. When chopped tissue was used the proportion of the two substances varied with the time of incubation. This indicates that at least one of them is labile and undergoes rapid metabolic changes during contact with the tissue. Only one of the two substances, the more polar one which elutes later from silica columns, was considered as SRS proper.

The chemical findings thus do not give much information about SRS-A beyond the statement that it consists of probably more than one acid, having modest to good lipidsolubility, and showing some rough relation to SRS-C in this respect.

Pharmacologically, BROCKLEHURST's and CHAKRAVARTY's preparations are similar, and whereas the chemical properties of CHAKRAVARTY's SRS are not incompatible with a prostaglandin, pharmacologically it appears to be a different entity. Thus SRS-A does not contract the hamster colon nor uterus preparations, but is active on organs desensitized to prostaglandin [22b].

The chromatographically purified SRS-A of ÄNGGARD et al. [2] differs from both these preparations. It has practically no action on the rabbit duodenum, even in concentrations which correspond to 100 times the threshold for the guinea-pig ileum. Such a selective action on guinea-pig ileum is quite unusual in the class of lipid-soluble acids.

An entirely different class of substances as possible carriers of SRS-A activity has been envisaged by SMITH [22a]. He concluded that SRS-A consisted of a mixture of neuraminic acid-containing substances, probably gangliosides. This conclusion was based partly on chemical analyses of purified material obtained from challenged guinea-pig lung, partly on the finding that sensitized guinea-pig lung loses gangliosides after challenge. The assumption seems doubtful, however, in the light of findings by ROBINSON *et al.* [21] according to which gangliosides do not stimulate smooth muscle.

Thus neither the chemical nor the pharmacological properties of SRS-A point to any known representative of lipid-soluble acids.

Another approach to the nature of SRS-A has been made by studying the conditions and the mechanism of its formation. In general, knowledge of the enzyme which generates a certain substance will give information about the class to which the substance belongs. Thus, the product of an action of trypsin is likely to be a peptide, and phospholipase A only cleaves fatty acids from phosphatides. However, a substance which like SRS-A is formed only from structurally intact tissue, poses more problems. An enzyme may liberate SRS or its blockade may interfere with the formation and release even if the enzyme itself is not involved chemically in the actual forming reaction. The enzyme may act as a trigger which initiates changes at or in the cells, and only subsequent to these changes endogenous enzymic processes may be activated to form SRS-A or to liberate histamine. This would mean a two-step process also in the formation of SRS-A, but different from that prevailing in the formation of SRS-C.

Certainly, the antigen-antibody reaction induces a sequence of enzymic processes which lead to the appearance of SRS-A. There exists an optimum of pH and temperature; Ca ions and oxygen are essential [11]: Heating the tissue to 45° prior to the challenge prevents the formation [10]. HÖGBERG and UVNÄS [15] have pointed out that some of the conditions are also favourable for the action of phospholipase A. They [14, 15] suggested that an endogenous phospholipase was activated in anaphylaxis. It was stressed, however, that the phospholipase acted merely indirectly by initiating other, unknown cellular processes. AUSTEN and BROCKLEHURST [3] suggested that a chymo-tryptic enzyme is involved in the anaphylactic release of SRS-A. Further, complement is essential [19]. It is of course impossible that these three entirely different enzymes or systems produce the same product directly from the same precursor. The conclusion seems justified that they only trigger a first step, the activation of SRS-producing cells. This is also suggested by the fact that – in the guinea pig at least – the conditions known to initiate SRS-A formation also lead to histamine release, and agents which block the SRS-A formation also block the release of histamine. As these two are entirely differ-ent processes, chemically, experimental procedures which impair or induce both histamine release and SRS formation are suspect of interfering with or inducing only the activation of the cells. They do not really throw light on the mechanism of formation of SRS-A and on its chemical nature.

Site of formation. As histamine and SRS-A normally appear together and their appearance can be blocked simultaneously, a correlation between the liberation of the two substances has been assumed. Since the release of histamine and SRS ran roughly parallel to the disruption of mast cells in guinea-pig lung Boreus and Chakravarty [6] assumed that the mast cells were responsible for both release of histamine and SRS-A. However, in rats Rapp [20] released SRS-A selectively, without histamine release or visible damage of the mast cells, under certain conditions. According to Orange *et al.* [19] the polymorphonuclear leucocytes are responsible for SRS-A generation in rats and these cells can be challenged selectively. Whether there are species differences regarding the origin of SRS-A is not known. When challenged with compound 48/80 rat mast cells do release a SRS which is indistinguishable from antigen-induced SRS of guinea-pig lung. Perfused lung tissue should not contain many leucocytes. On the other hand, leucocytes may also contribute to mast cell damage by releasing mast cell degranulating factors [17, 22].

For further details regarding the site of formation of SRS-A the reader is referred to the paper on SRS-A by Orange and Austen in this monograph. The important outcome of these investigations is that if not mast cells then other special cells, i.e. a small proportion of the tissue, seems to represent the site of SRS-A formation. If this were not the case it would appear strange that there should be one kind of cell injury, induced by venoms or exogenous phospholipase A, which creates conditions for the formation of prostaglandins, and another kind, induced by anaphylaxis or histamine liberators, which gives rise to SRS-A as a different entity. However, if the production of SRS-A is restricted to mast cells or other specific cells one can explain this diversity. Anaphylaxis would only activate the special system representing a small part of the tissue. In contrast venoms or exogenous phospholipase probably affect a large variety of cells releasing prostaglandin precursors everywhere. The phospholipase may, in addition, attack mast cells or leucocytes and trigger the formation of SRS-A; but the ubiquitous formation of prostaglandins would be overwhelming. As the amount of SRS-A which is released in anaphylaxis from guinea-pig lung is far less than that of SRS-C obtained after injection of cobra venom [16] the SRS-A may not have been detected in perfusates containing SRS-C but may actually be present. We would then envisage SRS-A as the specific product of activation of special cells, whereas SRS-C would be the product of a more unspecific and possibly ubiquitous cell injury.

Significance. SRS-C has been observed as such only after venomous poisoning. It could be responsible partly for the smooth muscle effects seen under such conditions – bronchial spasm, lung vessel constriction, etc. – although histamine is certainly of major significance. Of course, prostaglandins can be formed also by endogenous stimuli and therefore may have physiological functions. These are, however, outside the scope of this communication.

If SRS-A is specifically formed by an anaphylactic reaction then it could be significant only in that case. Among other possible actions it might contribute to bronchial spasm in asthma. If, on the other hand, the assumption is right that the same SRS is released by histamine liberators, then it is obvious that it can be released by various stimuli and its release under physiological conditions seems possible. Thus both types of SRS may not only appear under the pathological experimental conditions under which they have been found originally but may be physiological substances.

References

1. ÄNGGARD, E.: The isolation and determination of prostaglandins in lungs of sheep, guinea pig, monkey and man. Biochem. Pharmacol. *14:* 1507–1516 (1965).
2. ÄNGGARD, E.; BERGQVIST, U.; HÖGBERG, B.; JOHANSSON, K.; THON, I. L. and UVNÄS, B.: Biologically active principles occurring on histamine release from cat paw, guinea-pig lung and isolated rat mast cells. Acta physiol scand. *59:* 97–110 (1963).
3. AUSTEN, K. F. and BROCKLEHURST, W. E.: Anaphylaxis in chopped guinea-pig lung. I. Effect of peptidase substrates and inhibitors. J. exp. Med. *113:* 521–539 (1961).
4. BARTELS, J.; VOGT, W. and WILLE, G.: Prostaglandin release from and formation in perfused frog intestine. Naunyn-Schmiedebergs Arch. Pharm. exp. Path. *259:* 153–154 (1968).
5. BERGSTRÖM, S.; DANIELSSON, H. and SAMUELSSON, B.: The enzymatic formation of prostaglandin E_2 from arachidonic acid. Biochim. biophys. Acta *90:* 207–210 (1964).
6. BOREUS, L. O. and CHAKRAVARTY, N.: Tissue mast cells, histamine and 'slow reacting substance' in anaphylactic reaction in guinea pig. Acta physiol. scand. *48:* 315–322 (1960).
7. BROCKLEHURST, W. E.: The release of histamine and formation of a slow reacting substance (SRS-A) during anaphylactic shock. J. Physiol., Lond. *151:* 416–435 (1960).
8. BROCKLEHURST, W. E.: Slow reacting substance and related compounds. Progr. Allergy, Vol. 6., pp. 539–558 (Karger, Basel/New York 1962).
9. CHAKRAVARTY, N.: Observations on histamine release and formation of a lipid-soluble smooth-muscle stimulating principle ('SRS') by antigen-antibody reaction and compound 48/80 (Academic Thesis, Stockholm 1959).

10. CHAKRAVARTY, N.; HÖGBERG, B. and UVNÄS, B.: Mechanism of the release by compound 48/80 of histamine and of a lipid-soluble smooth-muscle stimulating principle ('SRS'). Acta physiol. scand. *45:* 255–270 (1959).

11. CHAKRAVARTY, N. and UVNÄS, B.: Histamine and a lipid-soluble smooth-muscle stimulating principle ('SRS') in anaphylactic reaction. Acta physiol. scand. *48:* 302–314 (1960).

12. FELDBERG, W.; HOLDEN, H. F. and KELLAWAY, C. H.: The formation of lysocithin and of a smooth-muscle-stimulating substance by snake venoms. J. Physiol., Lond. *94:* 232–248 (1938).

13. FELDBERG, W. and KELLAWAY, C. H.: Liberation of histamine and formation of lysocithin-like substances by cobra venom. J. Physiol., Lond. *94:* 187–226 (1938).

14. HÖGBERG, B. and UVNÄS, B.: The mechanism of the disruption of mast cells produced by compound 48/80. Acta physiol. scand. *41:* 345–369 (1957).

15. HÖGBERG, B. and UVNÄS, B.: Further observations on the disruption of rat mesentery mast cells caused by compound 48/80, antigen-antibody reaction, lecithinase A and decylamine. Acta physiol. scand. *48:* 133–145 (1960).

16. KELLAWAY, C. H. and TRETHEWIE, E. R.: The liberation of a slow-reacting smooth muscle-stimulating substance in anaphylaxis. Quart. J. exp. Physiol. *30:* 121–145 (1940).

17. KELLER, R.; MÜLLER-ECKHARDT, C.; KAYSER, F.-H. and KELLER, H. U.: Interrelations between different types of cells. I. A comparative study of the biological properties of a cationic polypeptide from lysosomes of polymorphonuclear leukocytes and other cationic compounds. Int. Arch. Allergy *33:* 239–258 (1968).

18. KUNZE, H.: (1968) to be published.

19. ORANGE, R. P.; VALENTINE, M. D. and AUSTEN, K. F.: Antigen-induced release of slow reacting substance of anaphylaxis (SRS-A rat) in rats prepared with homologous antibody. J. exp. Med. *127:* 767–782 (1968).

20. RAPP, H. J.: Release of a slow reacting substance (SRS) in the peritoneal cavity of rats by antigen-antibody interaction. J. Physiol. *158:* 35–36 P (1961).

21. ROBINSON, J. D.; CARLINI, E. A. and GREEN, J. P.: The effects of ganglioside preparations on smooth muscle. Biochem. Pharmacol. *12:* 1219–1223 (1963).

22. SEEGERS, W. and JANOFF, A.: Mediators of inflammation in leukocyte lysosomes. VI. Partial purification and characterization of a mast cell rupturing component. J. exp. Med. *124:* 833–849 (1966).

22a. SMITH, W. C.: Release of ganglioside from guinea-pig lung tissue during anaphylaxis. Nature, Lond. *209:* 1251 (1966).

22b. SWEATMAN, W. J. F. and COLLIER, H. O. J.: Effects of prostaglandins on human bronchial muscle. Nature, Lond. *217:* 69 (1968).

23. VAN DORP, D. A.; BEERTHUIS, R. K.; NUGTEREN, D. H. and VONKEMAN, H.: The biosynthesis of prostaglandins. Biochim. biophys. Acta *90:* 204–207 (1964).

24. VOGT, W.: Pharmacologically active substances formed in egg yolk by cobra venom. J. Physiol., Lond. *136:* 131–147 (1957).

25. VOGT, W.; MEYER, U.; KUNZE, H.; LUFFT, E. und BABILLI, S.: Entstehung von SRS-C in der durchströmten Meerschweinchenlunge durch Phospholipase A. Naunyn-Schmiedebergs Arch. Pharmak. exp. Path. *262:* 124–134 (1969).

Author's address: Dr. W. VOGT, Department of Biochemical Pharmacology, Max-Planck-Institute for experimental Medicine, *D-34 Göttingen* (Germany).

Cellular and Humoral Mechanisms in Anaphylaxis and Allergy, pp. 196–206
(Karger, Basel/New York 1969)

Slow Reacting Substance of Anaphylaxis in the Rat[1]

Robert P. Orange[2] and K. Frank Austen

Department of Medicine, Harvard Medical School
at the Robert B. Brigham Hospital
Boston, Mass.

In order to distinguish the slow reacting substance (SRS) appearing as the result of anaphylactic reactions in guinea pig lung from that extracted from normal tissues, Brocklehurst [7] termed the former material SRS-A. Since materials with similar pharmacologic characteristics have been released immunologically from other species, it seems appropriate to introduce a suffix to indicate the species from which the SRS-A has been obtained. Such a designation seems necessary until the chemical structure of these materials is established. At present, there is no way of knowing whether the SRS-A elaborated by different species is a single substance or whether it represents a family of closely related materials.

The Pharmacologic Characteristics of SRS-A^{rat}

As previously described [3] SRS-A^{rat} was obtained following the intraperitoneal (i.p.) injection of specific antigen into rats prepared 2 h previously by the i.p. injection of whole rat antiserum. SRS-A^{rat} demonstrates the properties previously described for SRS-A^{gp} [8] which include: the ability to produce a slow, prolonged contraction of the isolated guinea pig ileum in the presence of a potent antihistamine without producing tachyphylaxis (fig. 1 in ref. 13), little or no activity on the estrous rat uterus (table I), and resistance to inactivation by proteolytic enzymes such as chymotrypsin. Following

[1] Supported by grant AI-07722-02 from the National Institute of Allergy and Infectious Diseases.

[2] Postdoctoral Trainee supported by Training Grant AM-05076-11 from the National Institute of Arthritis and Metabolic Diseases.

Table I. Differential bioassay of SRS-A^{rat}[1]

| Compound tested | Smooth muscle preparation | | |
	Guinea pig ileum	Estrous rat uterus	Gerbil colon
SRS-A^{rat} (units/ml)[2]	1	50	50
Bradykinin (mug/ml)	15	0.05	2
PGE$_1$ (mug/ml)	25	4.0	6
PGF$_2a$ (mug/ml)	35	2.0	1

[1] All values refer to the concentration of test compound required to produce a contraction of equivalent amplitude to that produced by SRS-A^{rat} in that assay.

[2] SRS-A^{rat} preparation was ethanol-extracted and treated with chymotrypsin as described in the text. One unit of SRS-A^{rat} is arbitrarily defined as the concentration required to produce a contraction of the isolated guinea-pig ileum equal to that produced by 5 mug/ml of histamine base.

sedimentation of the cells in the rat peritoneal fluid, the supernatant containing SRS-A^{rat} was ethanol-extracted by the method of BROCKLEHURST [8], lyophilized, resuspended in buffer, and incubated at 37°C for 30 min with chymotrypsin, 5.0 mg/ml. Treatment with chymotrypsin had no effect on the activity of SRS-A^{rat} but completely inactivated 20 mug/ml of bradykinin treated in a similar fashion. Incubation of SRS-A^{rat} with pronase, 1.0 mg/ml, at 37°C for 150 minutes also failed to diminish its activity.

The report of AMBACHE [1] that the ascending colon of the gerbil was responsive to the prostaglandins and the finding of WEEKS et al. [21] that this preparation afforded the most readily quantitated bioassay led to the examination of an ethanol-extracted, chymotrypsin-treated preparation of SRS-A^{rat} for its activity on the ascending colon of the gerbil as compared with its activity on the guinea pig ileum and estrous rat uterus (table I). SRS-A^{rat} is very active on the isolated guinea pig ileum but it has little or no activity on the estrous rat uterus or ascending colon of the gerbil. The estrous rat uterus is very sensitive to bradykinin and serotonin, and the ascending colon of the gerbil is highly responsive to the prostaglandins, PGE$_1$ and PGF$_2a$. This profile of pharmacologic activity establishes further criteria for the identification of SRS-A^{rat} as a unique pharmacologic entity.

An ethanol-extracted, chymotrypsin-treated preparation of SRS-A^{rat} with no significant activity on the estrous rat uterus or gerbil colon was injected intradermally (I.D.) into guinea pigs and rats pretreated with antihistamine and antiserotonin agents (table II). This preparation produced a

Table II. Permeability studies with SRS-A[rat][1]

Compound tested	Concentration per site	Rat		Guinea pig	
SRS-A[rat] (units)	125	1+	8×8	4+	20×17
	50	1+	8×5	3+	18×15
	25	1+	3×3	3+	12×12
	5	Tr	4×3	2+	9×10
Serotonin (mug)	10	Tr	3×3	Tr	1×1
Histamine (mug)	10	Tr	3×3	Tr	2×2
Bradykinin (mug)	10	Tr	3×3	Tr	4×4
PGE$_1$ (mug)	10	1+	4×4	Tr	2×3
PGF$_2a$ (mug)	10	1+	4×5	Tr	1×2
Extracted peritoneal fluid[2] (dilution)	1:2	1+	3×3	Tr	3×3

[1] Each result represents the mean value for 3 animals. All animals were pretreated with mepyramine maleate, 50 mg/kg, and methysergide, 4 mg/kg, i.p., 30 min before the experiment. All sites were injected. i.d. with 0.1 ml volumes of test compounds and the animals were immediately injected i.v. with 1.0 ml 0.1 % Evan's blue dye. Thirty minutes later, the animals were sacrificed in ether, and the skin was reflected and transilluminated, and the size (mm) and intensity (0–4+) of the lesions recorded.

[2] Peritoneal fluid of rats injected i.p. with homologous antibody but not challenged with antigen. The fluid was extracted as for SRS-A[rat] as described in the text.

significant local increase in cutaneous permeability in the guinea pig at a dose of 5 units/site, and it demonstrated a dose-related response in the range of 5–125 units/site. This activity cannot be attributed to the presence of histamine and serotonin in the preparation, since these amines are eliminated in the extraction procedure as confirmed by bioassay. Furthermore, neither histamine nor serotonin in a dose of 10 mug/site elicited a significant response in test animals pretreated with antagonists of these amines. Bradykinin also would not account for the permeability activity since the SRS-A[rat] preparation is treated with chymotrypsin to destroy bradykinin as demonstrated by bioassay on the estrous rat uterus; in addition, bradykinin in a dose of 10 mug/site was inactive. The material was essentially free of the prostaglandins, PGE$_1$ and PGF$_2a$, as assessed by bioassay on the gerbil colon, and these materials proved to be inactive in guinea-pig skin in a dose of 10 mug/site. Finally, a control preparation isolated from the peritoneal cavity of rats prepared with homologous antiserum but not challenged with antigen was extracted for SRS-A[rat] as described, but it contained no mediators as assessed by bioassay and exhibited no activity in guinea-pig skin.

Thus, the immediate permeability-producing activity of the functionally pure SRS-A^{rat} preparation in guinea-pig skin can be attributed to its content of SRS-A^{rat}. It is noteworthy that the threshold for eliciting a change in cutaneous permeability in the rat is more than 10 times that required in the guinea pig.

Prerequisites for the Release of SRS-A^{rat}

The Immunoglobulins Involved in the Immunologic Release of SRS-A^{rat}

STECHSCHULTE et al. [20] observed that SRS-A^{rat} release was not a function of the entire population of precipitating rat antibodies but rather was associated with the IgG fraction or a subpopulation thereof. MORSE et al. [11, 6] have demonstrated that the hapten-specific antibodies of the IgG$_a$ class mediated the antigen-induced release of SRS-A^{rat}. This biologic property of rat IgG$_a$ was stable to heating at 56°C for 4 h and correlated with its hemolytic activity. During the course of these investigations, it was observed that rat IgG$_a$ was also capable of mediating the immunologic release of histamine in vivo in the rat [12]. The apparent association of the IgG$_a$ fraction of rat antisera with the capacity to prepare the rat for the immunologic release of two mediators, histamine and SRS-A^{rat}, was further investigated. This fraction was devoid of other species of immunoglobulins as assessed by: radioimmunoelectrophoretic analysis which revealed IgG$_a$ but not IgG$_b$, IgA, or IgM; the appearance of a single protein peak on analytical ultracentrifugation; and the elicitation of an antibody in guinea pigs which reacted with the Fc fragment of IgG$_a$ but not that of the other rat immunoglobulins as assessed by immunoelectrophoresis [12]. It seems likely that the IgG$_a$ fraction contains a single class of heat stable antibodies with three biologic activities: complement fixation, mast cell sensitization, and SRS-A^{rat} release. The heat stable IgG$_a$ antibodies are distinguished from the rat homocytotropic antibodies [10, 4] which sensitize rats for histamine but not SRS-A^{rat} release by the following criteria: thermostability, latent period for in vivo 'sensitization', and elution characteristics on DE52 cellulose chromatography [12].

The Cellular Elements Involved in the Immunologic Release of SRS-A^{rat}

The requirement for the polymorphonuclear (PMN) leukocyte in the antigen-induced release of SRS-A^{rat} has been established on the basis of the following observations: SRS-A^{rat} release is suppressed in rats by the depletion of circulating PMN leukocytes using either nitrogen mustard or a rabbit anti-rat PMN leukocyte antiserum (Ra anti-RPMN); partial restoration of SRS-A^{rat} release is associated with the intravenous (i.v.) injection of PMN leukocytes into leukopenic rats; and a marked enhancement of SRS-A^{rat} release is observed in the presence of an increased number of PMN leukocytes in the peritoneal cavities of rats at the time of antigen-antibody interaction [14, 15]. Reconstitution of the PMN leukocyte population of leukopenic rats proved difficult using the intravenous route of administration, and attention was directed towards achieving reconstitution within the peritoneal cavity. As shown in table III, the pretreatment of rats with Ra anti-RPMN so as to produce a marked neutropenia and decrease in the intraperitoneal PMN-leukocyte population was associated with a reduction in SRS-A^{rat} release from 605 to 86 units/rat. When the depleted rats received the peritoneal exudate cells elicited in normal rats by the i.p. injection of glycogen [15], subsequent antigen challenge revealed a 53 % restoration of the capacity to release SRS-A^{rat}. Further evidence that the PMN leukocyte is a prerequisite for the antigen-induced release of SRS-A^{rat} is derived from preliminary experiments in which the PMN leukocyte exudates from actively sensitized rats were passively transferred to the peritoneal cavity of unsensitized rats, and SRS-A^{rat} release was obtained upon subsequent challenge with specific

Table III. Partial restoration of SRS-A^{rat} release in rats pretreated with Ra anti-RPMN[1]

Modifying procedure	Absolute PMN leukocyte count/mm^3		Mean SRS-A^{rat} Release (units/rat)
	Peripheral blood	Peritoneal fluid	
–	4,355	10,656	605
Ra anti-RPMN	200	683	86
Ra anti-RPMN + PMN leukocytes i.p.[2]	966	14,630	320

[1] Each result represents the mean value for 3 rats in that group. 3.0 ml of Ra anti-RPMN was injected i.p. into 6 rats 16 h before the experiment. All rats were prepared for the antigen-induced release of SRS-A^{rat} by the i.p. injection of 1.0 ml rat anti-bovine serum albumin (BSA) (2.2 mg of specific antibody protein/ml); and 2 h later, they were challenged i.p. with 2.0 mg BSA in 5.0 ml Tyrode's solution containing heparin (50 μg/ml).

[2] 3.2×10^7 rat PMN leukocytes, obtained from normal rats injected i.p. 16 h previously with 20 ml 0.1 % oyster glycogen in 0.15 M saline, were injected i.p. into each rat 1 h after administration of antiserum and 1 h before antigen challenge.

Table IV. A comparison of the antigen-induced release of SRS-A^{rat} in the presence of peritoneal exudates consisting predominantly of neutrophils and eosinophils[1]

Peritoneal exudate	Peritoneal fluid Mean absolute cell counts/mm^3		Mean SRS-A^{rat} release (units/rat)
	Neutrophils	Eosinophils	
–	2,058	441	308
Neutrophils	30,876	498	895
Eosinophils	3,385	6,604	183

[1] Each result represents the mean value for 3 rats in that group. The peritoneal exudates containing neutrophils were induced by the i.p. injection of 20 ml 0.1% oyster glycogen in 0.15 M saline 16 h before the experiment. The peritoneal exudates containing eosinophils were induced by peritoneal lavage with 50 ml 0.15 M saline repeated 4 times at 3-day intervals [2]. All rats were prepared for the antigen-induced release of SRS-A^{rat} by the i.p. injection of 1.0 mg of rat anti-BSA (3.8 mg of specific antibody protein/ml) and 2 h later, they were challenged with 2.0 mg BSA in 5.0 ml Tyrode's solution containing heparin (50 μg/ml).

antigen [15]. This release could not be attributed to passive sensitization by free antibody because the latent period was too brief and the supernatant, following sedimentation of the cells, was inactive even when the appropriate latent period was used.

The possible contribution of the eosinophilic leukocyte to the antigen-induced release of SRS-A^{rat} was investigated by comparing the enhancement of SRS-A^{rat} release achieved in the presence of peritoneal exudates containing predominantly neutrophilic or eosinophilic leukocytes (table IV). As noted previously, the presence of an intraperitoneal PMN leukocyte exudate significantly enhanced the immunologic release of SRS-A^{rat} (table IV). In contrast, the presence of a greater than 10-fold increase in peritoneal eosinophils resulted in almost a 50% reduction in SRS-A^{rat} release. Whether the inhibition observed with peritoneal eosinophilia is due to an effect of this cell on the antibody, on the antigen-antibody complexes, or on the released SRS-A^{rat} remains to be determined.

The Role of Serum Complement in the Immunologic Release of SRS-A^{rat}

The precise role of serum complement in the reaction sequence leading to the formation and release of SRS-A^{rat} has not been clearly established. De-

Table V. Cutaneous immunologic reactions in the rat in the presence of various inhibitors[1]

Pretreatment procedure	PCA Dilutions of rat antiserum								Ra anti-RMC Dilutions of Ra anti-RMC			
	1:2		1:4		1:8		1:16		1:25		1:50	
None	4+	18	3+	15	2+	12	1+	10	4+	14	4+	12
Disodium cromoglycate	1+	12	1+	9	Tr	5	0	0	4+	12	4+	11
Diethylcarbamazine	3+	17	2+	13	2+	11	1+	7	4+	12	4+	10
Disodium cromoglycate + diethylcarbamazine	Tr	8	Tr	3	Tr	2	0	0	4+	13	3+	10
Mepyramine maleate + methysergide	1+	11	Tr	8	Tr	7	Tr	4	Tr	2	Tr	2
Mepyramine maleate + methysergide + diethylcarbama- zine	0	0	0	0	0	0	0	0	Tr	2	Tr	2

[1] Each result represents the mean value for 3 rats in that group. Rat anti-dinitrophenyl bovine gamma globulin (DNP-BγG) containing 3.4 mg of antibody/ml was injected i.d. in various dilutions into the dorsal skin of rats. Four hours later, the same rats were injected i.d. with 2 dilutions of Ra anti-RMC, and immediately thereafter they were challenged with 1.0 mg DNP-BSA in 1.0 ml 0.5 % Evan's blue dye i.v. The mean intensity (0–4+) and diameter (mm) of reactions for 3 rats in each group are described. Diethylcarbamazine, 20 mg/kg i.v., and disodium cromoglycate, 50 mg/rat i.v., were injected 30 sec before challenge with specific antigen. Mepyramine maleate, 50 mg/kg i.p., and methysergide, 4 mg/kg i.v., were administered 30 min before challenge.

complementation of rats achieved by pretreatment with either a non-toxic fraction of the venom from the cobra (Naja haje) [15] or with heat-aggregated human gamma globulin (HAHGG) [12] is associated with a marked suppression of the antigen-induced release of SRS-A^{rat}. However, cobra venom releases a slow reacting substance from guinea-pig lungs [9] and thus may produce substrate depletion when used in the rat. HAHGG may not only decomplement the animal but in so doing may also activate the pathway to the formation and release of SRS-A^{rat} and thus effect substrate depletion. The present data do not permit a conclusion as to whether the inhibitory action of cobra venom factor and of HAHGG is due to a complement requirement or is merely the result of substrate depletion and unrelated to a complement requirement.

Selective Pharmacologic Inhibition of the Immunologic Release of SRS-A[rat]

Diethylcarbamazine (Hetrazan, Lederle) effectively inhibits the immunologic release of SRS-A[rat] from the peritoneal cavity of the rat [16]. This agent does not appear to inhibit antigen-antibody interaction *in vitro* or *in vivo* [15, 16], and it does not block the activity of SRS-A[rat] on the smooth muscle in the bioassay [16]. A study of the chemical analogs of diethylcarbamazine revealed that the subgroups within the molecule required for optimal inhibitory activity included the carboxamide grouping and a saturated or unsaturated ring containing nitrogen [17]. Diethylcarbamazine and its analogs do not appear to interfere with the PMN leukocyte or serum complement *in vivo* or *in vitro* [17, 15]. These agents appear to act at some step in the reaction sequence leading to the formation and release of SRS-A[rat] subsequent to antigen-antibody interaction. Their action at this site permits the tissue to become desensitized because the antibody is utilized in a non-productive reaction [15].

Diethylcarbamazine appears to be selective in its action in that it inhibits the IgG_a-mediated release of SRS-A[rat] but not of histamine in the same animal [12]; it also fails to prevent the release of histamine mediated by the heat labile homocytotropic antibodies [17]. Conversely, disodium cromoglycate (Intal, Fison's Pharmaceuticals) inhibits the immunologic release of histamine mediated by either homocytotropic antibody or rat IgG_a, but it has no effect on the elaboration of SRS-A[rat] [12, 17]. The finding that disodium cromoglycate inhibits the immunologic release of histamine mediated by two classes of rat immunoglobulins is consistent with the view that the pathways involved share a similar or common step.

Inhibition of Passive Cutaneous Anaphylaxis (PCA) in the Rat

Rat antiserum devoid of heat labile homocytotropic antibody, or the IgG_a fraction therefrom, is not only capable of mediating the intraperitoneal release of SRS-A[rat] and histamine but also prepares rat skin for PCA after a 4 h but not a 48 h latent period [20]. In contrast, rat homocytotropic antibodies mediate a PCA reaction in the rat with an optimal latent period of 48–72 h [5]. The PCA reactions mediated by these two classes of rat antibody can be compared with the dermal blueing response mediated by rabbit antiserum against rat mast cells (Ra anti-RMC) in terms of the effect of various pharmacologic inhibitors. It has previously been reported that disodium cromoglycate, 50 mg/rat i.v., is capable of producing virtually complete suppression of the 48 h PCA reaction in the rat mediated by homocytotropic antibody, whereas diethylcarbamazine, 20 mg/kg i.v., is ineffective [17]. Pretreatment of rats with a combination of histamine and serotonin antagonists also completely suppressed the 48 h PCA reaction in the rat. As shown in table V, these inhibitors, alone and in combination, were also studied for their ability to inhibit the PCA reaction at 4 h mediated by antisera devoid of homocytotropic antibody and the dermal response to Ra anti-RMC. Disodium cromoglycate produced partial suppression of the PCA reaction at 4 h in the rat while diethylcarbamazine alone was without effect. However, the combination of these two inhibitors virtually abolished the reaction without significantly affecting the response to Ra anti-RMC. Pretreatment with mepyramine maleate (Neo-Antergan, Merck, Sharp and Dohme) and methysergide (UML-491, Merck, Sharp and Dohme) effected a marked suppression of the PCA reaction at 4 h and the addition of diethylcarbamazine to this regimen completely eliminated this reaction. The requirement of diethylcarbamazine for the complete suppression of the PCA reaction at 4 h mediated by rat antisera devoid of homocytotropic antibody and the ability of disodium cromoglycate alone, or the combination of histamine and serotonin antagonists, to completely abolish the PCA reaction at 48 h mediated by homocytotropic antibody suggests that the former reaction involves an additional mediator. Although functionally pure SRS-A[rat] is not particularly active in producing a local increase in cutaneous permeability in the rat (table II), the possibility that its presence increases the response to the amines requires investigation. Such an effect may account for the finding that diethylcarbamazine is required for the complete suppression of the PCA reaction at 4 h mediated by antisera devoid of homocytotropic antibody. The finding that disodium cromoglycate fails to block the blueing response in rat skin produced by Ra anti-RMC indicates that this agent is not a direct antagonist of either histamine or serotonin and that it has no effect on cytotoxic pathways to cell injury.

Concluding Comments

The passive sensitization of normal human lung tissue with whole antisera containing reaginic antibody (IgE) results in the antigen-induced release of histamine and SRS-A[hu] [18, 19], but this does not establish that IgE prepares the tissue for the release of both mediators; comparable studies using isolated immunoglobulin fractions have not been carried out. In the guinea pig [20] and in the rat [11] the immunologic release of SRS-A is not mediated by a heat labile homocytotropic antibody analogous to human reagin but rather by a distinctly different, heat stable antibody which is of the γ_1 class in the guinea pig and is associated with the IgG_a class of the rat.

Diethylcarbamazine and disodium cromoglycate are unique pharmacologic inhibitors in that they act at some point subsequent to antigen-antibody interaction but prior to the release of the chemical mediators. Their action at this site permits the tissue to become desensitized in the absence of inflammation because antigen-antibody interaction does not lead to the release of the chemical mediators. Their inhibitory activity appears to be remarkably selective; and the use of these agents or their chemical analogs, perhaps in combination, may provide a new therapeutic approach to the immunologic tissue injury associated with immediate-type hypersensitivity.

Acknowledgments

The authors gratefully acknowledge the advice of Dr. J. Weeks (The Upjohn Co., Kalamazoo, Michigan) concerning the bioassay of the prostaglandins. The authors also note appreciatively the excellent technical assistance of Mrs. C. R. Wesley and Miss A. Lunan.

References

1. Ambache, N.: Biological characterization of, and structure action studies on smooth-muscle-contracting hydroxy-acids. Mem. Soc. Endocr. *14:* 19–28 (1966).
2. Archer, G. T. and Hirsch, J. G.: Isolation of granules from eosinophil leukocytes and study of their enzyme content. J. exp. Med. *118:* 277–285 (1963).
3. Austen, K. F.; Orange, R. P. and Valentine, M. D.: Antibodies and cells involved in the antigen-induced release of slow reacting substance of anaphylaxis (SRS-A[rat]) in the rat; in K. F. Austen and E. L. Becker, eds., Biochemistry of the Acute Allergic Reactions, p. 283 (Blackwell Scientific Publications, Ltd., Oxford 1968).
4. Becker, E. L. and Austen, K. F.: Mechanism of immunologic injury of rat peritoneal mast cells. I. The effect of phosphonate inhibitors on the homocytotropic antibody-mediated histamine release and the first component of rat complement. J. exp. Med. *124:* 379–395 (1966).
5. Bloch, K. J.: The anaphylactic antibodies of mammals including man. Progr. Allergy Vol. 10, pp. 84–150 (Karger, Basel/New York 1967).
6. Bloch, K. J.; Morse, H. C. and Austen, K. F.: Biologic properties of rat antibodies. I. Antigen binding by four classes of anti-DNP antibodies. J. Immunol. *101:* 650–657 (1968).
7. Brocklehurst, W. E.: The release of histamine and the formation of a slow reacting substance (SRS-A) during anaphylactic shock. J. Physiol. *151:* 416–435 (1960).
8. Brocklehurst, W. E.: Slow reacting substance and related compounds. Progr. Allergy, Vol. 6, pp. 539–558 (Karger, Basel/New York 1962).

9. FELDBERG, W. and KELLAWAY, C. H.: Liberation of histamine and formation of a lecithin-like substance by cobra venom. J. Physiol. *94:* 187–226 (1938).
10. MOTA, I.: The mechanism of anaphylaxis. I. Production and biological properties of 'mast cell sensitizing' antibody. Immunology *7:* 681–699 (1964).
11. MORSE, H. C.; BLOCH, K. J. and AUSTEN, K. F.: Biologic properties of rat antibodies. II. Time-course of appearance of antibodies involved in the antigen-induced release of slow reacting substance of anaphylaxis (SRS-A[rat]); association of this activity with rat IgG . J. Immunol. *101:* 658–663 (1968).
12. MORSE, H. C.; AUSTEN, K. F. and BLOCH, K. J.: Biologic properties of rat antibodies. III. Histamine release mediated by two classes of antibodies J. Immunol. (in press).
13. ORANGE, R. P.; VALENTINE, M. D.; MORSE, H. C.; STECHSCHULTE, D. J. and AUSTEN, K. F.: *In vivo* inhibition of the immunologic release of slow reacting substance of anaphylaxis (SRS-A[rat]) in the rat. Proceedings of the VI. International Congress of Allergology (in press).
14. ORANGE, R. P.; VALENTINE, M. D. and AUSTEN, K. F.: Release of slow reacting substance of anaphylaxis in the rat: Polymorphonuclear leukocyte. Science *157:* 318–319 (1967).
15. ORANGE, R. P.; VALENTINE, M. D. and AUSTEN, K. F.: Antigen-induced release of slow reacting substance of anaphylaxis (SRS-A[rat]) in rats prepared with homologous antibody. J. exp. Med. *127:* 767–782 (1968).
16. ORANGE, R. P.; VALENTINE, M. D. and AUSTEN, K. F.: Inhibition of the release of slow reacting substance of anaphylaxis in the rat by diethyl-carbamazine. Proc. Soc. exp. Biol., N.Y. *127:* 127–132 (1968).
17. ORANGE, R. P. and AUSTEN, K. F.: Pharmacologic dissociation of immunologic release of histamine and SRS-A[rat]. Proc. Soc. exp. Biol., N.Y. *129:* 836–841 (1968).
18. PARISH, W. E.: Release of histamine and slow reacting substance with mast cell changes after challenge of human lung sensitized passively with reagin *in vitro*. Nature *215:* 738–739 (1967).
19. SHEARD, P.; KILLINGBACK, P. G. and BLAIR, A. M. J. N.: Antigen-induced release of histamine and SRS-A from human lung passively sensitized with reaginic serum. Nature, Lond. *216:* 283–284 (1967).
20. STECHSCHULTE, D. J.; AUSTEN, K. F. and BLOCH, K. J.: Antibodies involved in the antigen-induced release of slow reacting substance of anaphylaxis (SRS-A) in the guinea pig and rat. J. exp. Med. *125:* 127–147 (1967).
21. WEEKS, J. R.; SCHULTZ, J. R. and BROWN, W. E.: Evaluation of smooth muscle bioassays for prostaglandins E_1 and F_{1a} (submitted for publication).

Authors' address: ROBERT P. ORANGE, M.D., and K. FRANK AUSTEN, M.D., Department of Medicine, Harvard Medical School, at the Robert B. Brigham Hospital, *Boston, Mass.* (USA).

Cellular and Humoral Mechanisms in Anaphylaxis and Allergy, pp. 207–214
(Karger, Basel/New York 1969)

The Kinin System – A Review[1]

MARION E. WEBSTER

Experimental Therapeutics Branch, National Heart Institute, Bethesda, Md.
and
The Departamento de Bioquimica e Farmacologia, Escola Paulista de Medicina,
Sao Paulo, S.P.

Within the last year or two a number of books and reviews [12, 29, 13, 27, 28] have been published detailing various components of the kinin system. The three main components of this system are shown in figure 1. The *kallikreins*, the enzymes, act on the substrates, the *kininogens*, to release the pharmacologically active polypeptides, the *kinins*. The kallikreins, due to their different properties, have been separated into two classes – those derived from glandular sources and those derived from plasma. Most glandular tissues which have been investigated, with the notable exception of the liver, contain a kallikrein. This enzyme is usually secreted by the gland in an active form and is thus found in urine, saliva, sweat, feces, pancreatic juice, etc. Plama kallikrein, on the other hand, exists in plasma as on inactive precursor called prekallikrein. Each kallikrein derived from different sources or different species can be distinguished by in its response to proteolytic inhibitors or to antibody and consequently varies in structure. All of the kallikreins, however, act on one or the other of the kininogens in plasma to release the pharmacologically active kinins.

At present three classes of kininogens have been found in human plasma. The low molecular weight kininogens (LMW) [26] in most species represent the major kininogen content of plasma. They have a molecular weight around 50,000 and either the glandular kallikreins or trypsin will form kinins from these substrates. The high molecular weight kininogens-a (HMW-a) have a molecular weight around 200,000 and in common with other plasma proteins of this size are not normally found in lymph. Kinins are formed from these substrates by plasma kallikrein as well as the glandular kallikreins

[1] Supported in part by Fundaçao de Amparo à Pesquisa do Estado de Sao Paulo. Grant No. 68/638.

and trypsin. These kininogens, therefore, in most species except the guinea pig [17], represents the only substrate for plasma kallikrein. The high molecular weight kininogens-b (HMW-b) have only recently been found [WEBSTER, JACOBSEN and PIERCE, to be published] and little is known of their exact molecular weight or the structure of the kinin which is formed. Present evidence suggests that the kinins which are generated are different from those released from the other substrates. Trypsin is the only enzyme known to form a kinin from this substrate. Kallidin, a decapeptide (fig. 1), is the kinin formed by the action of human urinary kallikrein on LMW kininogens or HMW-a kininogens. Bradykinin, a nonapeptide, differing from kallidin by a single N-terminal lysine group, is the kinin formed by the action of human plasma kallikrein and trypsin on HMW-a or the action of trypsin on LMW kininogens.

Control over the generation of kinins under physiological and pathological conditions is mediated by inhibitors to the kallikreins which are found in plasma and in various body tissues. Also, there are kininases which cleave the kinins at various peptide bonds thus destroying their biological activity. There are at least two kininases in human plasma [31] – a carboxypeptidase N which cleaves the C-terminal arginine from the kinin moiety (fig. 1) and a peptidase which cleaves the Pro-Phe bond releasing the dipeptide Phe-Arg. A single passage through the circulation inactivates up to 90% of infused bradykinin [15] and a half life of around 16 sec has been found in the blood of dogs [24]. It is apparent, therefore, that the concentration of kinin is closely regulated under normal physiological conditions.

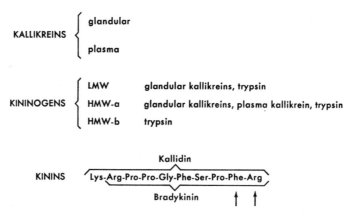

Fig. 1. The three main components of the kinin system. Arrows indicate bonds split by the two known kininases in human plasma.

Another method by which control can be exercised over kinin formation is by altering the concentration of the enzymes which activate the kallikreins. Little is known of the enzymes if any, which activate the glandular kalli-kreins. The glandular kallikreins, themselves, have been found in subcellular particles in the kidney [6] and in the submaxillary gland [3, 14], suggesting that these kallikreins may be stored in an active form. Our knowledge of the mechanism of activation of human plasma kallikrein is also still fragmentary and open to revision [30]. Figure 2 summarizes current knowledge in this field. At least five enzymes are thought to be involved in the activation of human plasma kallikrein and these enzymes are currently depicted as a series of preenzyme to enzyme conversions – each enzyme in succession activating the next. Hageman factor (factor XII in blood clotting terminology) is thought to initiate the present series of reactions as well as those involved in blood clotting. This enzyme in turn activates either Enzyme V, III or II – the order of their activation being still unknown. Enzyme II has been tentatively identified as PF-dil (permeability factor/dilute of MILES and WILHELM) since it, like plasma kallikrein, is an arginine esterase. It must be emphasized, however, that further purification and characterization of these enzymes is necessary before they can be considered unequivocally to be specific entities. Also, evidence has been presented recently [25] that in bovine plasma Hage-man factor may act directly on prekallikrein. Further studies with isolated enzymes are indicated.

The kinins reproduce some, although not all, of the manifestations of anaphylactic shock and, therefore, are candidates – like histamine, serotonin, slow-reacting substance and biologically active fragments of complement – for playing a central role in this condition. The possible role of the kinins as

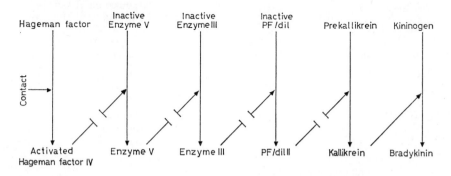

Fig.2. Current concept of mechanism of activation of human plasma kallikrein.

mediators of anaphylactic shock has been studied by a number of investigators. These authors have determined whether production of this type of shock caused an increase in kinin levels, a decrease in kininogen levels, release of a kallikrein or a decrease in kinin formation as measured by activation of the plasma. As shown, the current evidence appears to be overwhelmingly in favour of the thesis that the kinin system is indeed activated under these experimental conditions. In all species studied, i.e. dogs, guinea pigs, rabbits and rats and in isolated guinea pig lung preparations, some evidence could usually be found that the kinins had been liberated. Direct measurement of kinin levels in blood appears to be the most sensitive method for measurement of this activation as two investigators [7, 9] – one using the dog and the other the rat – could measure increased kinin levels

Table I. Evidence for formation of kinins during anaphylactic shock

Species	Percent of animals showing alteration in				References
	Kinin	Kininogen	Kalli-krein	Kinin Formation[1]	
Dog	40				BERALDO [2]
	100				BACK et al. [1]
	66	0			CIRSTEA et al. [7]
		66			DINIZ et al. [11]
Guinea pig	100	100			BROCKLEHURST and LAHIRI [4, 5]
		30			CIRSTEA et al. [7]
		100			KELLETT [19]
		100			GREEF et al. [16]
				100	KONOPKA and TCHORZEWSKI [20]
Rabbit		100			LECOMTE [22]
	100				BROCKLEHURST and LAHIRI [4]
		100			DINIZ and CARVALHO [10]
		100			LECOMTE and SALMON [23]
					LAMBERT et al. [21]
	50	75			CIRSTEA et al. [7]
Rat	100				BROCKLEHURST and LAHIRI [4]
	100	0	100		DAWSON et al. [9]
Guinea pig Lung			100		BROCKLEHURST and LAHIRI [4, 5]
			100		JONASSON and BECKER [18]
	100[2]				COLLIER and JAMES [8]

[1] Capacity of plasma to form kinins by activation (i.e. glass).
[2] Presence of kinins as demonstrated by specific tachyphylaxis.

but were unable to demonstrate a decrease in kininogen. This may in part have been due to their use of trypsin as the kinin-forming enzyme rather than plasma kallikrein. This latter enzyme might be a more specific enzyme for the substrate which was involved. In the rat, however, an increase rather than the expected decrease in kininogen levels was found and this despite the observations that the plasma obtained after shock contained increased levels of a kinin-forming enzyme as measured against an acid-treated heat-denatured substrate. In blood-free guinea-pig lung preparations *in vitro*, two groups of investigators [4, 5, 18] have clearly demonstrated that after the induction of anaphylaxis, a kallikrein appears in the perfusates. Current evidence suggests that the kallikrein activated by this antigen-antibody reaction is guinea-pig plasma kallikrein and it has been suggested that the prekallikrein from the plasma is adsorbed to endothelial cells or to other pulmonary tissues and is activated by a process involving Hageman factor [18]. Also, the presence of kinins as demonstrated by specific tachyphylaxis has been shown *in vivo* using the Konzett-Rossler preparation of guinea-pig lungs [8]. There appears to be little doubt, therefore, that the kinins are formed during anaphylactic shock.

The exact contribution of the kinins to anaphylactic shock is less clearly established. BROCKLEHURST and LAHIRI [4] reported a peak in the blood kinin levels 2 ½ min after challenge with soluble antigen in the guinea pig and 5 min after challenge in the rat and rabbit. COLLIER and JAMES [8], by inducing tachyphylaxis to bradykinin or slow-reacting substance have estimated the contribution of the kinins to bronchoconstriction of guinea-pig lungs *in vivo*. A reduction in the bronchoconstriction occurred with a maximum approximately two minutes after challenge. These data again suggest that the kinins contribute to the early phases of anaphylaxis in this species. Also LAMBERT *et al.* [21] as shown in figure 3 have presented evidence that, in the rabbit, kinins may play a role in the initial hypotension induced by anaphylaxis. In these experiments injection of antigen into a sensitized animal (left side of figure) caused an immediate fall in blood pressure, a marked decrease in kininogen content as measured with human salivary kallikrein and an increase in plasmin activity. However, when the animals were injected with a specific immune precipitate (right side of figure) – seventy-five minutes before challenge, the drop in blood pressure following injection of antigen was delayed and no decrease in kininogen was found even though the concentration of plasmin was still increased. These results, after confirmation by other investigators, illustrate at least two important points. First, activation of plasmin does not appear to be involved in this *in*

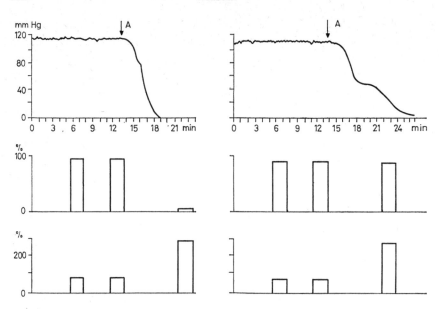

Fig. 3. The contribution of the kinins to anaphylactic shock. Upper panel shows response of blood pressure following injection of antigen (A) (arrow) into a sensitized rabbit (left) and into a rabbit which had received a prior injection of a specific immune precipitate (right). Middle and lower panels give the per cent decrease or increase in kininogen and plasmin, respectively, in the plasma samples [reproduced with permission from LAMBERT *et al.*, Int. Arch. Allergy *24:* 27–34 (1964).]

vivo activation of the kinin system. Second, the prior injection of a specific immune precipitate in some manner blocks the subsequent activation of the kinin system. This blockade does not appear to be due to exhaustion of the endogenous kinin-forming system by the initial injection of a specific immune precipitate as no alteration of kininogen levels was observed following this treatment. It is more likely that some substance required for activation of this system such as complement, leucocytes, Hageman factor etc., has been exhausted. Also, the delay in the drop in blood pressure need not be due solely to blockade of kinin release, as injection of an immune precipitate prior to anaphylaxis could cause the depletion of more than one factor. Nevertheless, it is by studies such as these that the contribution of the many factors involved in anaphylactic shock can be delineated. The use of multiple agents to block the various proposed mediators as employed by COLLIER and JAMES [8] will undoubtedly aid in determining their relative roles in the pathology of this condition.

References

1. BACK, N.; MUNSON, A. E. and GUTH, P. S.: Anaphylactic shock in dogs. Role of fibrinolysin and vasoactive polypeptide systems. J. Amer. med. Ass. *183:* 260–263 (1963).
2. BERALDO, W. T.: Formation of bradykinin in anaphylactic and peptone shock. Amer. J. Physiol. *163:* 283–289 (1950).
3. BHOOLA, K. D. and OGLE, C. W.: The subcellular localization of kallikrein, amylase and acetylcholine in the submaxillary gland of the guinea pig. J. Physiol., Lond. *184:* 663–672 (1966).
4. BROCKLEHURST, W. E. and LAHIRI, S. C.: The production of bradykinin in anaphylaxis. J. Physiol., Lond. *160:* 15–16 (1962).
5. BROCKLEHURST, W. E. and LAHIRI, S. C.: Formation and destruction of bradykinin during anaphylaxis. J. Physiol., Lond. *165:* 39–40 (1963).
6. CARVALHO, I. F. and DINIZ, C. R.: Kinin-forming enzyme (kininogenin) in homogenates of rat kidney. Biochim. biophys. Acta *128:* 136–148 (1966).
7. CIRSTEA, M.; SUHACIU, G. et BUTCULESCU, I.: Evaluation du rôle de la bradykinine dans le choc anaphylactique. Arch. int. Pharmacodyn. *159:* 18–33 (1966).
8. COLLIER, H. O. J. and JAMES, G. W. L.: Humoral factors affecting pulmonary inflation during acute anaphylaxis in the guinea pig *in vivo*. Brit. J. Pharmacol. Chemother. *30:* 283–301 (1967).
9. DAWSON, W.; STARR, M. S. and WEST, G. B.: Inhibition of anaphylactic shock in the rat by antihistamines and ascorbic acid. Brit. J. Pharmacol. Chemother. *27:* 249–255 (1966).
10. DINIZ, C. R. and CARVALHO, I. F.: A micro method for determination of bradykininogen under several conditions. N.Y. Acad. Sci. *104:* 77–88 (1963).
11. DINIZ, C. R.; CARVALHO, I. F.; DOS REIS, M. L. and CORRADO, A. P.: Bradykininogen in some experimental conditions; In International Symposium on Vaso-Active Polypeptides: Bradykinin and related kinins. M. ROCHA e SILVA and H. A. ROTHSCHILD, eds., pp. 15–20 (Edart Livraria Editôra Ltda., Sao Paulo, 1967).
12. ERDÖS, E. G.: Hypotensive peptides: bradykinin, kallidin and eledoisin. Adv. Pharmacol. *4:* 1–89 (1966).
13. ERDÖS, E. G.; BACK, N. and SICUTERI, S. (eds.): Hypotensive peptides (Springer, New York 1966).
14. ERDÖS, E. G.; TAGUE, L. L. and MIWA, I.: Kallikrein in granules of the submaxillary gland. Biochem. Pharmacol. *17:* 667–674 (1968).
15. FERREIRA, S. H. and VANE, J. R.: The disappearance of bradykinin and eledoisin in the circulation and vascular beds of the cat. Brit. J. Pharmacol. *30:* 417–424 (1967).
16. GREEF, K.; SCHARNAGEL, K.; LUHR, R. und STROBACK, H.: Die Abnahme des Kiningengehaltes des Plasmas beim toxischen, anaphylaktischen und anaphylaktoiden Schock. Arch. exp. Path. Pharmakol. *253:* 235–245 (1966).
17. JACOBSEN, S.: Substrates for plasma kinin-forming enzymes in rat and guinea-pig plasmas. Brit. J. Pharmacol. *28:* 64–72 (1966).
18. JONASSON, D. and BECKER, E. L.: Release of kallikrein from guinea-pig lung during anaphylaxis. J. exp. Med. *123:* 509–522 (1966).
19. KELLETT, D. N.: On the mechanism of the anti-inflammatory activity of hexadimethrine bromide. Brit. J. Pharmacol. *26:* 351–357 (1966).
20. KONOPKA, P. and TCHORZEWSKI, H.: Serotonin metabolism and kininforming activity of plasma during anaphylactic shock in guinea pigs and their modification after E-amino-caproic acid and Trasylol administration. Experientia *24:* 469–470 (1968).

21. LAMBERT, P. H.; OTTO-SERVAIS, M.; SALMON, J. et LECOMTE, J.: Sur le rôle du complément dans le choc anaphylactique du lapin. Int. Arch. Allergy *24:* 27–34 (1964).
22. LECOMTE, J.: Consommation des kininogènes plasmatiques au cours du choc anaphylactique du lapin. C. R. Soc. Biol. *155:* 1411–1413 (1961).
23. LECOMTE, J. et SALMON, J.: Rôle de la fibrinolyse dans le choc anaphylactique du lapin. Int. Arch. Allergy *22:* 378–387 (1963).
24. MCCARTHY, D. A.; POTTER, D. E. and NICOLAIDES, E. O.: An *in vivo* estimation of the potencies and half-lives of synthetic bradykinin and kallidin. J. Pharmacol. exp. Therap. *148:* 117–122 (1965).
25. NAGASAWA, S.; TAKAHASHI, H.; KOIDA, M. and SUZUKI, T.: Partial purification of bovine plasma kallikreinogen, its activation by the Hageman factor. Biochem. biophys. Res. Comm. *32:* 644–649 (1968).
26. PIERCE, J. V.: Structural features of plasma kinins and kininogens. Fed. Proc. *27:* 52–57 (1968).
27. ROCHA e SILVA, M. and ROTHSCHILD, H. A. (eds.): International Symposium on vasoactive polypeptides: Bradykinin and Related Kinins (Edart Livraria Editôra Ltda., Sao Paulo 1967).
28. SYMPOSIUM ON VASOACTIVE PEPTIDES. Fed. Proc. *27:* 49–99 (1968).
29. WEBSTER, M. E.: The kallikrein-kininogen-kinin system. Arth. Rheum. *9:* 473–482 (1966).
30. WEBSTER, M. E.: Human plasma kallikrein, its activation and pathological role. Fed. Proc. *27:* 84–89 (1968).
31. YANG, H. Y. T. and ERDÖS, E. G.: Second kininase in human blood plasma. Nature, Lond. *215:* 1402–1403 (1967).

Author's address: MARION E. WEBSTER, Ph.D., Experimental Therapeutics Branch, National Heart Institute, *Bethesda, Md.* (USA).

Cellular and Humoral Mechanisms in Anaphylaxis and Allergy, pp. 215–223
(Karger, Basel/New York 1969)

The Demonstration of Permeability Factors and of two Kinin-forming Enzymes in Plasma[1]

Henry Z. Movat[2], Mary P. Treloar, Nancy L. DiLorenzo,
John W. Robertson and Harold B. Sender

Division of Experimental Pathology, Department of Pathology
University of Toronto, Toronto

Several potent chemical mediators have been implicated in anaphylaxis and in the vascular phenomena of inflammation. A great deal is known regarding the mechanism of release of histamine and serotonin from cells. On the other hand, relatively little can be said on the mode of generation of kinins. This publication deals with biologically active substances which are generated when antigen-antibody precipitates come in contact with non-glass contacted serum. Probably the same substances are formed when serum is contacted with glass, kaolin and other surface active agents. The *in vitro* model chosen probably has *in vivo* significance.

Activation of the Kinin-forming System by Ag-Ab Precipitates

When washed precipitates of bovine serum albumin – anti bovine serum albumin are incubated with non-glass contacted guinea-pig, rabbit or human serum, the serum becomes 'activated' [6, 7]. The properties of such activated serum are shown in table I.

Both rabbit and guinea pig γG-antibody (the latter either electrophoretically slow i.e. γ_2 or fast i.e. γ_1) caused activation of the serum. The immune precipitates incubated with 1 ml non-glass contacted serum contained 100 μg Ab N.

[1] Supported by the Ontario Heart Foundation and Medical Research Council of Canada.

[2] Dr. Movat is a research associate of the MRC.

Fractionation of Ag-Ab Activated Serum

Activated serum, primarily guinea pig in origin, was fractionated by starch block electrophoresis, DEAE-cellulose, DEAE-Sephadex or QAE-Sephadex chromatography, sucrose density gradient ultracentrifugation and gel filtration on Sephadex G-200. The fractions were tested for their ability to enhance vascular permeability and for their kinin generating capacity. Enhanced vessel permeability was tested in antihistamine treated guinea pigs by injecting intravenously Evans blue (20 mg/kg) together with I^{125}-labeled human serum albumin (20 μc/kg). Punched out lesions (blue spots) were measured in a γ-scaler and expressed as counts per minute per lesion [7, 11]. Subsequently, the skin lesions were extracted with formamide and the extra-vasated dye measured spectrophotometrically [7]. The chromatographic fractions were tested for their kinin forming capacity. The following substrates were used: (a) heated plasma (61°C for 90 min), (b) boiled plasma (100°C for 10 min), (c) acidified and boiled plasma [2], (d) acidified and re-neutralized plasma [3] (in the presence of 1 mg/ml of hexadimethrine bromide), (e) fresh plasma. 8-hydroxyquinoline (1 mg/ml, final conc.) or o-phenanthroline HCl (0.5 mg/ml, final conc.) served as a kinin protective agent. After the chromatographic fractions and the appropriate substrate were incubated for 5–30 min, the mixture was boiled for 20 min and the precipitate spun out. The supernatant was tested on the atropinized rat uterus, as previously described [7, 8], using synthetic bradykinin (Sandoz) as standards. Most of the chromatographic studies were done with guinea pig serum, but more recently Ag-Ab activated rat and human serum were also chromatographed. The chromatographic fractions were tested for purity by agarose zone and immunoelectrophoresis and by analytical acrylamide electrophoresis.

Figure 1 shows a comparison of the bluing obtained with electrophoretic fractions of normal and Ag-Ab activated guinea pig serum. Three zones of activity can be discerned, the difference between normal and activated serum being only quantitative. It is known that starch and most other materials used for fractionation cause contact-activation of serum.

Better separation was obtained by fractionating activated guinea pig serum on DEAE-cellulose. Bluing, kinin-forming and esterolytic activity eluted in two regions: (a) with the low ionic strength starting buffer and (b) with high ionic strength buffers after the amin albumin peak [8]. With some columns slight bluing activity was also obtained with the fractions eluting before the main albumin peak. As reported previously [7], the Ag-Ab precipi-

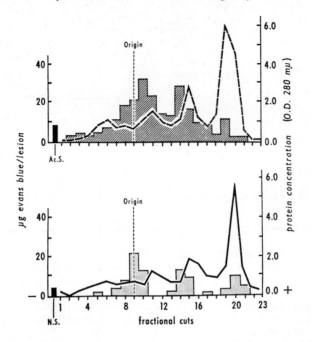

Fig. 1. Starch block electrophoresis of antigen-antibody activated guinea-pig serum (top) and normal guinea-pig serum (bottom) (from Movat, H. Z.; DiLorenzo, N. L. and Treloar, M. P., Lab. Invest. *19:* 201 (1968).

tates which had been used to activate the non-glass contacted serum had adsorbed some activity (bluing and clot-promoting), which could be readily eluted with Tyrode solution or better still with 1M NaCl. When these eluates were concentrated, dialysed and added to the original activated serum and then chromatographed, intense bluing activity was present in the fractions eluting from the column before the main albumin peak. However, these prealbumin fractions did not form kinin from any of the denatured substrates, but they were capable of generating kinin when added to fresh plasma.[3] As shown in figure 2, by anion exchange chromatography three regions of bluing activity can be eluted from Ag-Ab activated guinea-pig serum to which the washings (eluates) of the immune precipitates have been added. Not shown in figure 2 is the fact that the same fractions which induce

[3] More recent studies disclosed that the prealbumin fraction also generated kinin from heated plasma (61°C – 30 min), the precipitates formed during heating being not discarded but suspended in the heated plasma substrate.

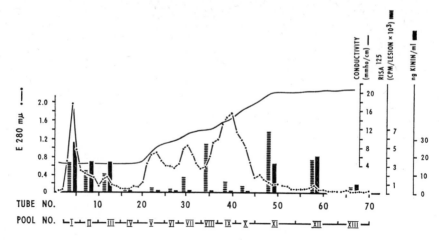

Fig.2. Fractionation of antigen-antibody activated guinea-pig serum on DEAE-Sephadex equilibrated with 0.1 M Tris HCl (pH 8.0). Elution was performed with 0.1 M Tris HCl and a linear gradient consisting of this buffer plus 0.2 M NaCl. Vascular permeability is expressed as counts per minute (CPM) per lesion. Kinin-forming activity is shown as bradykinin equivalent, released from 1 ml heated (61° for 90 min) guinea-pig plasma by 1 ml fraction (concentrated to ½ of sample volume). Note two areas of kinin-forming and three areas of bluing activity.

bluing are also capable of generating kinin from fresh plasma. On the other hand, as in the first runs, kinin was readily generated from denatured plasma substrate by fractions eluting with the low ionic strength starting buffer (pools I-III in fig. 2) and in the post albumin peaks with high ionic strength buffers (pools XI and XII). We have, therefore, tentatively designated the former as enzyme I or *kininogenase-I* and the latter as enzyme II or *kininogenase-II*. The pre-albumin fractions, possessing marked bluing activity and forming kinin only from fresh but not from denatured plasma were designated Pf/dil [16, 5].

Observations similar to those in the guinea pig were obtained recently with rat serum [10] and with human serum. Bluing experiments with rat serum fractions were performed in rats treated with mepyramine and BOL-148. The human serum fractions were tested in mepyramine treated guinea pigs. Rat serum behaved almost like guinea-pig serum. The bulk of both bluing and kinin-forming activity of human serum resided in the initial fractions (kininogenase-I). The kininogenases obtained with human serum may represent the two enzymes described by VOGT [12, 13, 14]; kininogenase-I possibly representing plasma kallikrein [15]. The fractions corresponding to human Pf/dil eluted in a manner previously described by others [1, 15]. However, it would appear that kininogenase-II has not been separated before from either human, guinea-pig or rat plasma. In human plasma BECKER and KAGEN [1] have described two permeability inducing substances, but did not find active fractions eluting after the albumin peak.

Whether the two kininogenases act on their own specific substrate remains to be investigated. Having used heat denatured plasma as substrate, the existence of an activatable pro-enzyme in the substrate could be excluded. WEBSTER [15] found an active fraction eluting after the albumin peak, but it generated kinin only from fresh plasma. It is likely that kininogenase-II does not generate kinin readily from denatured, but only from fresh substrate. Thus further studies along the lines initiated by JACOBSEN and KRIZ [4] and PIERCE and WEBSTER [9] seem pertinent.

Studies using sucrose density gradient ultracentrifugation and molecular sieve chromatography indicate that the kinin system may be more complex than hitherto suspected. Sucrose density gradient ultracentrifugation of some of the active DEAE-cellulose fractions of guinea-pig serum showed that most of the activity resides in low molecular weight (∞ 45,000) fractions [8]. When the above mentioned active fractions obtained with rat and human serum were centrifuged, most of the bluing activity sedimented in low density fractions, but some activity sedimented in fractions of higher density.

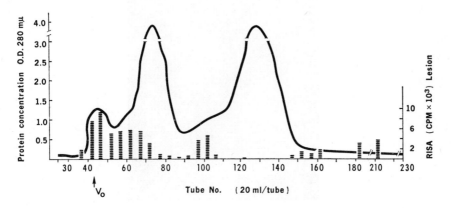

Fig. 3. Molecular sieve chromatography of antigen-antibody activated guinea-pig serum on a Sephadex G-200 superfine column, 10 × 88 cm (K 100/100 Pharmacia). Equilibrating and eluting fluid was 0.1 M Tris HCl (pH 8) plus 1.0 M NaCl. Each pool consisted of 5 tubes except the last three which consisted of 20 and the first which consisted of 15. RISA = I125-labeled human serum albumin. CPM = counts per minute. Enhanced vascular permeability was measured as described in the text.

When fractionated by gel filtration on Sephadex G-200, activated guinea-pig serum (containing the washings of the immune precipitates) had three well defined zones of bluing activity: (a) in the macroglobulin peak, (b) in a region intermediate between the 7S and the 4S peaks and (c) in the descending limb and trailing portion of the 4S peak (fig. 3). All fractions which induced enhanced vessel permeability also generated kinin.

There is evidence that kinins are generated when one of the substrates is incubated with the described chromatography fractions. The reaction product of substrate and kininogenase containing chromatographic fractions causes contraction of the rat uterus which is inhibited by carboxypeptidase-B (fig. 4). When added to the rat duodenum these same reaction products induce relaxation [8].

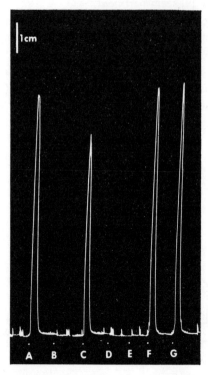

Fig.4. Kymograph tracing of contractions obtained with the rat uterus. A = mixture of a fraction (identical to Fr. XII, fig. 2) with a suspension of boiled guinea-pig plasma; B = same mixture incubated with 500 ng carboxypeptidase-B; C = 0.5 ng synthetic brady-kinin; D = mixture in 'A' incubated with 100 ng carboxypeptidase-B; E = 1 ng synthetic bradykinin incubated with 100 ng carboxypeptidase-B; F = same as A; G = 1 ng synthetic bradykinin.

Summary and Conclusions

Non-glass contacted guinea-pig, rabbit, rat or human serum becomes activated when incubated with antigen-antibody (Ag-Ab) precipitates, acquiring properties outlined in table I. The Ag-Ab precipitates adsorb some of the vascular permeability and most of the clot-enhancing activity and this can be eluted from the precipitates by repeated washings with Tyrode solution or 1M NaCl.

When Ag-Ab activated serum (containing the washings) is fractionated by anion exchange chromatography three major active components are obtained. All cause enhanced vascular permeability when injected intra-dermally and generate kinin from fresh plasma, but only two generate kinin from denatured plasma (see fig. 2). The last two (eluting with low and high ionic strength buffers respectively) have been tentatively designated as kininogenases-I and II. The third component which causes bluing and generates kinin from fresh but not from denatured plasma was designated Pf/dil.

Further studies, using gel filtration (Sephadex G-200) indicate that the kinin-forming system may be more complex, containing low, ($< 4S$) inter-mediate and large molecular size ($\sim 19S$) kinin-forming enzymes.

The present state of knowledge of the kinin system can probably be compared to the complement or blood clotting systems as they were known some years ago. In order to elucidate the entire system and the sequence in which the components interact it will be essential to obtain activated and unactivated components (pro-enzymes, pro-accelerators). Then it should be possible to test which active component acts on which unactivated compo-

Table I. Properties of Ag-Ab activated guinea-pig serum

1. Increase in vascular permeability (intra-dermal bluing test)	6. Inhibitors:
	(a) Hexadimethrine bromide (before incubation with Ag-Ab)
2. Contraction of guinea pig ileum and rat uterus; inhibited by carboxypeptidase-B	(b) DFP, Trasylol, C′ 1-esterase inhibitor (before or after incubation with Ag-Ab)
3. Hypotension (i.v. injection)	
4. TAME-esterase activity	
5. Enhanced clotting of recalcified plasma	7. Enhancing agents:
	(a) Diethyldithiocarbamate
	(b) 8-Hydroxyquinoline
	(c) o-Phenanthroline

nent and thereby elucidate the interaction sequence. Hexadimethrine bromide with diisoprophyl-fluorophosphate or ethylenediamine tetraacetate prevent the activation of Hageman factor during chromatography and permit the isolation of kininogens. Preliminary data in our laboratory indicate that pro-kininogenases can also be isolated in this manner and that factor XII of the rat can activate pro-kininogenase II. Whether this requires an intermediary (possibly Pf/dil), present in the pro-kininogenase II fractions, remains to be ascertained.

References

1. Becker, E. L. and Kagen, L.: The permeability globulins of human serum and the biochemical mechanism of hereditary angioneurotic edema. Ann. N.Y. Acad. Sci. *116:* 866 (1964).
2. Diniz, C. R. and Carvalho, I. F.: A micromethod for determination of brady-kininogen under several conditions. Ann. N.N. Acad. Sci. *104:* 77 (1963).
3. Eisen, V.: Effect of hexadimethrine bromide on plasma kinin formation, hydrolysis of p-tosyl-L-arginine methyl ester and fibrinolysis. Brit. J. Pharmacol. *22:* 87 (1964).
4. Jacobsen, S. and Kriz, M.: Some data on two purified kininogens from human plasma. Brit. J. Pharmacol. *29:* 25 (1967).
5. Mason, B. and Miles, A. A.: Globulin permeability factors without kininogenase activity. Nature, Lond. *196:* 587 (1962).
6. Movat, H. Z.: Activation of the kinin system by antigen-antibody complexes. International Symposium on Vasoactive Polypeptides: Bradykinin and Related Kinins, M. Rocha e Silva and H. A. Rothschild, eds., (Soc. Bras. Farmacol. São Paulo 1967).
7. Movat, H. Z. and DiLorenzo, N. L.: Activation of the plasma kinin system by antigen-antibody aggregates. I. Generation of permeability factor in guinea-pig serum. Lab. Invest. *19:* 187 (1968).
8. Movat, H. Z.; DiLorenzo, N. L. and Treloar, M. P.: Activation of the plasma kinin system by antigen-antibody aggregates. II. Isolation of permeability-enhancing and kinin-releasing fractions from activated guinea-pig serum. Lab. Invest. *19:* 201 (1968).
9. Pierce, J. V. and Webster, M. E.: The purification and some properties of two different kallidinogens from human plasma; in *Hypotensive Peptides*, G. E. Erdös, N. Bach, and F. Sicuteri, eds. (Springer, New York 1966).
10. Robertson, J. W.; Takeuchi, Y. and Movat, H. Z.: The demonstration of permeability factors and of two kinin-forming enzymes in rat serum.
11. Udaka, K.; Takeuchi, Y. and Movat, H. Z.: Simple physicochemical assay for quantitation of enhanced vascular permeability (to be published).
12. Vogt, W.: Demonstration of the presence of two separate kinin-forming systems in human and other plasma; in Hypotensive Peptides, e.g. Erdös, E. G.; Bach, N. and Sicuteri, F., eds. (Springer, New York 1966).
13. Vogt, W.; Garbe, G. und Schmidt, G.: Untersuchungen zur Existenz zweier verschiedener kininbildender Systeme in menschlichem Plasma. Arch. Pharmak. exp. Path. *256:* 127 (1967).

14. Vogt, W. und Wawretschek, W.: Weitere Untersuchungen zur Existenz zweier kininbildender Systeme in menschlichem Plasma. Arch. Pharmak. exp. Path. *260:* 223 (1968).
15. Webster, M. E.: Human plasma kallikrein, its activation and pathological role. Feder. Proc. *27:* 84 (1968).
16. Wilhelm, D. L.; Miles, A. A. and Mackay, M. E.: Enzyme-like globulins from the serum reproducing the vascular phenomena of inflammation. II. Isolation and properties of the permeability factor and its inhibition. Brit. J. exp. Path. *36:* 82 (1955).

Author's address: Dr. Henry Z. Movat, Division of Experimental Pathology, Medical Sciences Building, University of Toronto, *Toronto, Ont.* (Canada).

Cellular and Humoral Mechanisms in Anaphylaxis and Allergy, pp. 224–225
(Karger, Basel/New York 1969)

Kinin Generation Caused by two Immunologic Systems (Human IgG – Rheumatoid Factor Complex and Endotoxin – Antibody – Complement Complex)

Kenneth L. Melmon, Wallace Epstein, Margaret Tan and Alan S. Nies

Division of Clinical Pharmacology, Departments of Medicine and Pharmacology
Cardiovascular Research Institute
University of California, San Francisco Medical Center, San Francisco, Calif.

The early phase of endotoxin shock in man and in unanesthetized primates is characterized by hypotension without changes in cardiac output. The decreased peripheral vascular resistance correlates in time with a rising blood concentration of kinin. We have previously shown that human granulocyte-endotoxin interaction which can result in kinin production is *not* dependent on the 19S antibody to endotoxin. However, the kinin generation produced by endotoxin – plasma interaction appears related to distinctly different requirements.

The mechanism of kinin formation by endotoxin was investigated *in vitro* in normal adult human plasma, decomplemented plasma, Hageman factor deficient plasma and human newborn plasma. Endotoxin was found to activate plasma kinin-forming enzymes and deplete plasma kininogen only in the presence of complement and the naturally occurring antibody to endotoxin. The plasma-endotoxin interaction was inhibited by soybean trypsin inhibition but not by ovomucoid trypsin inhibitor. This pattern of inhibition implicates plasma kallikrein or plasmin as the enzymes responsible for kininogen conversion to kinin in this system. Normal Hageman factor *was not* necessary for kinin formation. Salicylates in pharmacological concentrations were able to block kinin formation by endotoxin but cortisol was not. We conclude that endotoxin reacts with antiendotoxin antibody and complement to activate plasma kallikrein or plasmin and that this can be effectively inhibited by salicylates but not hydrocortisone.

To determine whether kinin could be generated by endotoxin – plasma interaction only, another immunologic system was tested. Circulating rheumatoid factor is a regular concomitant of rheumatoid arthritis. There are no established mechanisms by which such a factor might initiate or sustain an inflammatory response. In the present study, the macroglobulin fraction of sera from 10 patients with rheumatoid arthritis and from 11 normals was isolated and individually combined with either aggregated or non-aggregated normal human IgG, and the mixture was added to fresh normal plasma. The kininogen content (trypsin-released kinin minus kinin in nontrypsinized plasma) was determined at 0 and 10 min. An average fall of $47.2 \pm 9.2\%$ in plasma kininogen resulted from the addition of aggregated IgG combined with rheumatoid macroglobulin. A significant difference $(P < 0.01)$ was found when normal macroglobulin plus aggregated IgG caused a decrease of only $9.1 \pm 6.8\%$. Combination of nonaggregated IgG with rheumatoid or normal macroglobulin resulted in kininogen depletion of 9.8% and 5.5% respectively. Controls of normal or rheumatoid macroglobulin or of aggregated or nonaggregated IgG individually added to normal plasma caused a kininogen fall of less than 5%. Naturally occurring 22S complex isolated from two rheumatoid sera caused the depletion of 38% and 40% of plasma kininogen. The 7S and 19S gamma globulins dissociated from the 22S complex were incapable of generating kinin, but their recombination restored this ability. Although the several rheumatoid macroglobulin fractions were high in rheumatoid factor hemagglutinating activity, the mixture of rheumatoid macroglobulin with aggregated IgG capable of kinin generation is itself devoid of such activity. These findings indicate that the antigen-antibody complex of aggregated IgG and rheumatoid factor also is capable of initiating kinin production.

Thus our data associated with investigations of other laboratories tends to indicate that a 'pathological' mechanism for kinin production may be intimately associated with the presence of abnormal immunologic systems.

Authors' address: KENNETH L. MELMON, M.D., WALLACE EPSTEIN, M.D., MARGARET TAN, M.D. and ALAN S. NIES, M.D., Department of Medicine, University of California, San Francisco Medical Center, *San Francisco, Calif.* (USA).

Cellular and Humoral Mechanisms in Anaphylaxis and Allergy, pp. 226–232
(Karger, Basel/New York 1969)

Radioimmunoassay for Bradykinin with an Iodinated Bradykinin Analog and Dextran-coated Charcoal[1]

Richard C. Talamo, Jocelyn Spragg, Edgar Haber and K. Frank Austen

Department of Medicine, Harvard Medical School at the Robert B. Brigham and Massachusetts General Hospitals Boston, Mass.

A meaningful assessment of the specific activation of the kinin system requires demonstration of depletion of the substrate (kininogen), activation of the kinin-forming enzyme (kallikrein) and production of the biologically-active nonapeptide bradykinin. The methods used should be highly specific and avoid denaturation of the native materials being measured. In order to develop functional assays for kininogen and kallikrein, it is first necessary to have a sensitive and specific method for the measurement of bradykinin and thus, our attention has been directed to the development of a radioimmunoassay for bradykinin [4, 7, 8].

Development of a radioimmunoassay for bradykinin involves the determination of the most appropriate immunogen, radioactive hapten, and the procedure by which antibody-bound radioactivity is separated from unbound. The first radioimmunoassay for bradykinin, developed by Spragg, Austen and Haber [4] (table I), involved the use of bradykinin linked to polylysine by toluene diisocyanate (BK-TC-PL+) as immunogen, an extrinsically-labeled radioactive hapten, [3H]-acetyl-N-bradykinin, and Sephadex G-25 gel filtration for the separation procedure. The sensitivity of this assay is in the 10 to 100 mμg range. A more sensitive assay has recently been developed [8], in the range of 0.1 to 10 mμg, employing bradykinin linked to ovalbumin via toluene diisocyanate (BK-TC-OA) as immunogen, an iodinated 8-tyrosine derivative of bradykinin as hapten and dextran-coated charcoal as a means of separating free from antibody-bound radioactivity.

[1] Supported by grants AI-07722–02 and AI-04967 from the National Institute of Allergy and Infectious Diseases and 60-094 from the Heart and Lung Foundation of the Harvard University Medical School.

Table I. Bradykinin radioimmunoassay

	SPRAGG, AUSTEN, HABER [4]	TALAMO, SPRAGG, AUSTEN, HABER [8]
Immunogen	BK-TC-PL	BK-TC-OA
Hapten	[^{3}H]-Ac-N-BK	[^{125}I]-tyr^8-BK
Separation procedure	Gel filtration	Dextran-charcoal
Sensitivity	10 mμg	0.1 mμg

Choice of Immunogen

Eight bradykinin-carrier compounds were prepared and employed for immunization of rabbits and monkeys in order to select the immunogen which most reliably elicited the production of antibody to bradykinin suitable for radio immunoassay [7]. Bradykinin was linked to three different polypeptide carriers by two different methods: The amino terminal of bradykinin was linked via toluene diisocyanate to the epsilon amino side chain groups of polylysine (BK-TC-PL$^+$), as previously described [4]. In order to obtain a bradykinin-carrier compound with a different net charge, the amino terminal of bradykinin was linked by carbodiimide condensation to the carboxyl groups of succinylated polylysine (BK-SUCC-PL$^-$). Because others had found a polyalanine, polylysine multichain co-polymer useful in rendering various polypeptides immunogenic [9], the amino terminal of bradykinin was coupled via toluene diisocyanate to the polyalanine side chains of this co-polymer (BK-TC-ALA-LYS$^+$).

These three compounds were complexed with protein molecules of considerable net opposite charge in the preparation of three additional materials for immunization. Horseshoe crab hemocyanin was succinylated (HCy-SUCC$^-$), in order to give it a net negative charge, and then complexed with the positively-charged molecules of either BK-TC-PL$^+$ or BK-TC-ALA-LYS$^+$. Positively-charged methylated bovine serum albumin (MeOBSA) was complexed with negatively-charged bradykinin polylysine succinate (BK-SUCC-PL$^-$).

Bradykinin was also linked to two different protein carriers: To ovalbumin via toluene diisocyanate (BK-TC-OA) and to rabbit serum albumin with a carbodiimide method previously employed by GOODFRIEND, LEVINE and FASMAN [1]. Toluene diisocyanate selectively couples the alpha-amino terminal of bradykinin to the amino side chains of the carrier molecule, resulting in an immunogen substituted in a relatively specific manner. The carbodiimide synthesis, on the other hand, allows coupling of several different side chains on both the peptide and the protein carrier, thus creating several different immunogenic configurations of the hapten.

Antibody activity was detected and followed at frequent intervals after immunization by binding of extrinsically-labeled [³H]-acetyl-N-bradykinin [7]. The peak response of individual animals and the time of the peak response were compared for the various methods of immunization which produced detectable binding of tritiated hapten. Bradykinin linked to ovalbumin via toluene diisocyanate (BK-TC-OA) elicited an antibody response in all 10 rabbits immunized. The response in a monkey was less than that observed in rabbits. Pre-immunization of rabbits with the carrier, ovalbumin, alone three weeks before giving the BK-TC-OA was not advantageous. The two complexes of bradykinin linked via toluene diisocyanate to either polylysine (BK-TC-PL⁺) or polyalanine-polylysine (BK-TC-ALA-LYS⁺) with hemocyanin-succinate (HCy-SUCC⁻) elicited minimal responses. There was no response to BK-SUCC-PL⁻ or to the complex of BK-SUCC-PL⁻ with MeOBSA; no response to BK-TC-PL⁺ was elicited in four rabbits or two monkeys in the comparative study of various bradykinin-carrier compounds [7], although one out of 12 rabbits has produced a useful level in another study [4, 5, 6].

Antiserum to the bradykinin-rabbit serum albumin conjugate (BK-RSA) bound a relatively large amount of [³H]-acetyl-N-bradykinin. However, this antiserum is not primarily directed against native bradykinin. In competitive binding studies, more than 1,000 times more unlabeled bradykinin was needed to achieve 50% inhibition of binding of [³H]-acetyl-N-bradykinin by anti-BK-RSA as compared to the amounts of unlabeled bradykinin needed for 50% inhibition with antisera against BK-TC-PL⁺ or BK-TC-OA. Further, binding curves performed with intrinsically-labeled [¹⁴C]-bradykinin demonstrated that rabbit anti-BK-RSA had a titer of 2.4 mcg/ml antibody protein and a binding affinity of 0.32×10^7 M^{-1}; anti-BK-TC-PL⁺ had a titer of 7.2 mcg/ml and a binding affinity of 0.75×10^7 M^{-1}; anti-BK-TC-OA had a titer of 22 mcg/ml antibody protein and a binding affinity of 0.65×10^7 M^{-1}.

Immunization of rabbits with bradykinin linked to the immunogenic carrier ovalbumin via toluene diisocyanate proved to be the method of choice for production of antibody to bradykinin for radioimmunoassay. The criteria governing this conclusion include immunogenicity of the compound used and the specificity and affinity of the antibody elicited.

Choice of Radioactive Hapten

The properties of an appropriate radioactive hapten for use in bradykinin radioimmunoassay would include the following: It must bind well with bradykinin antiserum and not with pre-immunization serum from the same rabbit; it must be displaced readily from antibody by native bradykinin; the hapten should have a high specific activity, so as to achieve the degree of sensitivity necessary for measurement of bradykinin; and it must be possible to prepare the radiolabeled hapten in relatively pure form, free of competing unlabeled hapten and labeled altered products.

The extrinsically-labeled hapten, [³H]-acetyl-N-bradykinin (fig. 1), as originally prepared by SPRAGG, AUSTEN and HABER [4], was found useful in the detection of the immune response to bradykinin [7], in the development of the initial radioimmunoassay for bradykinin [4], and in studies with structural analogs of bradykinin [5]. The specific activity of this hapten, 1500 mC/mM, allowed detection of bradykinin in the 10 to 100 mμg range. Because a greater degree of sensitivity was required, and because stored preparations of this hapten were found to contain impurities demonstrable by high voltage electrophoresis, attention was directed toward the development of other labeled haptens for the radioimmunoassay.

Intrinsically-labeled [¹⁴C]-bradykinin (fig. 1) was produced by the New England Nuclear Corp. in nearly pure form, with a specific activity of 250 mC/mM[2]. This hapten appeared stable in storage at −70°C in 0.1 N acetic acid. It has been employed along with analogs and fragments of bradykinin in determining the structural requirements for binding to anti-bradykinin

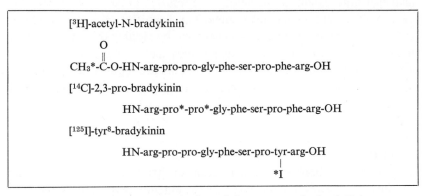

Fig. 1. Various radiolabeled haptens in the radioimmunoassay for bradykinin.

[2] Made available by the National Heart Institute.

antibody elicited by various immunogens [5, 6]. It has also been useful in studies of the titer and binding affinity of various antisera to bradykinin [7].

Since the amino acid sequence of native bradykinin (H-arg-pro-pro-gly-phe-ser-pro-phe-arg-OH) does not contain a tyrosine residue, it was necessary to consider structural analogs which contain tyrosine, in order to obtain a radioactive hapten containing a high specific activity isotope of iodine. Tyr[8]-bradykinin was obtained from the New England Nuclear Corp. and purified by carboxymethyl-Sephadex column chromatography. This analog differs from native bradykinin in that it has the added hydroxyl group of tyrosine, in the 8 position, usually occupied by phenylalanine. Tyr[8]-bradykinin inhibits the binding of [14C]-bradykinin to antibody prepared against BK-TC-OA 1/3 as well as native bradykinin, and has a biological activity 1/6 that of native bradykinin when assayed on the estrus rat uterus. [125I]-tyr[8]-bradykinin (fig. 1) was prepared by the method of GREENWOOD and HUNTER [8] and purified by high voltage electrophoresis and column chromatography with sulfoethyl-Sephadex C-25. This hapten has a specific activity of approximately 3,700 mC/mM, binds well to antibody-containing sera and not to pre-immunization sera, and is readily displaced by native bradykinin, permitting the radioimmuno assay of native bradykinin with a sensitivity in the 0.1 to 10 mμg range [8].

Choice of Method of Separation of Antibody-Bound Radioactivity

After incubation of antibody with labeled hapten and varying amounts of unlabeled bradykinin, gel filtration on Sephadex G-25 has been used for separation of antibody-bound radioactivity from free radiolabeled hapten [4, 5, 6, 7]. A standard curve was constructed by plotting the per cent inhibition of binding of radioactive hapten against the varying amounts of unlabeled bradykinin added. More than two hours are required to obtain each point on a standard inhibition curve and a separate column is run for each point.

A rapid method for solid phase adsorption of free radiolabeled hapten on dextran-coated charcoal has been used in the radioimmunoassay of insulin by HERBERT et al. [3]; this technique has been adapted for radioimmunoassay of bradykinin [8]. Dextran of 70,000 molecular weight fills the sites on charcoal particles which would otherwise adsorb antibody molecules, leaving sites available for adsorption of the small molecular weight hapten. [125I]-tyr[8]-bradykinin, antiserum and various amounts of

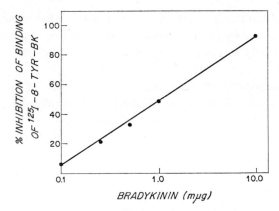

Fig. 2. Inhibition of binding of [^{125}I]-tyr^{8}-bradykinin to antibody by varying amounts of unlabeled bradykinin.

unlabeled bradykinin are incubated in the cold for two hours; binding of the labeled and unlabeled haptens to antibody takes place. A solution of dextran-coated charcoal is added, and the free hapten, both radioactive and un-labeled, is taken up immediately by the available small molecular sites on the charcoal. The mixture is centrifuged, leaving only the antibody-bound hapten in solution in the supernate. An aliquot of the supernate is removed for gamma counting and a standard curve is constructed by plotting the per cent inhibition of binding of radioactive hapten against the varying amounts of unlabeled bradykinin added (fig. 2). With increases of unlabeled brady-kinin over the range of 0.1 to 10 mμg there is an increase of inhibition of binding of the iodinated hapten to antibody from 6 to 92%. In comparison to gel filtration, the dextran-coated charcol method of separation of free radiolabeled hapten from that bound to antibody offers greater speed of preformance; an entire inhibition curve and several test samples can be run at once.

Conclusions

Immunization of rabbits with bradykinin linked to the immunogenic carrier ovalbumin via toluene diisocyanate has proved to be the method of choice for production of antibody for radioimmunoassay of bradykinin. The criteria governing this conclusion include immunogenicity of the compound used and the specificity and affinity of the antibody elicited.

[^{125}I]-tyr^{8}-bradykinin, an iodinated analog of bradykinin, is the radio-labeled hapten of choice for radioimmunoassay of bradykinin, because it binds well to antibody-containing sera and not to pre-immunization sera, is readily displaced by native bradykinin from binding to antisera, and has the specific activity necessary for measurement of bradykinin at the 0.1 mμg level.

The dextran-coated charcoal method of separation of antibody-bound radiolabeled hapten from free radiolabeled hapten offers greater speed of performance and reproducibility than gel filtration.

The radioimmunoassay for bradykinin has a sensitivity equivalent to that obtained in the biologic assay using the estrus rat uterus (0.1 mμg), but has the added advantages of specificity and ease of performing numerous determinations simultaneously.

Acknowledgments

The expert technical assistance of Mrs. ANN KITTELBERGER and Miss ADELE LUNAN is gratefully acknowledged.

References

1. GOODFRIEND, T.L.; LEVINE, L. and FASMAN, G.D.: Antibodies to bradykinin and angiotensin: A use of carbodiimides in immunology. Science 144: 1344–1345 (1964).
2. GREENWOOD, F.C. and HUNTER, W.M.: The preparation of ^{131}I-labeled human growth hormone of high specific radioactivity. Biochem. J. 89: 114–123 (1963).
3. HERBERT, V.; LAU, K.-S.; GOTTLIEB, C.W. and BLEICHER, S.J.: Coated charcoal immunoassay of insulin. J. clin. Endocrin. 25: 1375–1384 (1965).
4. SPRAGG, J.; AUSTEN, K.F. and HABER, E.: Production of antibody against bradykinin: Demonstration of specificity by complement fixation and radioimmunoassay. J. Immunol. 96: 865–871 (1966).
5. SPRAGG, J.; SCHRÖDER, E.; STEWART, J.M.; AUSTEN, K.F. and HABER, E.: Structural requirements for binding to antibody of sequence variants of bradykinin. Biochem. J. 6: 3933–3941 (1967).
6. SPRAGG, J.; TALAMO, R.C.; SUZUKI, K.; APPELBAUM, D.M.; AUSTEN, K.F. and HABER, E.: Structural requirements for binding of bradykinin to antibody. II. Studies with bradykinin fragments. Biochem. J. 7: 4086–4089 (1968).
7. TALAMO, R.C.; HABER, E. and AUSTEN, K.F.: Antibody to bradykinin: Effect of carrier and method of coupling on specificity and affinity. J. Immunol. 101: 333–341 (1968).
8. TALAMO, R.C.; SPRAGG, J.; AUSTEN, K.F. and HABER, E.: Radio-immunoassay of bradykinin; in Methods in Immunology and Immunochemistry. Vol. III (Academic Press, New York 1968).
9. SELA, M. and ARNON, R.A.: A specific synthetic polypeptide antigen. Biochim. Acta 40: 382–384 (1960).

Authors' address: RICHARD C. TALAMO, M.D., JOCELYN SPRAGG, EDGAR HABER, M.D., and K. FRANK AUSTEN, M.D., Dept. of Medicine, Harvard Medical School at the Robert B. Brigham and Massachusetts General Hospital, *Boston, Mass.* (USA).

Cellular and Humoral Mechanisms in Anaphylaxis and Allergy, pp. 233–236
(Karger, Basel/New York 1969)

The Kallikrein-kinin-kininase System

(Chairman's closing remarks)[1]

E. G. ERDÖS

Dept. of Pharmacology, University of Oklahoma School of Medicine,
Oklahoma City, Okla.

I should like to touch upon three aspects of the kinin problem.

Those of us who follow the progress of research on the kallikrein–kinin system are often perplexed and the unitiated outsiders are discouraged by the complexities of the system. In addition to the plethora of important factors involved in kinin release, blood plasma of man and some animals contains at least two different, parallel kallikrein-kinin systems. Activation of both systems results in kinin release and subsequent inactivation of the peptide. Thus besides the existence of a number of kallikrein activators, kallikrein, kallikrein inhibitor and kininogen occur in two or more forms in human plasma. Figures 1 and 2 present the evidence for the existence of two kininases [4]. Gel filtration of human plasma on Sephadex G-200 column revealed that in addition to carboxypeptidase N (kininase I) another enzyme is also responsible for the inactivation of kinins (fig. 1). The peptidase and esterase activities, as measured with HLL and HLAa substrates were found in a single protein peak. The kininase gave a broader peak, however, than the carboxypeptidase. When this plasma protein fraction containing the kininase activity was adsorbed on a DEAE-Sephadex A-50 column and eluted stepwise, two kininase were separated (fig. 2). One peak contained carboxypeptidase N (kininase I). This enzyme inactivated bradykinin by cleaving the C-terminal Arg[9]. The other peak contained an enzyme that split the Pro[7]-Phe[8] bond of bradykinin, thus removed the C-terminal phenylalanyl-arginine dipeptide. In this respect, it was similar to an enzyme called peptidase P that occurs in swine kidney microsomes [1].

[1] This work was supported in part by a grant No. HE-08764 from the National Institute of Health, U.S.P.H.S.

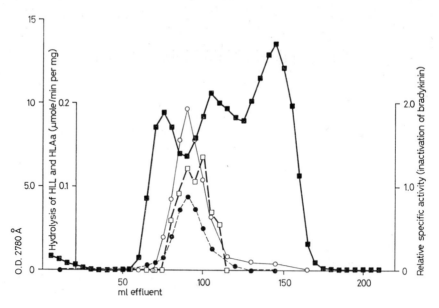

Fig. 1. 'Sephadex G-200' filtration of human plasma kininases. 15 ml of fresh heparinized human plasma was filtered through a 3.5 × 46 cm column. A 0.05 molar phosphate buffer, pH 7, containing 0.5 moles/l of sodium chloride was the eluent. 5 ml fractions were collected every 30 min. HLL, Hippuryl-L-lysine; HLAa, Hippuryl-L-argininic acid. ■———■, protein; □———□.hydrolysis of bradykinin; ▲······▲, hydrolysis of HLL; ○———○, hydrolysis of HLAa (from YANG and ERDÖS [4]).

Human blood plasma and that of various animals contains two kininases with different bond affinities and inhibition pattern. Very likely the two enzymes originate from different organs as well.

After having contributed to the complexity of the problem by showing the simultaneous existence of two kininases, I should like to urge you to seek ways to simplify the system. Obviously we need rapid, reliable and quantitative assays. It is also evident that all the factors cannot be measured simultaneously. Perhaps we should learn from studies on blood coagulation. Although some thirteen factors are involved in coagulation there are various tests designed to measure only one factor or just a few of them. In the kinin field we should aim also for establishing minimal assay systems, that take only a few of the available components into consideration. Such a simplified system could be based, for example, on assaying the amount of kinin released in plasma, when the kininase is inhibited and the plasma kallikrein is activated via the contact factor. Thus we would deal with only four com-

ponents in mammalian blood plasma: (1) a kallikrein activator. (2) prekallikrein. (3) kininogen and (4) kininase that can be inhibited by o-phenanthroline.
This system, which is similar to that used by Margolis years ago, would
measure the amount of kinin released when one of the plasma kininogenases
is activated by Hageman factor. The 'minimal system' described would
reflect the activation of an endogenous plasma kininogenase in mammals
in vitro and in some reptiles such as turtles or alligators. Birds which lack the
contact factor also release plasma kinin when the contact factor is transferred
from reptilian or mammalian plasma [2]. In other words avian plasma, that has
components 2, 3 and 4, can also be included here after the transfer of 1.

Similar simple standard tests based on taking a minimum number of
components into consideration should be devised for assaying links in the
kallikrein-kinin system.

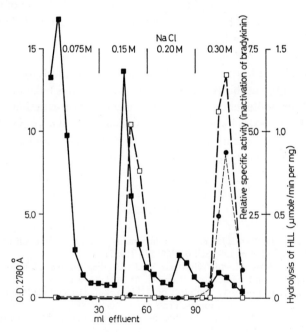

Fig. 2. Separation of the two kininases on a DEAE-'Sephadex A-50' column. 300 mg of
protein obtained after gel filtration was purified on a 1 × 30 cm column. Fractions were
eluted step by step by increasing the concentration of sodium chloride in a 0.02 molar
phosphate buffer, pH 6.8. 5 ml was collected every 30 min. The activity eluted with 0.3
molar sodium chloride contains kininase I (carboxypeptidase N). Kininase II moved with
the fraction that was eluted with 0.15 molar sodium chloride. HLL, Hippuryl-L-lysine.
■———■, protein; □———□, hydrolysis of bradykinin; ▲·······▲, hydrolysis of
HLL (from YANG and ERDÖS [4]).

Finally we may ask, what is the importance of the presence of the kalli-krein-kinin-kininase system in blood? Maybe we will find the answer when the evolution of the kallikreins, kinins and kininases will be studied in a variety of animals other than mammals. For example, frog skin contains free active kinin and wasp venom has active kinins. Snake venom is a rich source of kallikrein-like enzymes. We could not release kinin from native frog plasma or snake plasma, although relatively large amounts of the peptide are present in inactive form as kininogen in the blood of the so-called 'higher', phylo-genetically diversed animals, such as mammals, turtles, etc. Such plasma release active kinin upon activation of endogenous kininogenases. Since many tests showed bradykinin to be among the most potent endogenous materials – I am thinking here of pain, vascular permeability or vaso-dilation –, it might be a substance with a relatively simple function in 'lower' animals that has been included into a complex system in blood of mammals, etc. As kinin is released by various processes, it is also inactivated and remov-ed from the circulation [3]. Thus kinins may belong to those noxious sub-stances that are more important under pathological than under normal conditions. The kallikrein-kinin-kininase system is a carefully balanced one in blood of mammals, birds and some reptiles. When this balance is disturbed by the lack or malfunction of one component or over-reaction of another, the free kinin can exert its action, and contributes to a syndrome. Besides the pathological conditions mentioned in this volume, there are numerous other symptoms where this type of reactions may occur.

References

1. ERDÖS, E. G. and YANG, H. Y. T.: An enzyme in microsomal fraction of kidney that inactivates bradykinin. Life Sci. 6: 569–574 (1967).
2. ERDÖS, E. G.; MIWA, I. and GRAHAM, W. J.: Studies on the evolution of plasma kinins: reptilian and avian blood. Life Sci. 6: 2433–2439 (1967).
3. ERDÖS, E. G.: Hypotensive peptides: bradykinin, kallidin and eledoisin. Adv. Phar-macol. vol. 4, pp. 1–90 (Academic Press, New York 1966).
4. YANG, H. Y. T. and ERDÖS, E. G.: Second kininase in human blood plasma. Nature, Lond. 215: 1402–1403 (1967).

Author's address: E. G. ERDÖS, Department of Pharmacology, University of Oklahoma School of Medicine, Oklahoma City, Okla. (USA).

Anaphylatoxin and Biologically Active Fragments of Complement

Cellular and Humoral Mechanisms in Anaphylaxis and Allergy, pp. 237–252
(Karger, Basel/New York 1969)

Biologically Active Cleavage Products of Components of Complement[1]

IRWIN H. LEPOW, W. DIAS DA SILVA and RICHARD A. PATRICK[2]
Department of Pathology, Health Center, University of Connecticut, Hartford, Conn.

Among the many fascinating and gratifying facets of the development of modern immunology has been the effective, synergistic interplay among chemical, biological, pathobiological and clinical approaches to the solution of fundamental problems. Our present exciting stage of dynamic progress could not, of course, have been reached without a lag period between biological and medical observations and the emergence of biochemical concepts and techniques. With their emergence, however, this synergism soon became an important theme of immunological investigations. The patient with multiple myeloma sheds light on biological mechanisms of immunoglobulin synthesis and provides proteins which have contributed significantly to our understanding of the chemistry and genetics of immunoglobulins. This information, in turn, adds to our appreciation of the pathophysiology of the disease and, in part, suggests approaches to management. Conversely, biochemical description of IgA as a discrete class of immunoglobulins and biochemical and biological recognition of secretory IgA make possible rational insights into mechanisms of host resistance in infections of

[1] Original investigations were supported by Grant Nos. AI-01255 and AI-08251, National Institute of Allergy and Infectious Diseases, National Institutes of Health.

In accordance with recently adopted conventions of nomenclature, the nine components of complement, previously designated C'1 ... C'9 are now referred to as C1 ... C9. The subunits of C1, previously designated C'1q, C'1r and C'1s, are now referred to as C1q, C1r and C1s. Activated C1 and activated C1s̄, previously designated C'1a and C'1 esterase, are now referred to as C1̄ and C1s̄. Biologically active small fragments of C3 and C5, previously designated F(a)C'3 and F(a)C'5, are now referred to as C3a and C5a; the larger fragments are referred to as C3b and C5b. The larger fragment of C2 which is incorporated with C4 into 'C3 convertase' is referred to as C2a; C3 convertase is written C4̄,C2a.

[2] Research Fellow of the Connecticut Heart Association.

mucosal surfaces and fresh approaches to protection against these diseases by immunological means.

The pattern of evolution of complement research has followed a similar but, as yet, less fully developed course. The lag between initial biological and medical observations and the establishment of a biochemical base was lengthened by the complexity of the complement system, the lability and trace concentrations of some of the complement components, and the dependence on advances in immunoglobulin structure and function. However, the lag period is now well passed and the fruitful interaction among biochemists, biologists, pathologists and clinicians, as in the main-stream of immunology, is already clearly apparent. For example, purifi-cation of the components of complement has not only permitted study of biochemical mechanism of action but has also made possible preparation of specific antisera with which to detect individual components in experimental and clinical lesions and to measure components in pathological sera. Using basic information on the purification and immunogenicity of human C3 developed by MÜLLER-EBERHARD and his coworkers [39, 45], ALPER and ROSEN [1] observed a specific depletion of this component in sera of patients with progressive glomerulonephritis. Further study led to the conclusion that this was ascribable to decreased biosynthesis of C3, a finding which now requires biochemical explanation and emphasizes our current ignorance of control of synthesis of complement components.

A similar interplay, in this case initiated at the pathobiological and clinical level, is exemplified by the major subject of this paper: biologically active cleavage products of components of complement and the multiple nature of anaphylatoxin. An attempt will be made to approach the topic from this developmental perspective. Since Dr. VOGT will be presenting data suggesting that an anaphylatoxin may be derived from the action of a non-complement enzyme on a non-complement component substrate, we shall restrict ourselves to experiments bearing on the complement system.

Historical Background

The term 'anaphylatoxin' was introduced by FRIEDBERGER in 1910 to describe a property that induced a syndrome similar to anaphylactic shock in guinea pigs when homologous serum was exposed to immune precipitates [16]. Shortly thereafter, BORDET found that a similar property could be generated from guinea-pig serum with agar [5, 6] and NATHAN showed that starch and inulin were also effective [43, 44]. Generation of anaphylatoxin in rabbit and rat serum was reported by Novy and DE KRUIF in 1917 [46]. DALE and KELLAWAY observed contraction of guinea-pig ileum *in vitro* by anaphylatoxin in 1923 [9]. Following a rather protracted period of relative dormancy, interest in anaphylatoxin was renewed when HAHN and OBERDORF in 1950 [19], ROCHA E SILVA, BIER and ARONSON in 1951 [53], and MOTA in 1959 [36] published data indicating that the action of anaphylatoxin could be explained, at least in part, by its histamine-releasing properties.

FRIEDBERGER himself, in 1911, suggested that the complement system might be involved in anaphylatoxin formation [17] but the chemical base on which to explore this hypothesis was lacking. Indeed, at that time, knowledge of complement was restricted to two components: mittstück and endstück (midpiece and endpiece). The hypothesis was revived in the 1950's, by which time four components of complement were recognized and known to act in the sequence C1, C4, C2, C3. Within the context of this information, OSLER and his coworkers in 1959 made a major advance by investigating the effects of immune aggregates on fresh rat serum [47]. They demonstrated a direct relationship between loss in hemolytic activity of the serum, loss in activity of C3, and generation of an activity which, by virtue of contraction of smooth muscle with tachyphylaxis and enhancement of vascular permeability in guinea pig skin, closely resembled anaphylatoxin. This study was and is a landmark in the history of anaphylatoxin but further broadening and exploitation of the chemical base was necessary before a more definitive attack on the problem could be launched.

In the mid-1950's, the first biochemical information on the mechanism of action of complement began to emerge. Work by LEVINE [32], BECKER [3, 4], and PILLEMER, RATNOFF and LEPOW [26–29, 31, 51] indicated that C1 exists in serum as an enzyme precursor which is activated by complexes of antigen and complement-fixing antibody. The natural substrates for the active enzyme were shown to be C4 and C2 but esterolysis of selected amino acid esters was also demonstrated. Further work in our laboratory established that human C1 is a macromolecular complex of three different subunits, designated C1q, C1r and C1s, the integrity of which is maintained by Ca^{2+} [25, 42]; that the catalytic site of activated C1 resides on the C1s portion of the macromolecule [42]; that activated C1s (then referred to as C'1-esterase) could be highly purified and retain its enzymatic activity both on synthetic amino acid esters and on C4 and C2 in free solution [18]; and that a normal serum inhibitor of activated C1 or activated C1s exists and could be purified [24, 33, 48, 51].

It was at this point that a clinical observation was made which gave great impetus to the anaphylatoxin problem. DONALDSON and EVANS found that patients with hereditary angioneurotic edema had a genetic deficiency of the serum inhibitor of activated C1 [14]. It was further discovered that during attacks of edema these patients had circulating *active* C1 and essentially complete disappearance of hemolytically active C4 and C2 [15]. This *in vivo* pattern of complement component utilization was identical to that previously described from our laboratory in *in vitro* experiments. It led RATNOFF and LEPOW to speculate anew about the possible role of the complement system, and particularly activated C1, in initiating events leading to enhanced vascular permeability. With the availability of highly purified human activated C1s in our laboratory and Dr. RATNOFF's recent return from sabbatical leave in Dr. ASHLEY MILES' laboratory, it was a relatively simple matter to act on these speculations. In short, activated C1s was quickly shown to be a permeability factor in guinea-pig skin and its effect was referable to a mechanism involving histamine release [52]. Soon thereafter we were able to construct an *in vitro* system in which incubation of very small amounts of human C1s̄ with fresh guinea-pig serum led to generation of a permeability factor as a function of depletion of hemolytic complement [55], in a manner very similar to that reported earlier by OSLER and coworkers for immune aggregates [47]. The concept that C1s̄ might be an inducer of anaphylatoxin formation then emerged as a prime possibility. Indeed, DIAS DA SILVA and LEPOW soon showed that the activity generated from fresh guinea pig or rat serum by human C1s̄ satisfied available criteria for anaphylatoxin: in addition to enhancing vascular permeability in guinea pig skin, it contracted guinea pig ileum with tachyphylaxis, failed to contract rat uterus, and degranulated mast cells in guinea pig mesentery preparations. Furthermore, its activities were blocked by triprolidine, an anti-histaminic drug and cross-desensitization of guinea-pig ileum with rat agar anaphylatoxin was achieved [10]. It appeared highly probable, therefore, that anaphylatoxin might well be a product of the complement system. Parenthetically, it must be emphasized that, although this series of investigations was prompted by patients with hereditary angioneurotic edema, it is now quite clear that anaphylatoxin is not the mediator of edema formation in this disease.

Between 1962 and 1965, concurrently with the studies just described, the chemical base of the complement system was further broadened. C3 was shown by several groups to be first two, then three, then four and ultimately six components, now called C3, C5, C6, C7, C8 and C9. Human C4, C2, C3 and C5 were purified in MÜLLER-EBERHARD's laboratory [38, 39, 45, 49, 50] and human C2 was simultaneously purified in our laboratory [30]. Purified C1s̄ was already available [18]. The possible ingredients for direct examination of the anaphylatoxin problem were therefore at hand.

C3a: A Cleavage Product of Human C3 as an Anaphylatoxin

It was reasoned by Dias da Silva and Lepow that a free solution system of purified components of complement would be the experimental model of choice. The requirement for antigen-antibody complexes or other inducers of anaphylatoxin formation could be bypassed by using C1s̄ as the initiator of subsequent reactions of the complement cascade. Since the primary function of the immune complex with respect to complement is to effect activation of C1 to C1̄, purified C1s̄ could be employed as a means of entering the complement sequence at the point of completion of the first major reaction step. Examination of biological activities and biochemical events in such a system would be uncomplicated by possible uncertainties in the choice of antigen and antibody and the presence of an insoluble phase. Investigations were therefore begun on reaction mixtures consisting solely of purified components of human complement [11, 12].

Various combinations of early acting, purified components were incubated together in the presence of Mg^{2+} at pH 7.4, ionic strength 0.15 and tested for appearance of an activity which would contract guinea-pig ileum *in vitro*. No activity was observed with mixtures consisting of C1s̄, C4 and C2; C1s̄, C4 and C3; C1s̄, C2 and C3; or C2, C3 and C4. However, incubation of C1s̄, C4, C2 and C3 at 37°C resulted in very rapid appearance of a property which contracted guinea-pig ileum with tachyphylaxis. The concentrations of reactants which were required were all well within the normal physiological range of these components. In keeping with known mechanisms of the C2 step, Mg^{2+} was an absolute requirement for generation of biological activity. It was also of distinct interest that appearance of the smooth muscle-contracting property could be correlated with immunoelectrophoretic conversion of C3 from its characteristic position in the β_1-globulin region to anodically faster species, suggesting the possibility that the biologically active factor might be a product of the C3 step.

In addition to contracting guinea-pig ileum with tachyphylaxis, mixtures of C1s̄, C4, C2 and C3 possessed other biological properties which were consistent with identification as anaphylatoxin: failure to contract rat uterus, enhancement of vascular permeability in guinea-pig skin, degranulation of

mast cells in guinea pig mesentery preparations, and blocking of biological
activities by the anti-histaminic drug, triprolidine. There were, however, two
properties of this mixture of purified components of human complement
which were inconsistent with classical descriptions of anaphylatoxin:
release of histamine from *rat* peritoneal mast cells and failure to cross-
desensitize guinea pig ileum to rat or guinea pig anaphylatoxins generated by
incubation of the respective sera with agar or C1s̄. Although these observations gave pause concerning the identity of our activity with classical
anaphylatoxin, it was also admissable at that time that they might be
referable to special properties of *human* anaphylatoxin. Our index of sus-
picion was, however, raised that the anaphylatoxin problem might be more
complex than projected at the outset.

Attempts were then made to isolate the biologically active factor in
mixtures of C1s̄, C4, C2 and C3 and to determine its relationship to a
component of human complement. These experiments were initially thwarted
by failure to recover any biological activity following various separation
procedures performed at pH 7.4. Since recombination of fractions did not
restore activity, it was reasonable to assume that the isolated factor lost
activity rapidly under the conditions in use. At this point, an observation of
STEGEMANN, VOGT and FRIEDBERG was indepedently confirmed that
anaphylatoxin is stabilized at low pH values [57]. It then became possible to
incubate C1s̄, C4, C2 and C3 at pH 7.4 to generate biological activity, to
adjust pH to 3.5, to perform sucrose density gradient ultracentrifugations
and gel filtrations at pH 3.5, and to recover biological activity in fractions of
relatively low molecular weight. Thus, the property being sought was a
cleavage product of one or more reactants in the mixture of complement
components. Identification of the origin of the product was achieved by
performing experiments with components externally labeled with [125]I [13].

It was soon shown that C3 and only C3 was the component which was
cleaved to yield the biologically active fragment. When ^{125}I-C3 was employed
in reaction mixtures with the remaining three unlabeled components,
labeled fractions were obtained from the top of sucrose gradients and a
retarded region of Biogel P-60 columns which contracted guinea pig ileum
with tachyphylaxis. When C1s̄, C4 or C2 were labeled with ^{125}I in comparable
experiments, *unlabeled* fractions of low molecular weight were recovered
which had biological activity. Since the C3 used was pure by all available
criteria, the conclusion was clear that the ileum-contracting activity was a
property of a cleavage product of C3. The fragment, originally designated
F(a)C′3, is now referred to as C3a.

C3a had all of the biological properties originally observed in mixtures of C1s̄, C4, C2 and C3, including release of histamine from rat peritoneal mast cells and failure to cross-desensitize guinea-pig ileum to contraction by classical sources of anaphylatoxin. In more recent unpublished experiments, performed in collaboration with Dr. FRED S. ROSEN at the Childrens Hospital in Boston, we have observed that purified C3a is highly active in enhancing vascular permeability in *human* skin. Whereas intradermal injection of 1–2 μg of C3a into guinea pigs previously injected with Evans Blue produces a local lesion of blueing of about 4 mm diameter, maximal response in human skin is achieved at a dosage of 10–50 ng. The lesion consists of a wheal of 10–12 mm diameter, sometimes exhibiting pseudopodia, surrounded by an irregular zone of erythema. The total diameter of the lesion is 25–40 mm. Suppression of this response by pyribenzamine has also been observed. Thus, human C3a is not only active in human skin but is some two orders of magnitude more active than in guinea-pig skin.

The studies with mixtures of C1s̄, C4, C2 and C3 clearly demonstrated that biological properties at least in part consistent with anaphylatoxin were associated with a cleavage product of C3 having a molecular weight of about 6,800. At the time of these investigations, such a fragment had not been described as a product of the C3 step of complement action. Indeed, available evidence from direct studies by MÜLLER-EBERHARD and coworkers on the mechanism of immunoelectrophoretic conversion of C3 indicated that fragmentation of C3 did not occur [40]. The pathobiological approach, coupled with biochemical experiments, therefore contributed to understanding of fundamental mechanisms and led MÜLLER-EBERHARD'S group to a reinvestigation of the nature of immunœlectrophoretic conversion of C3 by prior acting components [41]. In an elegant series of experiments, they showed that C1s̄ acts on C4 and C2 to form a new enzyme, $\overline{C4, C2a}$, which in turn attacks C3. When the products of the C3 step were examined at low pH, a fragment with the previously described biological and physicochemical properties of C3a was found.

The mechanism of generation of C3a by C1s̄, C4, C2 and C3 may therefore be written:

$$C4 + C2 \xrightarrow{\ \text{C1s̄}\ } \overline{C4, C2a} + \text{Products}$$

$$C3 \xrightarrow{\ \overline{C4, C2a}\ } C3a + C3b$$

C3a is liberated to express potentially its biological properties relevant to histamine release. C3b, the large residual portion of the original C3 molecule, is incorporated into the antigen-antibody-complement complex. In the case of immune hemolysis, the complex formed is $EAC\overline{1}, C\overline{4}, \overline{C2a}, C3b$. This intermediate is not only reactive with the remaining components of complement in a sequence culminating in hemolysis but is, of itself, capable of entering into various secondary phenomena. These include immune adherence, immunoconglutination, conglutination and enhanced phagocytosis. The mechanism of C3 fragmentation is therefore uncommonly economical and sets the stage for diverse pathobiological phenomena [7].

An important concept follows from these considerations: at points short of full expression of the complement sequence terminating in cell membrane lesions and immune cytotoxicity, intermediate complexes and reaction products are formed which have their own pathobiological properties. Activities of the complement system, accordingly, are no longer to be viewed as an obligatory consequence of the action of all of the components. The generation and functioning of C3a represent a case in point.

An equally important concept has emerged from further studies on C3 fragmentation: components of complement may be utilized as substrates by enzymes which are entirely unrelated to the complement system. For example, a cleavage product of C3 with biological properties indistinguishable from C3a may be prepared by incubation of human C3 with small amounts of trypsin for very short periods of time [8, 23]. More prolonged incubation results in further degradation of both the a and b fragments. Plasmin can cleave a fragment of molecular weight 6,000 from C3; this product has marked chemotactic activity for polymorphonuclear leukocytes [59]. A purified constituent of cobra venom can form a complex with a serum protein unrelated to complement and then act on C3 to effect cleavage of a fragment with properties very similar to C3a [37]. These illustrative examples serve to demonstrate that the complement system may be entered at points beyond the earliest components by pathways which may be entirely independent of an immunological event. Activities of the complement system, accordingly, are no longer to be viewed as an obligatory consequence of the interaction of an antigen-antibody complex with C1, the formation of $C\overline{1}$, the subsequent formation of $C\overline{4}, \overline{C2a}$, etc. The potential role of complement as a mediator of inflammation is therefore not restricted to immunopathological insult.

C5a: A Cleavage Product of Human C5 as an Anaphylatoxin

Concurrently with the studies described above on human C3a, Jensen was investigating the role of components of guinea-pig complement in anaphylatoxin formation. Utilizing partially purified preparations of guinea pig components and inducing agents which included immune complexes, cobra venom and trypsin evidence was obtained that C5 was a source of anaphylatoxin [20, 21]. There was no reason to doubt the validity of either JENSEN's observations on guinea pig C5 or those on human C3. Although the apparent discrepancy could have been due to species differences, it was considered at least equally probable that both C3 and C5 might serve as anaphylatoxinogens. The latter view was particularly attractive in the light of previously cited unexpected properties of human C3a.

Prompted by JENSEN's experiments, COCHRANE and MÜLLER-EBERHARD in unpublished experiments in 1967 incubated purified human C5 with trypsin and obtained an activity which contracted guinea-pig ileum with tachyphylaxis. This observation was pursued in our laboratory and a fragment of C5 was soon obtained by gel filtration of incubated mixtures of human C5 and trypsin [23]. This product, previously designated F(a)C'5 and now referred to as C5a, was somewhat larger than C3a, emerging from Biogel columns close to the region of cytochrome c. In common with C3a, it contracted guinea-pig ileum with tachyphylaxis, failed to contract rat uterus, enhanced vascular permeability in guinea pig skin, degranulated mast cells in guinea pig mesentery preparations, and was blocked by triprolidine. However, it differed biologically from C3a in two noteworthy respects: it *failed* to liberate histamine from *rat* peritoneal mast cells and it was *active* in cross-desensitizing guinea-pig ileum to preparations of classical anaphylatoxin, such as rat serum incubated with agar. Thus, human C5a fulfilled all of the known criteria for classical anaphylatoxin. The special attributes of human C3a were therefore not referable to unique properties of human anaphylatoxin but rather to the existence of a previously undescribed activity. In these terms, C3a was a new anaphylatoxin and C5a was the classical anaphylatoxin of FRIEDBERGER.

As in so many comparable situations, reconciliation of apparently discordant results was achieved by Hegelian synthesis: more than one protein fragment possessed biological properties which, at least for the most part, were consistent with designation as anaphylatoxin. The question of whether or not to designate C3a as an anaphylatoxin is largely semantic. Historically and puristically, the term should be reserved for C5a. Conceptually and functionally, there is value in including C3a. In either event, it is clear that fragments of two different components of human complement share several biological properties which are of interest in the pathogenesis of the acute inflammatory response.

As in the case of C3, the pathobiological approach also contributed to knowledge of fundamental mechanisms of the C5 step. All of the observations on human C5a prepared by tryptic cleavage of C5 were concurrently being made by Cochrane and Müller-Eberhard [8]. In addition, they showed that incubation of EAC$\overline{1, 4, 2a}$, 3b with C5 resulted in cleavage of C5 with formation of a fragment biologically indistinguishable from C5a prepared with trypsin. This was the first demonstration of complement-mediated cleavage of C5 as a facet of the mechanism of action of this component. As in the case of C3 again, cleavage of C5 is also uncommonly economical, the larger fragment, C5b, apparently being incorporated into the antigen-antibody-complement complex.

Fragmentation of complement components is now recognized to be a major biochemical theme in their mechanism of action. Both guinea pig and human C2 are cleaved by C$\overline{1}$ or C1$\overline{s}$ [34, 35, 50, 58]. Cleavage of guinea pig C3 and C5 by complement-mediated reactions with formation of biologically active fragments has been reported [35, 54]. A C5 fragment very similar to or identical with C5a has also recently been obtained by incubation of serum with endotoxin [56]. It appears highly likely that further elaborations of this theme will emerge as definitive studies on the mechanism of other components are performed.

Serum Inactivator of Human C3a

It was an early observation in our laboratory that the biological activity of C3a, readily demonstrable in mixtures of highly purified C1$\overline{s}$, C4, C2 and C3, was undetectable when less purified components were employed. There are no reports in the literature, to our knowledge, of generation of an activity compatible with C3a by incubation of human serum with inducers of anaphylatoxin formation. In our own attempts to generate C3a from human serum with antigen-antibody complexes, zymosan, agar or C1$\overline{s}$, immunoelectrophoretic conversion of C3 has frequently been effected but biological activity of C3a has not been found. Similarly, in experiments with C1$\overline{s}$ and guinea-pig or rat serum, the anaphylatoxin generated had properties compatible with C5a, not C3a [10]. All of these findings and the previous absence of description of the existence of C3a were consistent with the hypothesis that serum contains an inactivator of the biological activity of C3a.

With Miss MARY CAROL CONROY, we have recently begun to investigate this hypothesis and have indeed found that normal human serum is a potent inhibitor of the smooth muscle-contracting activity of C3a. The activity of purified C3a containing 30 μg/ml is blocked within 2 min at 0°C by mixture with an equal volume of human serum diluted 1/40. In terms of the ability of nanagram quantities of C3a to enhance vascular permeability in man, this inhibitory effect of diluted serum on microgram concentrations of C3a is quite striking. It suggests that C3a must act quickly on cell receptors or come under control of the serum inactivator, a situation conceptually analogous to C1s̄ and its serum inhibitor [22].

The serum inactivator of C3a is heat labile, becoming undetectable after incubation of human serum at 56°C for 20 min. It is unstable upon exposure of serum for 1 h at 0°C to pH values of 4 and 9 but retains activity under these conditions of time and temperature at pH 5–8. It is non-dialyzable and does not require divalent cations for its activity. Addition of small amounts of human serum to mixtures of purified C1s̄, C4, C2 and C3 prevents the generation of biologically detectable C3a, although immunoelectrophoretic conversion of C3 still occurs. This observation is compatible with the hypothesis that C3a may be a transient product which is rapidly blocked by the serum inactivator. The inactivator is not present in highly purified human serum albumin; indeed albumin is now being employed as an effective stabilizer of purified C3a. Further descriptive characterization of the inactivator is in progress, preparatory to its isolation and physico-chemical characterization.

Preliminary studies bearing on the possible mechanism of inactivation have been performed. They have been severely compromised by the tendency of ^{125}I-C3a to adhere to surfaces and to the point of application to supporting media. However, in collaboration with Dr. FRED S. ROSEN, it has been found that ^{125}I-C3a mixed with human serum migrates in agarose electrophoresis with the slow β-globulins, whereas ^{125}I-C3a alone remains at the origin. In sucrose density gradient ultracentrifugation experiments with Miss JANE CHAPITIS, ^{125}I-C3a has appeared to sediment somewhat more rapidly in the presence of human serum than in its absence. These experiments suggest that the serum inactivator of C3a may be a relatively low molecular weight β-globulin which binds C3a but the technical problems associated with these studies are such that this is to be viewed only as a working hypothesis.

Regardless of the nature of the serum inactivator and its mechanism of action, its presence in normal human serum accounts, at least in part, for the failure to detect biological activity of C3a in whole serum or in mixtures of less highly purified C1s̄, C4, C2 and C3 under usual conditions of assay. It is of interest however that ARCHER was able to release histamine from *rat* peritoneal mast cells by addition of antigen to fresh immune rat serum in the simultaneous presence of rat mast cells. If antigen were incubated with fresh immune serum before addition of the mast cells, histamine release did not occur [2]. These observations are compatible with the concept that C3a is indeed capable of being generated in whole serum and expressing biological activity but that it rapidly comes under the control of the serum inactivator.

Concluding Remarks

An attempt has been made to trace the origins of our current knowledge of biologically active cleavage products of components of complement, stressing the historical interplay between pathobiological observations and the development of information on biochemical mechanisms. Particular emphasis has been placed on C3a and C5a, the low molecular weight fragments of C3 and C5. Evidence has been reviewed for the conclusion that C5a is the classical anaphylatoxin of FRIEDBERGER and that C3a is a new property which has biological activities both in common with and distinct from C5a. Accordingly, anaphylatoxin is a general term which is descriptive of more than one chemical entity.

Preliminary experiments have been presented bearing on the presence in normal human serum of an inactivator of C3a. Its possible relevance to the failure to detect biological activity of C3a in whole human serum has been discussed.

Although much is yet to be learned about the full range of pathobiological properties of C3a and C5a and their operation in specific examples of experimental and clinical disease, it is clear that they possess at least the potential for initiating such important features of the acute inflammatory response as smooth muscle contraction, enhanced vascular permeability and degranulation of mast cells with release of histamine. Subsequent papers in this Symposium will deal with the chemotactic activity of these fragments and of other products of the complement system. Thus, the complement system, activated at the C1 step by immune complexes, may serve as a mediator of inflammation in immunopathological injury. Furthermore, the existence of alternate pathways to the utilization of complement components as substrates by enzymes unrelated to the complement system provides the potential for consideration of complement as a mediator of inflammation initiated by non-immunological events.

References

1. ALPER, C. A. and ROSEN, F. S.: Studies of the *in vivo* behavior of human C'3 in normal subjects and patients. J. clin. Invest. *46:* 2021–2034 (1967).
2. ARCHER, G. T.: Release of histamine from mast cells by antigen-antibody reactions *in vitro*. Australian J. exp. Biol. Med. Sci. *38:* 147–151 (1960).
3. BECKER, E. L.: Inhibition of complement activity by di-isopropyl fluorophosphate. Nature, Lond. *176:* 1073 (1955).
4. BECKER, E. L.: Concerning the mechanism of complement action. I. Inhibition of complement activity by diisopropylfluorophosphate. II. The nature of the first component of guinea pig complement. V. Early steps in immune hemolysis. J. Immunol. *77:* 462–468, 469–478 (1956); ibid. *84:* 299–308 (1960).
5. BORDET, J.: Gélose et anaphylatoxine. Compt. rend. Soc. Biol. *74:* 877 (1913).
6. BORDET, J. et ZUNZ, E.: Production de l'anaphylatoxine dans le sérum traité par de l'agar épuré de son azote (parabine). Z. ImmunForsch. *23:* 42–48 (1914).
7. CINADER, B. and LEPOW, I. H.: The neutralization of biologically active molecules; in Antibodies to Biologically Active Molecules, pp. 1–24 (Pergamon Press, Oxford/New York 1966).
8. COCHRANE, C. G. and MÜLLER-EBERHARD, H. J.: The derivation of two distinct anaphylatoxin activities from the third and fifth components of human complement. J. exp. Med. *127:* 371–386 (1968).
9. DALE, H. H. and KELLAWAY, C. H.: Anaphylaxis and anaphylatoxins. Phil. Trans. Roy. Soc. London, Ser. B. *211:* 273–315 (1923).
10. DIAS DA SILVA, W. and LEPOW, I. H.: Anaphylatoxin formation by purified human C'1 esterase. J. Immunol. *95:* 1080–1089 (1965).
11. DIAS DA SILVA, W. and LEPOW, I. H.: Properties of anaphylatoxin prepared from purified components of human complement. Immunochemistry *3:* 497 (1966).
12. DIAS DA SILVA, W. and LEPOW, I. H.: Complement as a mediator of inflammation. II. Biological properties of anaphylatoxin prepared with purified components of human complement. J. exp. Med. *125:* 921–946 (1967).
13. DIAS DA SILVA, W.; EISELE, J. W. and LEPOW, I. H.: Complement as mediator of inflammation. III. Purification of the activity with anaphylatoxin properties generated by interaction of the first four components of complement and its identification as a cleavage product of C'3. J. exp. Med. *126:* 1027–1048 (1967).
14. DONALDSON, V. H. and EVANS, R. R.: A biochemical abnormality in hereditary angioneurotic edema: Absence of serum inhibitor of C'1-esterase. Amer. J. Med. *35:* 37–44 (1963).
15. DONALDSON, V. H. and ROSEN, F. S.: Action of complement in hereditary angioneurotic edema: The role of C'1-esterase. J. clin. Invest. *43:* 2204–2213 (1964).
16. FRIEDBERGER, E.: Weitere Untersuchungen über Eiweissanaphylaxie. IV. Mitteilung. Z. ImmunForsch. *4:* 636–689 (1910).
17. FRIEDBERGER, E. und ITO, T.: Über Anaphylaxie: XXI. Mitteilung. Näheres über den Mechanismus der Komplementwirkung bei der Anaphylatoxinbildung *in vitro*. Z. ImmunForsch. *11:* 471–478 (1911).

18. HAINES, A. L. and LEPOW, I. H.: Studies on human C′1-esterase. I. Purification and enzymatic properties. II. Function of purified C′1-esterase in the human complement system. III. Effect of rabbit anti-C′1-esterase on enzymatic and complement activities. J. Immunol. *92:* 456–467, 468–478, 479–490 (1964).
19. HAHN, F. und OBERDORF, A.: Antihistaminica und anaphylaktoide Reaktionen. Z. ImmunForsch. *107:* 528–538 (1950).
20. JENSEN, J.: Formation of anaphylatoxin. Immunochemistry *3:* 498 (1966).
21. JENSEN, J.: Anaphylatoxin in its relation to the complement system. Science *155:* 1122–1123 (1967).
22. LEON, M. A. and LEPOW, I. H.: Interaction of a serum inhibitor of C′1 esterase with intermediate complexes of the immune haemolytic system. II. Kinetics and mechanism of the interaction. Immunology *5:* 235–244 (1962).
23. LEPOW, I. H.; DIAS DA SILVA, W. and EISELE, J. W.: Nature and biological properties of human anaphylatoxin; in Biochemistry of the Acute Allergic Reactions, pp. 265–282 (Blackwell, Oxford/Edinburgh 1968).
24. LEPOW, I. H. and LEON, M. A.: Interaction of serum inhibitor of C′1-esterase with intermediate complexes of the immune haemolytic system. I. Specificity of inhibition of C′1 activity associated with intermediate complexes. Immunology *5:* 222–234 (1962).
25. LEPOW, I. H.; NAFF, G. B.; TODD, E. W.; PENSKY, J. and HINZ, C. F., Jr.: Chromatographic resolution of the first component of human complement into three activities. J. exp. Med. *117:* 983–1008 (1963).
26. LEPOW, I. H. and PILLEMER, L.: Studies on the mechanism of inactivation of human complement by plasmin and by antigen-antibody aggregates. II. Demonstration of two distinct reaction stages in complement fixation. J. Immunol. *75:* 63–70 (1955).
27. LEPOW, I. H.; RATNOFF, O. D. and LEVY, L. R.: Studies on the activation of a proesterase associated with partially purified first component of human complement. J. exp. Med. *107:* 451–474 (1958).
28. LEPOW, I. H.; RATNOFF, O. D. and PILLEMER, L.: Elution of an esterase from antigen-antibody aggregates treated with human complement. Proc. Soc. exp. Biol. med. *92:* 111–114 (1956).
29. LEPOW, I. H.; RATNOFF, O. D.; ROSEN, F. S. and PILLEMER, L.: Observations on a proesterase associated with partially purified first component of human complement. Proc. Soc. exp. Biol. Med. *92:* 32–37 (1956).
30. LEPOW, I. H.; TODD, E. W.; SMINK, R. D., Jr. and PENSKY, J.: Purification of the second component (C′2) of human complement. Fed. Proc. *24:* 446 (1965).
31. LEPOW, I. H.; WURZ, L.; RATNOFF, O. D. and PILLEMER, L.: Studies on the mechanism of inactivation of human complement by plasmin and by antigen-antibody aggregates. I. The requirement for a factor resembling C′1 and the role of Ca^{++}. J. Immunol. *73:* 146–158 (1954).
32. LEVINE, L.: Inhibition of immune hemolysis by diisopropylfluorophosphate. Biochem. biophys. Acta *18:* 283–284 (1955).
33. LEVY, L. R. and LEPOW, I. H.: Assay and properties of serum inhibitor of C′1-esterase. Proc. Soc. exp. Biol. med. *101:* 608–611 (1959).
34. MAYER, M. M. and MILLER, J. A.: Inhibition of guinea pig C′2 by rabbit antibody. Quantitative measurement of inhibition, discrimination between immune inhibition and complement fixation, specificity of inhibition and demonstration of uptake of C′2 by EAC′1a, 4. Immunochemistry *2:* 71–93 (1965).
35. MAYER, M. M.; SHIN, H. S. and MILLER, J. A.: Fragmentation of guinea pig complement components C′2 and C′3c; in Protides of the Biological Fluids, pp. 411–417 (Elsevier Publishing Co., Amsterdam 1967).

36. MOTA, I.: The mechanism of action of anaphylatoxin. Its effect on guinea pig mast cells. Immunology 2: 403–413 (1959).
37. MÜLLER-EBERHARD, H. J.: Mechanism of inactivation of the third component of human complement (C'3) by cobra venom. Fed. Proc. 26: 744 (1967).
38. MÜLLER-Eberhard, H. J. and BIRO, C. E.: Isolation and description of the fourth component of human complement. J. exp. Med. 118: 447–466 (1963).
39. MÜLLER-EBERHARD, H. J.; NILSSON, U. and ARONSSON, T.: Isolation and characterization of two β-glycoproteins of human serum. J. exp. Med. 111: 201–215 (1960).
40. MÜLLER-EBERHARD, H. J.; POLLEY, M. J. and CALCOTT, M. A.: Formation of the C'4, C'2a complex in cell-free solution and its effect on C'3. Immunochemistry 3: 500 (1966).
41. MÜLLER-EBERHARD, H. J.; POLLEY, M. J. and CALCOTT, M. A.: Formation and functional significance of a molecular complex derived from the second and the fourth component of human complement. J. exp. Med. 125: 359–380 (1967).
42. NAFF, G. B.; PENSKY, J. and LEPOW, I. H.: The macromolecular nature of the first component of human complement. J. exp. Med. 119: 593–613 (1964).
43. NATHAN, E.: Über Anaphylatoxinbildung durch Stärke. Z. ImmunForsch. 18: 636–650 (1913).
44. NATHAN, E.: Über Anaphylatoxinbildung durch Inulin (zugleich ein Beitrag über die Bedeutung des physikalischen Zustandes für die Anaphylatoxinbildung. Z. ImmunForsch. 23: 204–220 (1914).
45. NILSSON, U. R. and MÜLLER-EBERHARD, H. J.: Isolation of β1F-globulin from human serum and its characterization as the fifth component of complement. J. exp. Med. 122: 277–298 (1965).
46. NOVY, F. G. and DeKRUIF, P. H.: Anaphylatoxin and anaphylaxis. III. Agar anaphylatoxin: Rabbit serum. IV. Agar anaphylatoxin: Rat serum. J. Infect. Diseases 20: 566–588, 589–617 (1917).
47. OSLER, A. G.; RANDALL, H. G.; HILL, B. M. and OVARY, Z.: Studies on the mechanism of hypersensitivity phenomena. III. The participation of complement in formation of anaphylatoxin. J. exp. Med. 110: 311–339 (1959).
48. PENSKY, J.; LEVY, L. R. and LEPOW, I. H.: Partial purification of serum inhibitor of C'1-esterase. J. Biol. Chem. 236: 1674–1679 (1961).
49. POLLEY, M. J. and MÜLLER-EBERHARD, H. J.: Isolation of the second component of human complement and the effect of iodoacetamide on its activity. Fed. Proc. 24: 446 (1965).
50. POLLEY, M. J. and MÜLLER-EBERHARD, H. J.: The second component of human complement: its isolation, fragmentation by C'1 esterase, and incorporation into C'3 convertase. J. exp. Med. 128: 533–551 (1968).
51. RATNOFF, O. D. and LEPOW, I. H.: Some properties of an esterase derived from preparations of the first component of complement. J. exp. Med. 106: 327–343 (1957).
52. RATNOFF, O. D. and LEPOW, I. H.: Complement as a mediator of inflammation. Enhancement of vascular permeability by purified human C'1 esterase. J. exp. Med. 118: 681–698 (1963).
53. ROCHA E SILVA, M.; BIER, O. and ARONSON, M.: Histamine release by anaphylatoxin. Nature, Lond. 168: 465–466 (1951).
54. SHIN, H. S.; PICKERING, R. J.; MAYER, M. M. and COOK, C. T.: Guinea pig C'5. Abstracts of the Complement Workshop. J. Immunol. 101: 813 (1968).
55. SMINK, R. D., Jr.; ABERNETHY, R. W.; RATNOFF, O. D. and LEPOW, I. H.: Enhancement of vascular permeability by mixtures of C'1-esterase and normal serum. Proc. Soc. exp. Biol. med. 116: 280–283 (1964).

56. Snyderman, R.; Gewurz, H. and Mergenhagen, S. E.: Interactions of the complement system with endotoxic polysaccharide. Generation of a factor chemotactic for polymorphonuclear leukocytes. J. exp. Med. *128:* 259–275 (1968).
57. Stegemann, H.; Vogt, W. and Friedberg, K. D.: Über die Natur des Anaphylatoxins. Hoppe-Seylers Z. physiol. Chem. *337:* 269–276 (1964).
58. Stroud, R. M.; Mayer, M. M.; Miller, J. A. and McKenzie, A. T.: C′2a^d, an inactive derivative of C′2 released during decay of EAC′4,2a. Immunochemistry *3:* 163–176 (1966).
59. Ward, P. A.: A plasmin-split product of C′3 as a new chemotactic factor. J. exp. Med. *126:* 189–206 (1967).

Authors' addresses: Irwin H. Lepow and Richard A. Patrick, Dept. of Pathology, Health Center, *Hartford, Conn.* (USA); W. Dias da Silva, Dept. of Physiology, Universidade Federal de Minas Gerais, *Belo Horizonte* (Brazil).

Cellular and Humoral Mechanisms in Anaphylaxis and Allergy, pp. 253–259
(Karger, Basel/New York 1969)

Pharmacology of Anaphylatoxin

H. Giertz

Pharmacological Institute, University of Freiburg, Freiburg i. Br.

In 1910 Friedberger [12] demonstrated that fresh guinea-pig serum or plasma which has been incubated with immune precipitates *in vitro* becomes toxic for guinea pigs. Since the fatal effect of this plasma-born poison is very similar to anaphylaxis, Friedberger called it anaphylatoxin and thought it to be the mediator substance responsible for the anaphylactic symptoms.

Four findings in allergy research let Friedberger's theory fall into oblivion for at least 20 years. First, Schultz [37] and Dale [6] showed that anaphylactic reactions can be elicited in isolated organs also in the absence of blood or plasma. Second, Bordet [4] and other (for references see Giertz and Hahn, ref. 16) succeeded in producing anaphylatoxin by incubation of serum with various polysaccharides instead of immune precipitates. Third, Dale and Kellaway [8] observed some principle differences between anaphylatoxin effects and anaphylactic symptoms. Fourth, Bartosch, Feldberg and Nagel in 1932 [2] proved that histamine is released in guinea pig-anaphylaxis, and so supported by their experiments Dale's [7] histamine theory which fits the data of anaphylaxis better than Friedberger's anaphylatoxin theory.

However, there was a rebirth of anaphylatoxin research in the fifty's by the discovery that anaphylatoxin is a histamine liberator in the guinea pig [30, 35, 34, 26, 22]. This fact raised anew the question whether anaphylatoxin could play some supplementary role in anaphylaxis, especially in anaphylactic histamine release in the intact guinea pig. As long as the chemical nature of anaphylatoxin is a matter of discussion and as long as direct proof of anaphylatoxin production in anaphylaxis is not possible, the question of anaphylatoxin participation in immune reactions can be answered foremost by a careful comparison of anaphylatoxin effects and anaphylactic symptoms. Most of the results detailed in this paper were gained by the use of rat serum anaphylatoxin produced by incubation of fresh rat serum with dextran [16]. The effects of anaphylatoxin were compared to histamine shock and to active anaphylaxis with ovalbumen as antigen.

Above all anaphylatoxin shock and anaphylaxis have in common that the tissue mast cells are damaged and disappear [33, 13]. At that they pour out their histamine and heparin. In contrast, histamine does not affect the mast cells, though it produces a comparable inflation of the lungs.

The histamine release is responsible for the bronchoconstriction induced by anaphylatoxin or anaphylaxis. Rising doses of an antihistamine inhibit the bronchospasm, measured with the Konzett-Rössler method in the intact animal, as well as in histamine as in anaphylatoxin or anaphylactic shock to about the same degree [19, 26a]. That histamine action is essentially involved in the fatal outcome of anaphylatoxin and anaphylactic shock, may also be seen from the rough parallelism between death rate and plasma histamine level, using different doses of anaphylatoxin or antigen [22, 26a]. A further consequence of the histamine liberation seems to be the increase of the plasma potassium level which is about the same in histamine, ana- phylatoxin, or anaphylactic shocks of comparable lethality. This increase is reduced by an antihistamine as well as in histamine as in anaphylactic shock [24], but with this respect the anaphylatoxin shock has not been investigated.

Since sublethal anaphylatoxin doses protect guinea pigs against lethal doses subsequently applied, several authors postulated that such a state of anaphylatoxin tachyphylaxis should protect the guinea pigs against ana- phylaxis if anaphylatoxin played any essential role therein [16, 27]. In contrast to some previous findings HALPERN and co-workers [31, 32] described an inhibition of anaphylactic shock in guinea pigs which were tachyphylactic against anaphylatoxin. But FRIEDBERG and co-workers [9, 10, 11] could not confirm these observations. However, without regard to anaphylatoxin participation in anaphylactic phenomena, an inhibiting effect of high anaphylatoxin doses on subsequent anaphylaxis has to be expected, because anaphylatoxin depletes the histamine stores. Indeed, by repeatedly giving higher than lethal doses of anaphylatoxin in animals pretreated with mepyramine we succeeded in reducing the lethality of subsequent anaphy- lactic shock [26a, 27]. It was further proved that the decrease in the anaphylact- ic death rate after anaphylatoxin pretreatment runs parallel with a decrease in plasma histamine level. Control experiments showed that injections of heat inactivated serum or saline instead of anaphylatoxin have no effect on the lethality in subsequent anaphylaxis.

The fact that the desensitization remains submaximal may indicate that the extent to which single organs (e.g. the lungs) contribute to the total histamine release into the plasma, is different in anaphylatoxin shock and anaphylaxis [26a].

The amount of heparin released in anaphylatoxin or anaphylactic shock of guinea pigs is not sufficient to inhibit blood coagulation [21, 25], in contrast to dog anaphylaxis. In the guinea pig, however, heparin is a strong histaminase liberator [19]. Exactly as in the case of the anaphylactic dog the increased heparin level in plasma of anaphylatoxin treated or anaphylactic guinea pigs is to be referred back to heparin release from the liver [29]. The histaminase liberated by heparin also originates from the liver [36]. After anaphylatoxin injection into the iugular or portal vein, the increases of heparin and histaminase levels in plasma from systemic circulation or from liver veins run roughly parallel (GIERTZ, HAHN and MITZE, to be published).

The amount of plasma histaminase liberated in anaphylatoxin or anaphylactic shock is much lower than the amount released by injection of high heparin doses. It is limited, because only a small part of the total liver heparin is liberated in shock, which is true for liver histamine, too, as has to be expected since both substances originate from mast cells [25].

The similarities between the pharmacological effects of anaphylatoxin and anaphylaxis and the results of the desensitization experiments are based on the effect of anaphylatoxin and anaphylaxis on the tissue mast cells. A more detailed analysis reveals some differences between anaphylatoxin shock and anaphylaxis. Whereas in histamine and anaphylatoxin shock the occurrence of acute death can be almost completely reduced by antihistamine doses as minute as 10 μg mepyramine maleate per kg, in anaphylactic shock considerably higher doses are needed for inhibition of the acute fatal outcome. The emphysema reducing capacity of mepyramine runs parallel to the inhibition of acute death [19] so that in all three shock types the animal survives if the emphysema is reduced to the same extent, but in anaphylaxis for this reduction much more mepyramine is needed. This means, with regard to the fact that mepyramine induces an equally potent broncholysis in all three shock types, that in the anaphylactic animal a much higher degree of broncholysis is required for survival or reduction of the emphysema than in anaphylatoxin or histamine shock. The factor which is, besides bronchoconstriction, involved in anaphylactic emphysema is the cardiac dyspnoe which is caused by heart failure induced by a strong anaphylactic constriction of the pulmonary and, probably, the coronary vessels.

This constriction which is resistant against mepyramine and is lacking in anaphylatoxin and histamine shock, is the cause of another phenomenon which can be observed only in anaphylaxis. About half of the anaphylactic animals die due to a protracted type of shock [17] even after very high mepyramine doses. Whereas in acute anaphylaxis the inflation of lungs is the main pathological symptom, in protracted shock the lung emphysema is only slight or completely lacking, but there is a strong dilation of the right heart ventricle and a congestion of the intestines and the liver. In these animals a strong spasm of the lung arteries can be observed histologically (GIERTZ, HAHN and OEHLERT, to be published).

The data given up to this point show that in the intact animal anaphylatoxin behaves like a histamine liberator, whereas in anaphylaxis some shock symptoms cannot be explained by histamine liberation alone. However, they do not speak against a supplementary role of anaphylatoxin in anaphylactic histamine liberation. To prove or disprove participation of anaphylatoxin in anaphylaxis further experiments are necessary.

The simple question whether plasma intensifies the anaphylactic histamine liberation from isolated guinea-pig lungs must be denied. Some experiments with positive results [38] could not be confirmed [5].

Since the precursors of anaphylatoxin are consumed by anaphylatoxin production [15], it is of interest that in serum from anaphylactic animals the capacity of anaphylatoxin production is not diminished. This finding is the more decisive as in another shock type, the Forssman shock, a decrease of this capacity occurs [20, 26a]. Another argument against participation of anaphylatoxin in anaphylaxis and in favor of its involvement in Forssman shock is the following: The injection of huge heparin doses into guinea pigs abolishes the capacity to produce anaphylatoxin in the serum from these animals. The same doses of heparin are not able to reduce significantly the anaphylactic death rate, whereas the Forssman shock is completely suppressed even by lower doses (GIERTZ, HAHN and EBNER, to be published). Further, in anaphylatoxin and, even more, in Forssman shock the number of blood platelets is diminished, whereas anaphylactic shock has no significant effect on the platelet number [22]. In heart lung preparations the Forssman shock can only be produced if the preparation is perfused with whole blood, Forssman antibodies are not effective using a blood cell suspension in saline as perfusion fluid [28]. Of course, the humoral factor which is involved in this shock type may be, but need not be anaphylatoxin.

Despite such indications of an involvement of anaphylatoxin in Forssman shock, there are some arguments against the decisive role of anaphylatoxin in this shock type. For, in Forssman shock the histamine liberation is only small [14, 22], an inhibitory effect of antihistamines does not exist [1, 30], and in contrast to anaphylatoxin shock extensive lung edema occurs.

Another problem can only be touched on: Are the effects of anaphylatoxin exclusively or only partially caused by histamine liberation? This question concerns not only the effects in the intact animals but also in isolated organs or in the guinea-pig skin. Certainly, the anaphylatoxin effect on white blood cells is no consequence of histamine release. In VOGT's laboratory several effects of purified hog anaphylatoxin preparations, especially on the respiration [3], could be observed only a part of which can be explained by histamine liberation. Further, some anaphylatoxin effects in isolated organs cannot be explained by histamine release [16].

Summary and Conclusions

The pharmacological effects of anaphylatoxin on the guinea pig are mainly, but not exclusively caused by its action on mast cells. In spite of the close similarities between the pharmacological effects of anaphylatoxin and anaphylactic symptoms, and, again, in spite of the indications of an involvement of anaphylatoxin in certain immunological reactions, a definite proof of the biological significance of anaphylatoxin is lacking up to now.

References

1. ARBESMANN, C.E.; NETER, E. and BECKER, C.F.: The effect of pyribenzamine, neohetramine, and rutin on reversed anaphylaxis in guinea pigs. J. Allergy *21:* 25–33 (1950).
2. BARTOSCH, R.; FELDBERG, W. und NAGEL, E.: Das Freiwerden eines histaminähnlichen Stoffes bei der Anaphylaxie des Meerschweinchens. Pflügers Arch. ges. Physiol. *230:* 129–153 (1932).
3. BODAMMER, G.: Untersuchungen zum Mechanismus der Atemwirkung des Anaphylatoxins. Naunyn-Schmiedebergs Archiv *260:* 16–25 (1968).
4. BORDET, J.: Gélose et anaphylatoxine. C.R. Soc. Biol. *74:* 877–878 (1913).
5. BROCKLEHURST, W.E.: The release of histamine and formation of a slow-reacting substance (SRS-A) during anaphylactic shock. J. Physiol. *151:* 416–435 (1960).
6. DALE, H.H.: The anaphylactic reaction of plain muscle in the guinea pig. J. Pharmacol. *4:* 167–223 (1913).
7. DALE, H.H.: Some chemical factors in the control of the circulation. Lecture III. Local vasodilator reactions. – Histamine (cont.). – Acetylcholine. – Conclusion. Lancet *216:* 1285–1290 (1929).
8. DALE, H.H. and KELLAWAY, C.H.: Anaphylaxis and anaphylatoxins. Philos. Trans. (A/B) *211:* 273–315 (1922).

9. Friedberg, K.D. und Bauer, U.: Anaphylaktischer Schock nach passiver Sensibilisierung am anaphylatoxinvorbehandelten Meerschweinchen. Naunyn-Schmiedebergs Archiv 250: 171–172 (1965).

10. Friedberg, K.D.; Engelhardt, G. und Meineke, F.: Über die Tachyphylaxie der Anaphylatoxinreaktion und ihre Bedeutung für die Anaphylaxie. Int. Arch. Allergy 22: 166–169 (1963).

11. Friedberg, K.D.; Engelhardt, G. und Meineke, F.: Untersuchungen über die Anaphylatoxin-Tachyphylaxie und über ihre Bedeutung für den Ablauf echter anaphylaktischer Reaktionen. Int. Arch. Allergy 25: 154–181 (1964).

12. Friedberger, E.: Weitere Untersuchungen über Eiweissanaphylaxie. IV. Mitteilung. Z. Immunforsch. 4: 636–689 (1910).

13. Gemählich, M.; Frenger, W. und Scheiffarth, F.: Untersuchungen zur Morphologie der Mastzellen im Anaphylatoxinschock beim Meerschweinchen. Int. Arch Allergy 13: 370–376 (1958).

14. Giertz, H. und Hahn, F.: Die inverse Anaphylaxie vom Standpunkt der Histamintheorie der Anaphylaxie. Int. Arch. Allergy 6: 23–44 (1955).

15. Giertz, H. und Hahn, F.: Weitere Untersuchungen über die Bildung und die Natur des Anaphylatoxins. Int. Arch. Allergy 19: 94–111 (1961).

16. Giertz, H. und Hahn, F.: Makromolekulare Histaminliberatoren. (Eiklar, Dextran, Polyvinylpyrrolidon, Tween 20, Anaphylatoxin). Handb. exp. Pharmakol. 18/I pp. 481–568 (1966).

17. Giertz, H. und Hahn, F.: Über die Wirkung von Mepyramin und Papaverin auf den anaphylaktischen Schock des Meerschweinchens mit besonderer Berücksichtigung des protrahierten Schocks. Naunyn-Schmiedebergs Archiv 258: 11–23 (1967).

18. Giertz, H. and Hahn, F.: Mechanism of histaminase liberation in guinea pig anaphylaxis. Int. Arch Allergy (in press 1968).

19. Giertz, H.; Hahn, F. and Bernauer, W.: On the cause of the different sensitivity to antihistaminics (mepyramine) of anaphylactic, histamine, and anaphylatox in shock. Naunyn-Schmiedebergs Archiv 259: 172–173 (1968).

20. Giertz, H.; Hahn, F.; Jurna, I. und Lange, A.: Zur Frage der Beteiligung des Anaphylatoxins im anaphylaktischen Schock. Int. Arch. Allergy 13: 201–212 (1958).

21. Giertz, H.; Hahn, F.; Krull, P. and Albert, U.: Histaminase liberating and anticoagulant activity of heparin released in anaphylactic shock in the guinea pig. Int. Arch. Allergy 33: 306–312 (1968).

22. Giertz, H.; Hahn, F.; Schmutzler, W. und Kollmeier, J.: Plasma- und Bluthistamin bei verschiedenen Schockformen des Meerschweinchens. Int. Arch. Allergy 25: 26–45 (1964).

23. Giertz, H.; Hahn, F.; Seseke, G. und Schmutzler, W.: Über die Wirkung von Heparin und Aminoguanidin auf den anaphylaktischen, Anaphylatoxin- und Histaminschock des Meerschweinchens. Naunyn-Schmiedebergs Archiv 256: 26–39 (1967).

24. Giertz, H. und Krakó, K.: Der Plasmakaliumspiegel bei verschiedenen Schockformen. Naunyn-Schmiedebergs Archiv 260: 120–121 (1968).

25. Giertz, H.; Mitze, R. und Mészáros, E.: Heparin und Histaminase in der Leber anaphylaktischer Meerschweinchen. Naunyn-Schmiedebergs Archiv (in press 1968).

26. Hahn, F.: Zur Anaphylatoxinfrage. Naturwissenschaften 41: 465–470 (1954).

26a. Hahn, F.: Anaphylatoxin and anaphylaxis. Excerpt Med. Int. Congr. Ser. No. 162, Proc. VIth Congr. Int. Ass. Allergol., Montreal, 1967, pp. 145–159.

27. Hahn, F.; Ebner, C. and Giertz, H.: Anaphylatoxin tachyphylaxis and anaphylaxis. Int. Arch. Allergy (in press, 1968).

28. Hahn, F. und Giertz, H.: Pharmakologische Aspekte der Allergie. Naunyn-Schmiedebergs Archiv 250: 105–111 (1965).

29. HAHN, F.; GIERTZ, H. und KRULL, P.: Die Heparinfreisetzung im anaphylaktischen Schock des Meerschweinchens und ihre Beziehung zur anaphylaktischen Histaminaseliberierung. Naunyn-Schmiedebergs Archiv 256: 430–438 (1967).
30. HAHN, F. und OBERDORF, A.: Antihistaminica und anaphylaktoide Reaktionen. Z. Immunforsch. 107: 528–538 (1950).
31. HALPERN, B.N. et LIACOPOULOS, P.: Protection du cobaye contre le choc anaphylactique mortel par l'anaphylatoxine et son mécanisme. C. R. Soc. Biol. 150: 108–112 (1956).
32. HALPERN, B.N.; LIACOPOULOS, P. et BRIOT, M.: Mécanisme de protection du cobaye contre le choc anaphylactique mortel par l'anaphylatoxine. Acta allerg. 10: 9–14 (1956).
33. MOTA, I.: Action of anaphylactic shock and anaphylatoxin on mast cells and histamine in rats. Brit. J. Pharmacol. 12: 453–456 (1957).
34. ROCHA E SILVA, M. and ARONSON, M.: Histamine release from the perfused lung of the guinea pig by serotoxin (anaphylatoxin). Brit. J. exp. Path. 33: 577–586 (1952).
35. ROCHA E SILVA, M.; BIER, O. and ARONSON, M.: Histamine release by anaphylatoxin. Nature, Lond. 168: 465–466 (1951).
36. SCHMUTZLER, W.; HAHN, F.; SESEKE, G. und BERNAUER, W.: Über die Herkunft der Plasmahistaminase im anaphylaktischen Schock des Meerschweinchens. Naunyn-Schmiedebergs Archiv 252: 332–338 (1966).
37. SCHULTZ, W.H.: Physiological studies in anaphylaxis. I. The reaction of smooth muscle of the guinea pig sensitized with horse serum. J. Pharmacol. 1: 549–567 (1910).
38. UNGAR, G. and DAMGAARD, E.: Tissue reactions to anaphylactic and anaphylactoid stimuli; proteolysis and release of histamine and heparin. J. exp. Med. 101: 1–15 (1955)

Author's address: H. GIERTZ, M.D., Pharmacological Institute, University of Freiburg, D–78 Freiburg im Breisgau (Germany).

Cellular and Humoral Mechanisms in Anaphylaxis and Allergy, pp. 260–264
Karger, Basel/New York 1969)

Anaphylatoxin Formation, Problems of its Relation to Complement and Identity in Various Species

W. VOGT

Department of Biochemical Pharmacology, Max-Planck-Institute for Experimental Medicine, Göttingen

The formation of AT has been studied mainly in rat plasma which is one of the classical sources known to give the best yield. Our results seemed rather to contradict the participation of complement. By the time it has however become extremely difficult to disprove as well as to prove its involvement.

Lastly the endogenous formation of AT is an enzymic process. This we have shown by separating from rat plasma an enzyme fraction which acts catalytically, and a substrate fraction which limits the amount of product formed [8]. The enzyme – however complex it may be – can be adsorbed to well-known AT-inducing agents, for example Sephadex or zymosan. Zymosan incubated with rat or human plasma and washed afterwards with saline is a convenient source of AT-forming enzyme, free of substrate. The substrate – anaphylatoxinogen – has been partly purified by chromatographic methods.

If the enzyme is part of complement then it should consist of the complex C' 1, 4, 2 or C' 1, 4, 2, 3 [1, 4, 5]. One approach to investigate the role of complement is to eliminate functionally or materially one or the other of its components. This has been done by OSLER et al. [6], earlier; a parallelism between elimination of single complement components and inactivation of the AT-forming system was described. We found that deionization or treatment with ammonia of rat plasma did not interfere with its ability to form AT on incubation with contact agents, although the total complement activity was reduced to often less than 5%, as measured by immune haemolysis [8]. C' 1 and 2 or 4 should have been largely inactivated by these methods. However, it is nearly impossible to rule out these components entirely. Traces left may be sufficient to still generate AT, as they act catalytically. We therefore looked for conditions under which the complement reaction would start or proceed but AT would not be formed.

One method was to incubate rat plasma with human aggregated γ-globulin. It is known that soluble contact agents do not well form AT when dissolved in the plasma but do so when added as solid. When rat plasma was incubated with aggregated γ-globulin for 30 or even 60 min at 37°, 70 to nearly 90% of the total complement activity was lost but only 10 to 20% of the available anaphylatoxinogen was converted to AT. When a contact agent (Sephadex) was added subsequently the bulk of AT was formed although only little complement activity was left. Thus complement consumption and AT formation did not run parallel. This is no definite proof against complement representing the AT-forming enzyme, but if complement were engaged one could conclude that the complex C' 1, 4, 2 (or C' 1, 4, 2, 3) has varying properties dependent on whether it is fixed at surfaces or formed in solution. It seems that it acts on anaphylatoxinogen efficiently only in the adsorbed state.

DIAS DA SILVA and LEPOW [4], COCHRANE and MÜLLER-EBERHARD [1] obtained AT-like activity from human C' 3 by incubating it with the complex C' 1, 4, 2 in solution. In rat plasma C' 3 is not anaphylatoxinogen. OSLER et al. [6] have earlier shown that phloridzin strongly inhibits AT formation by immune aggregates in rat plasma and we have confirmed this observation using other contact agents as activators. Phloridzin does not inhibit the cleavage of $C'3$ by $C'_{1, 4, 2}$ [2, 5a, 6a]. Further, rat plasma treated with hydrazine yielded as much AT on incubation with the cobra enzyme as did a control although 60% of C' 3 were destroyed by the treatment. Conversely, anaphylatoxinogen was destroyed to more than 95% by heating to 62° for 20 min at pH 7.5, although this treatment left 80% or more of C' 3 intact. This means that a cleavage product of C' 3 could at most contribute to a very small percentage of the total activatable AT of rat plasma.

JENSEN [5] found evidence that in guinea-pig serum C' 5 represents anaphylatoxinogen. This could hold also for rat plasma. Our purified anaphylatoxinogen fraction does contain C' 5. Both C' 5 and anaphylatoxinogen are destroyed at 62° and also the inhibition by phloridzin would be compatible with the identity.

However, the consumption of C' 5 and formation of AT in rat plasma incubated with aggregated human γ-globulin did not run parallel. Although more than 50% of C' 5 (and C' 3) were consumed in 30 min, only 8–10% of AT were formed. Subsequent incubation with zymosan released the remaining 90% AT although less than 50% C' 5 were left for further consumption, measured by immune haemolysis. Further, we found large discrepancies between the relations of C' 5 content to anaphylatoxinogen content in rat plasma and purified anaphylatoxinogen fractions.

If the postulate that C' 5 is anaphylatoxinogen is right then it follows that the complement activity of C' 5 is not essential for contact-activation of AT or that the formation of AT is not a simple or the only cleavage process occurring at C' 5. Apparently C' 1, 4, 2, 3 can inactivate C' 5 in a reaction which does not give rise to the appearance of AT. The reaction does not interfere, on the other hand, with subsequent AT formation. Again, it seems that for efficient AT formation the enzyme needs to be adsorbed, whereas inactivation of C' 5 as a complement factor proceeds reasonably well in solution.

How may rat AT be related to human AT, for which seemingly other conditions of formation prevail? As regards the human C' 3 cleavage product [1, 3]. I think it is justified to say that this is not AT in the original sense. Unlike AT its formation and action cannot be demonstrated in whole plasma. It originates from a different precursor and has different properties. Above other differences it does not produce cross-tachyphylaxis with rat and guinea-pig anaphylatoxin. This is an indication that it acts at different receptor sites, hence by a different mechanism and thus has a different principal structure.

The AT-like compound obtained more recently from human C' 5 by the same authors could be identical or related. Formation of AT from C' 5 would also be in accordance with the findings of JENSEN [5] about guinea-pig AT. However, the attempt of DIAS DA SILVA et al. [3] to produce AT by interaction of human C' 5 with human C' 1, 4, 2, 3 complex failed, possibly because the enzyme acted in solution. In fact, COCHRANE and MÜLLER-EBERHARD [1] succeeded in producing weak AT activity by reacting human C' 5 with EAC' 1, 4, 2, 3. The product of this reaction did, however, not produce cross-desensitization with guinea-pig AT.

We have recently been able to prepare human AT by incubating human plasma with yeast and purifying the product according to the method used before for hog AT [7]. We obtained reasonably active preparations one of which contracted the guinea-pig ileum maximally, at concentrations of 0.3 μg/ml and which did produce cross-tachyphylaxis with rat, hog and guinea-pig ATs prepared by contact activation or cobra venom, purified or unpurified.

We don't see any indication for differences of ATs from various sources but they all appear chemically and biologically related if not identical. This in turn suggests that also the mechanism of formation is the same in different species.

The product of human C' 3 seems to be a new biologically active compound. In order to avoid confusion one should not call this an AT. This would blur the term AT which actually is quite well defined. Primarily AT is the shock-producing, histamine-liberating and smooth-muscle-contracting principle which forms and is stable in guinea-pig serum after incubation with contact agents. If other conditions or systems for the formation are chosen the identity with or relation to the original AT of the product obtained needs to be demonstrated. This has been done with all ATs obtained by contact activation or with cobra enzyme, from rat, hog and human plasma. None of these ATs shows indications of qualitative differences.

Conclusion

Since all ATs show the same properties they are intimately related and most likely are the products of the same process. Since there is such strong evidence that guinea-pig AT originates from C' 5 this component may also function as anaphylatoxinogen in human and rat plasma. However, as regards human AT, the crucial experiment, the formation by purified complement components in a manner as efficient as in whole plasma, remains to be demonstrated; and as regards rat AT, some discrepancies between complement reactions and AT formation remain to be explained.

References

1. COCHRANE, C. G. and MÜLLER-EBERHARD, H. J.: The derivation of two distinct anaphylatoxin activities from the third and fifth components of human complement. J. exp. Med. *127:* 371–386 (1968).
2. COOPER, N. R. and BECKER, E. L.: Complement associated peptidase activity of guinea-pig serum. I. Role of complement components. J. Immunol. *98:* 119–131 (1968).
3. DIAS DA SILVA, W.; EISELE, J. W. and LEPOW, I. H.: Complement as a mediator of inflammation. III. Purification of the activity with anaphylatoxin properties generated by interaction of the first four components of complement and its identification as a cleavage product of C' 3. J. exp. Med. *126:* 1027–1048 (1967).
4. DIAS DA SILVA, W. and LEPOW, I. H.: Complement as a mediator of inflammation. II. Biological properties of anaphylatoxin prepared with purified components of human complement. J. exp. Med. *125:* 921–946 (1967).

5. Jensen, J.: Anaphylatoxin in its relation to the complement system. Science *155:* 1122–1123 (1967).
5a. Müller-Eberhard, H.-J.; Dalmasso, A. P. and Calcott, M. A.: The reaction mechanism of β-1c-globulin (C′3) in immune hemolysis. J. exp. Med. *123:* 33–54 (1966).
6. Osler, A. G.; Randall, H. G.; Hill, B. M. and Ovary, Z.: Studies on the mechanism of hypersensitivity phenomena. J. exp. Med. *110:* 311–339 (1959).
6a. Shin, H. S. and Mayer, M. M.: The third component of the guinea-pig complement system. III. Effect of inhibitors. Biochemistry *7:* 3003–3006 (1968).
7. Vogt, W.: Preparation and some properties of anaphylatoxin from hog serum. Biochem. Pharmacol. *17:* 727–733 (1968).
8. Vogt, W. and Schmidt, G.: Formation of anaphylatoxin in rat plasma, a specific enzymic process. Biochem. Pharmacol. *15:* 905–914 (1966)

Author's address: Dr. W. Vogt, Department of Biochemical Pharmacology, Max-Planck-Institute for Experimental Medicine, *D–34 Göttingen* (Germany).

Cellular and Humoral Mechanisms in Anaphylaxis and Allergy, pp. 265–278
(Karger, Basel/New York 1969)

Chemotactic Activity, a Property of Guinea Pig C'5-Anaphylatoxin[1]

J. A. Jensen, R. Snyderman and S. E. Mergenhagen

Department of Microbiology, University of Miami, School of Medicine, and Variety
Children's Research Foundation, Miami, Fla. and
Immunology Section, National Institute of Dental Research, National Institutes of Health,
Bethesda, Md.

Introduction

Two years ago we demonstrated that the 'classical' anaphylatoxin (AT) generated by treatment of whole guinea-pig (g. p.) serum with immune precipitates, Zymosan, cobra venom factor, Sephadex, agar or immune complexes was closely associated with the fifth component of the guinea pig complement system (C' 5). The active materials not only showed the typical delayed but abrupt contraction of the isolated guinea-pig ileum, which could be depressed by antihistamine, but they also exhibited crossed tachyphylaxis among themselves and with anaphylatoxins generated in a similar manner in rat serum. In addition, it could be shown for the first time that AT was generated if highly purified C' 5 was acted upon by the immune complex EAC' 1a, 4, 2a, 3, or by low concentrations of trypsin (5 μg/ml at 30°C for 10 min) [3]. In the meantime these observations have been confirmed and extended by other laboratories and early discrepancies concerning the identity of the anaphylatoxinogen have been explained by the fact that in the human system C' 5 *and* C' 3 give rise to biologically active fragments with similar but not identical properties [5, 2, 1]. It is now agreed upon by those concerned that the singular term anaphylatoxin is inadequate and that one has to specify which AT is under consideration. This report is concerned with the properties of g. p. C' 5-AT or, following Lepow's suggestion [2] the fragment of g. p. C' 5 with the properties of AT: F(a)C' 5. Table I is a sum-

[1] This investigation was supported in part by research grant No. T-381 from the American Cancer Society by General Research Support Grants No. FR-5516 and FR-5363-05 from the National Institutes of Health, U.S. Public Health Service, and by the Howard Hughes Medical Institute.

Table I. Conditions for the formation of g. p. C' 5-anaphylatoxin

	Reaction mixtures	Incubation-time and temp.	Anaphylatoxin generation
Ia	'Venom factor' + C'		+
b	'Venom factor' + C' s C' 5		−
c	'Venom factor' + C' 5	30' 30° C	−
d	'Venom factor' + C' 5 + cofactor		+
IIa	Trypsin (5 µg ml) + C' 5		+[1]
b	Trypsin (5 µg ml) + all other components	10' 25° C	−
c	Trypsin (5 µg ml) + C' 5 (inactivated)		+[1]
IIIa	Immune-ppt. + C'		+
b	Immune-ppt. + C' s C' 1		−
c	Immune-ppt. + C' 1		−
d	Immune-ppt-C' 1 + C' s C' 1	30' 30° C	+
e	Immune-ppt-C' 1 + C' s C' 1 s C' 5		−
f	Immune-ppt-C' 1 + same + C' 5		+
IVa	EAbC' 14 + C' 2 + C' 3		−
b	EAbC' 1423 + C' 5		+
c	EAbC' 1423 + C' 5 (inactivated)	20' 30° C	−
d	EAbC' 143 + C' 5		−
e	EAbC' 143 + C' 5 + C' 2		+

[1] Prevented by crystalline soybean trypsin inhibitor. s = without.

mary of our earlier work, showing the various ways in which C' 5 AT could be generated.

Since that time we have tried to answer three major questions: [1] is the AT, generated by immune complexes identical with that generated by the cobra venom factor (CVF) or by trypsin [2]. What is the biological role and significance of AT, and [3] is there any other specific, reliable and quantitatively measurable activity associated with AT, other than the contraction of the isolated g. p. ileum. The guinea-pig ileum contraction appears to be specific but quite unreliable and impossible to quantitate unless one is dealing with very potent preparations. In order to answer any one of these questions the active materials had to be isolated from other serum constituents and purified.

Experimental: A. Purification and characterization of C' 5-AT. Whole g. p. serum was incubated for 60 min at 30°C with an immune precipitate consisting of bovine serum albumin (BSA) and rabbit anti-BSA formed in the

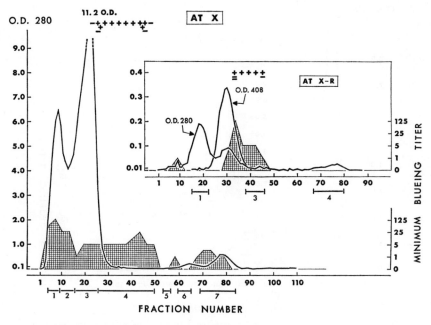

Fig. 1. Gelfiltration (Sephadex G-100) of immune precipitate treated guinea pig serum on 4.5 × 55 cm column at 4°C. See text for details. (+) indicates fractions with anaphylatoxin activity (ileum contraction), hatched areas: fractions causing increase of vascular permeability. Pool 4 (fractions 26–50) from Col AT-X was concentrated to 50 ml and again passed through the same column (Col AT-X-R) see insert.

presence of EDTA and thoroughly washed. In preliminary experiments it
was established that an amount of immune precipitate representing 320 μg
7S-Ab-N per ml of serum would generate a maximal amount of AT. Forty
ml of treated serum were applied to a 4.5×55 cm Sephadex G-100 column,
equilibrated with 0.15 M; NaCl-phosphate buffer pH 7.5; 10 ml fractions were
collected after discarding the void volume. The fractions were tested for
AT-activity on the isolated g. p. ileum and for their ability to increase
vascular permeability in the g. p. skin. The latter activity was expressed in
minimal skin blueing units obtained by testing 5-fold fraction dilutions.
Figure 1 shows the profile of this column (AT-X) and as an insert (AT-X-R)
the results of rechromatography of the anaphylatoxin-active pool from
AT-X through the same column after concentration (Diaflo, membrane #1).
In figure 2, (AT-XII) which is almost identical with figure 1, the same G-100
column was used for the filtration of 40 ml guinea pig serum treated for
60 min at 30°C with partially purified cobra venom factor in amounts

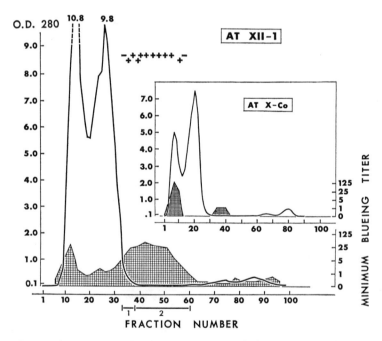

Fig. 2. Same as figure 1 except that the serum was treated with cobra venom factor. Insert:
Normal, untreated guinea pig serum (20 ml) passed through the same column. Note the
small peak of skin blueing activity in the same area where anaphylatoxin appears on Col
AT-X and AT-XII. This peak possibly represents anaphylatoxin, generated by contact
with Sephadex on the column, but too weak to cause ileum contraction.

sufficient to generate maximal AT-reactivity. The insert of this figure shows the profile of 27 ml of untreated serum, passed through the same column (ATX-Co).

A comparison of the two figures shows that the ileum reactive material indicated by (+) appeared in both cases in the same well defined area eluting later than albumin and just after the hemoglobin (insert fig. 1). No other fractions caused the typical ileum contraction, but earlier and sometimes, later eluting fractions exhibited strong skin blueing activity. On further purification non-AT associated vascular permeability factors could be well separated from anaphylatoxin. However, even our purest anaphylatoxin preparations with high specific activity always caused a strong increase of vascular permeability that could be depressed by antihistamines, and could not be separated from the ileum contracting activity. It seemed therefore reasonable to assume that one of the characteristics of purified anaphylatoxin was its ability to increase vascular permeability in the g. p. skin, especially since this was also found to be characteristic of AT generated by trypsin treatment of purified C′ 5. Purified anaphylatoxin preparations of CVF- and immune precipitate treated serum and trypsin treated C′ 5 were submitted to sucrose density gradient ultracentrifugation. Figure 3 depicts two typical runs. The antibodies and the C′ 5 were titrated in microtiter

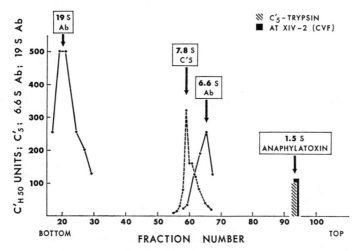

Fig. 3. Sucrose density gradient ultracentrifugation (10–40%) of a purified anaphylatoxin preparation (AT-XIV-2; CVF generated) and of trypsin treated purified C′ 5. The markers 6.6-S and 19-S Ra-anti sheep E antibodies and C′ 5 were titrated hemolytically in microtiter plates; the anaphylatoxin activity in the guinea pig skin. Total number of fractions: 111.

plates, the AT was tested in the g. p. skin using its capillary permeability increasing activity as indicator. All three materials, at different times and represented by different preparations had calculated S-values of 1.5–1.65.

Rabbit antiserum against purified AT (generated by CVF) was thoroughly dialysed to remove the serum histamine and was then tested for its inhibitory action in comparison with normal rabbit serum. The ileum contracting activity of the three purified anaphylatoxins was completely abolished if one part serum was mixed with nine parts AT and incubated for 30 min at 30°C. The normal rabbit serum had no such effect.

In view of their similar elution characteristics from Sephadex G-100, and their similar S-values, it appears that the C′ 5-anaphylatoxins generated by immune precipitate, CVF and trypsin are very closely related if not identical materials. In addition, the inactivation of the various AT preparations tested by one anti-AT serum strengthens this hypothesis.

B. Relation of g. p. C′ 5-AT to a major chemotactic factor generated in g. p. serum. A factor chemotactic for polymorphonuclear leukocytes (PMN's) can be generated in fresh guinea pig serum by the interaction of endotoxic lipopolysaccharide (LPS) and the complement system [7]. Figure 4 shows the

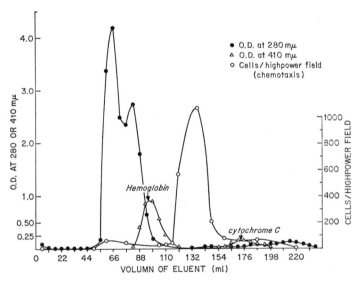

Fig. 4. G-100 Sephadex separation of fresh guinea pig serum-LPS reaction mixture. The peak of chemotactic factor activity lies between the previously calibrated hemoglobin and cytochrome c peaks (taken from SNYDERMAN *et al.*, J. exp. Med. *128:* 259, 1968).

elution profile that was obtained when 2.0 ml of guinea pig serum incubated with 45 μgm LPS for 45 min at 37°C was chromatographed on a G-100 Sephadex column (2.5 × 45 cm). From its position between hemoglobin and cytochrome c on gel filtration and on sucrose density gradient ultracentrifugation (fig. 5) the S-value of the major chemotactic factor activity was estimated at 1.5. A comparison of figure 1, 2, and 3, with figure 4 and 5 reveals a striking similarity: anaphylatoxin- and chemotactic reactivity appeared to belong to materials with identical elution characteristics and S-values.

When this similarity was recognized in April 1968, our two laboratories decided to exchange materials. The objective of this exchange was to

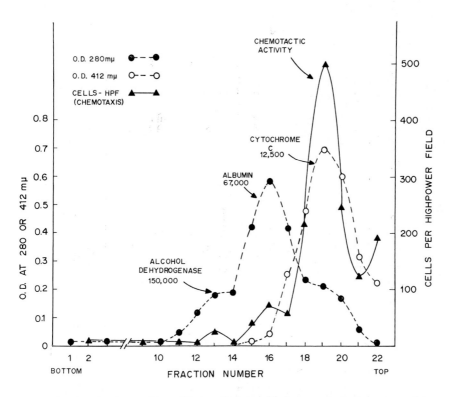

Fig. 5. Sucrose density gradient ultracentrifugation of chemotactic factor generated by LPS in guinea pig serum. The chemotactically active material was the peak of activity from a G-100 Sephadex column concentrated ten times. A 5% to 20% sucrose density gradient was used. The chemotactic factor and markers were centrifuged simultaneously at 35,000 rpm for 18 h in a SW 41 rotor.

Table II. Comparison of ileum contracting and chemotactic activities of various preparations

Active material	Generation[3]	Purification	Ileum contraction	Chemotaxis
Chemotactic factor	Endotoxin	$(NH_4)_2SO_4$, G-100	+[1]	+[1]
Purified C' 5 (both hemolytically active and inactive forms)	Trypsin		+[1]	+[1]
AT-X-R Pool 1	Immune Ppt.[2]	G-100 rechromatography	−	−
AT-X-R Pool 3	Immune Ppt.[2]	of active fractions	+	+
AT-X-R Pool 4	Immune Ppt.[2]	off G-100 column	−	−
AT-XII-1	Cobra venom factor	2X G-100	+[1]	+[1]
AT-XIV-2	Cobra venom factor	2X G-100	+	+
AT-VI-1 Effl. 1	Cobra venom factor	DEAE-cellulose (pH 7.5 μ 0.002)	+	+
AT-VI-1 Effl. 2	Cobra venom factor	DEAE-cellulose (pH 7.5 μ 0.002)	+	+
AT-VIII-P	Cobra venom factor	3X G-100	Initially + but activity lost on storage	−

[1] Activity inhibited by rabbit-anti-AT. (The other materials were not tested.)
[2] BSA-rabbit-anti-BSA (320 μg AB-N/ml guinea-pig serum).
[3] In guinea-pig serum.

investigate whether the two biological activities might be properties of one and the same fragment of C′ 5. Table II is a summary of the results of this exchange. It can be seen 1. that all AT preparations, purified and crude showed strong chemotactic activity; 2. that LPS-generated, chromatographed chemotactic factor showed typical ileum contraction; 3. that anti-AT neutralized the ileum and the chemotactic reactivity not only of the AT preparations but also of the chemotactic factor (fig. 6). It is furthermore noteworthy that AT-negative fractions eluting before and after the AT-peak were also negative regarding chemotactic activity. In consideration of these results one can hardly avoid to conclude that chemotactic activity is a property of g. p. C′ 5 anaphylatoxin. This view is strongly supported by Shin's recent findings concerning a C′ 5 fragment obtained by reacting highly purified C′ 5 at high concentration with EAC′ 1a, 4, 2a, 3. This fragment also had ileum contracting and chemotactic activity and an S-value of 1.5 [6]. Furthermore, using radioactively labelled complement components, it has been shown that the major chemotactic factor generated in whole guinea pig serum upon interaction with LPS is derived as a split product from C′ 5 [8]. If anaphylatoxin, as we believe, is endowed with the ability to attract polymorphonuclear leukocytes, its generation in immune reactions

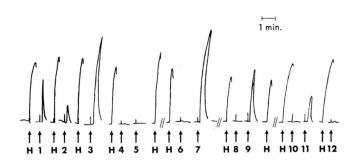

Fig. 6. Composite tracing of guinea pig ileum contractions. Organ bath: 8 ml; Tyrode solution, 37°C with aeration. Contractions recorded by electrically writing kymograph. //to// one ileum piece. H) 0.12 μg histamine (base). As AT-positive control (+ Co) material served CVF treated guinea pig serum, diluted 1:5 in saline. 1. Chemotactic factor 0.4 ml; 2. + Co, 0.2 ml; 3. chemotactic factor 1.0 ml; 4. + Co. 0.4 ml; 5. chemotactic factor 1.0 ml; 6. chemotactic factor + anti-AT 1.0 ml; 7. same + normal rabbit serum 1.0 ml; 8. + Co + anti-AT 0.5 ml; 9. same + normal rabbit serum; 10. C′ 5 + trypsin inhibitor + trypsin 0.5 ml; 11. C′ 5 + trypsin (10 min 30°C) + trypsin inhibitor; 12. + Co, 0.3 ml.

involving the complement system would allow a meaningful answer to our second question concerning the biological role of AT provided that such activity can be observed also *in vivo*.

C. In vivo chemotaxis studies. Chemotactically-active fractions from a G-100 column and other fractions from the same column containing more protein but little or no *in vitro* chemotactic activity were pooled individually. Each pool was concentrated to 1/5 its original volume and 0.2 ml of each was injected intradermally into New Zealand white rabbits. In addition, 5 μg LPS, 10 μg Kallidin, or buffered saline were injected intradermally in 0.2 ml volumes. In certain rabbits Pelikan dye was injected intravenously to localize areas of increased vascular permeability. Biopsies for histological examination were taken at 4 and 24 h. All injection sites, except those receiving buffered saline showed increased vascular permeability. Histological examination revealed little or no inflammatory exudate at 4 cr 24 h after injection of chemotactically-negative pools (fig. 7), kallidin (fig. 8), or saline. Tissue sections from sites receiving LPS showed a small number of PMN's at 4 h with a greater number of lymphocytes and macrophages (fig. 9) appearing at 24 h. However, skin sites receiving the chemotactically-active pool showed a marked accumulation of PMN's at 4 h with the exudate predominately consisting of PMN's (fig. 10) persisting at 24 h. It appears therefore that the chemotactic factor generated in guinea pig serum by LPS in addition to its *in vitro* activity, leads to an early and marked accumulation of PMN's after intradermal injection in rabbits.

In addition, in preliminary experiments, purified guinea pig C' 5, treated with trypsin as previously described, was injected intradermally into rabbits. C' 5 alone as well as trypsin and soybean trypsin inhibitor were used as controls. The trypsin treated C' 5 material lead to the accumulation of PMN's *in vivo* at both 4 and 24 h whereas the controls did not.

Fig. 7. Section of rabbit skin into which 0.2 ml of pooled chemotactically inactive fractions from G-100 Sephadex chromatography was injected 24 h previously. Hematoxylin and eosin X 400.

Fig. 8. Section of rabbit skin into which 0.2 ml of kallidin (10 μg) (kindly supplied by Sandoz Pharmaceuticals) was injected 24 h previously. Hematoxylin and eosin X 400.

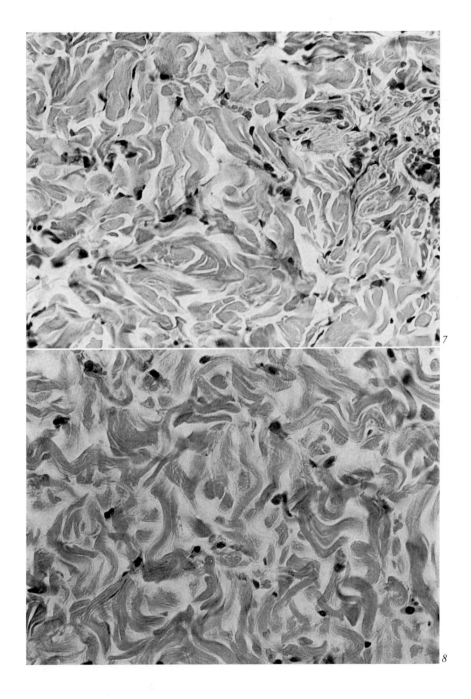

7

8

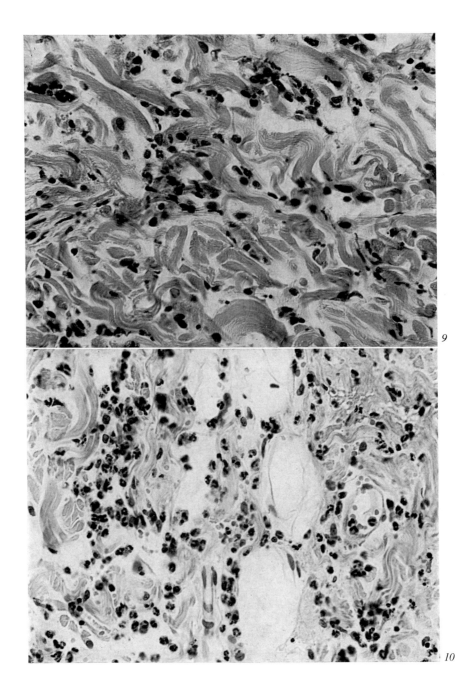

9

10

Conclusion

The presented evidence suggests that an important biological activity, namely, that of *in vitro* and *in vivo* chemotaxis be recognized as a property of guinea pig C' 5-anaphylatoxin. Together with its ability to strongly increase vascular permeability this property gives a new meaning to the complement dependent generation of AT, that presumably takes place wherever complement fixing antibody, antigen and complement interact. In contrast to its ileum contracting activity the chemotactic property of AT can be relatively easily quantitated; this will be of importance in regard to the many unanswered questions concerning the generation of AT. We have observed for instance (a) that hemolytically inactive C' 5 (heated or repeatedly frozen) would still give rise to AT upon trypsin treatment but not in the hemolytic sequence [3]; (b) that the trypsin treatment can be so mild that AT is produced with apparently no or very little loss of C' 5 hemolytic reactivity and (c) that during AT generation with CVF or immune complexes the C' 5 hemolytic reactivity was little affected [4]. Further studies of these and other problems require quantitation of AT and independence from the cumbersome and often frustrating ileum contraction assay.

Acknowledgements

Dr. JEAN MAILLARD, formerly Visiting Investigator, Howard Hughes Medical Institute, participated in the purification of various anaphylatoxin preparations and did most of the vascular permeability studies. The technical assistance of Miss ELENA IGLESIAS, Mr. BERNARD ALLER, Mrs. JEAN K. PHILLIPS and Mr. JOHN B. KENNEDY is gratefully acknowledged. We would also like to acknowledge Miss CHERYL BURG for the preparation of the histological sections.

Fig. 9. Section of rabbit skin into which 5 μg endotoxin was injected 24 h previously. Note predominance of lymphocytes and monocytes with a smaller number of PMN's. Hemotoxylin and eosin X 400.

Fig. 10. Section of rabbit skin into which 0.2 ml of pooled chemotactically active fraction from G-100 Sephadex chromatography was injected 24 h previously. Note predominance of PMN's. Hematoxylin and eosin × 400.

References

1. COCHRANE, C. G. and MÜLLER-EBERHARD, H. J.: The derivation of two distinct anaphylatoxin activities from the third and fifth component of human complement. J. exp. Med. *127:* 371 (1968).
2. DIAS DA SILVA, W.; EISELE, J. W. and LEPOW, I. H.: Complement as a mediator of inflammation. III. Purification of the activity with anaphylatoxin properties generated by interaction of the first four components of complement and its identification as a cleavage product of C' 3. J. exp. Med. *126:* 1027 (1967).
3. JENSEN, J.: Anaphylatoxin in its relation to the complement system. Science *155:* 1222 (1967).
4. JENSEN, J.: Unpublished data.
5. LEPOW, I. H.; DIAS DA SILVA, W. and EISELE, J. W.: Nature and biological properties of human anaphylatoxin. International Symposium on the Biochemistry of the Acute Allergic Reactions. Punta Ala, Italy, June 5–7, 1967 (in press) (Blackwell 1968).
6. SHIN, H. S.; SNYDERMAN, R.; FRIEDMAN, E.; MELLORS, A. and MAYER, M. M.: A chemotactic and anaphylatoxic fragment cleaved from guinea pig C' 5 by EAC' 1 a, 4, 2a, 3. Science *162:* 361 (1968).
7. SNYDERMAN, R.; GEWURZ, H. and MERGENHAGEN, S. E.: Interactions of the complement system with endotoxic lipopolysaccharide: Generation of a factor chemotactic for polymorphonuclear leukocytes. J. exp. Med. *128:* 259 (1968).
8. SNYDERMAN, R.; SHIN, H. S.; GEWURZ, H. and MERGENHAGEN, S. E.: Chemotactic factor derived from the fifth component of complement upon interaction of endotoxin with guinea-pig serum. Federation Proc. *28:* 361 (1969).

Authors' addresses: J. A. JENSEN, M. D., Dept. of Microbiology, University of Miami, School of Medicine, and Variety Children Research Foundation, *Miami, Fla.* (USA): S. E. MERGENHAGEN, M. D., and SNYDERMAN, R., M. D., Immunology Section, National Institute of Dental Research, National Institutes of Health, *Bethesda, Md.* (USA).

Cellular and Humoral Mechanisms in Anaphylaxis and Allergy, pp. 279–288
(Karger, Basel/New York 1969)

The Heterogeneity of Chemotactic Factors for Neutrophils Generated from the Complement System[1]

Peter A. Ward

Immunology Branch, Armed Forces Institute of Pathology
Washington, D. C.

Introduction

Chemotaxis of polymorphonuclear leukocytes (neutrophils) due to factors generated from the complement system seems to be a well established fact [16, 17, 14, 15, 12]. That several chemotactic factors can be generated from the complement system is not altogether surprising in view of the multiplicity of bioactive products produced from interaction of the 9 complement components [10]. In addition, it is becoming increasingly clear that all factors chemotactic for neutrophils are not necessarily complement-associated. Many species of bacteria elaborate into the culture medium in the absence of serum a chemotactic factor of low molecular weight [6, 18]. There is some suggestion that chemotactic factors can be generated in fresh serum without the participation of complement, as determined by conventional complement fixation assays [5]. The purpose of this paper is to emphasize the heterogeneity of chemotactic factors for neutrophils that can be generated from the complement system.

Materials and Methods

Chemotactic assay. This has been performed using rabbit neutrophils obtained from a glycogen-induced peritoneal exudate, and employing modified Boyden chambers [1] with micropore filters of 650 mμ. All techniques have been described in detail elsewhere [16, 17].

Complement preparations. Highly purified human third component of complement (C3) and fifth component (C5) were obtained according to the method of Nilsson and Müller-

[1] This work was supported by the National Institutes of Health, Bethesda, Md., Grant AI-07291-AIA.

EBERHARD [11]. In general, this consists of isoelectric precipitation of the euglobulin, ion exchange chromatography, followed by elution from hydroxyl-apatite. $C(5,6,7)_a$, the complement associated chemotactic factor of high molecular weight, was prepared according to procedures listed in earlier reports [16].

Enzymes. Crystalized trypsin (Mann Research Laboratories, New York, N.Y.) was dissolved in phosphate buffered saline (pH 7.3) before use. Conditions of the enzyme reactions are described in the appropriate experiments. The trypsin reaction was terminated by the addition of soybean trypsin inhibitor (Worthington Co., Freehold, N.J.) in an amount double that of trypsin.

Antibody to C6. Antibody to C6 (kindly donated by Dr. PETER LACHMANN, University of Cambridge) was obtained from appropriately immunized rabbits[2] genetically deficient in C6. The antibody was present in a lyophilized IgG preparation and was dissolved in phosphate buffered saline. Reconstitution in saline was made to the equivalent concentration of IgG in the original serum. The anti C6 reacted readily with human and rabbit C6 to block the hemolytic activity in serum and to give precipitin bands in Ouchterlony analysis. Increasing amounts of anti C6 were added to 0.1 ml activated rabbit serum. In order to activate rabbit serum and render it chemotactically active, an immune precipitate made with 100 μgN rabbit antibody (as IgG) to bovine serum albumin (BSA), with BSA added at equivalence, was added to each 0.1 ml serum, followed by incubation at 37°C for 1 h. The precipitate was then removed by centrifugation.

Sucrose density gradient ultracentrifugation. As previously described chemotactically active preparations were ultracentrifuged in tubes containing linear density gradients of 7.3–35% or 10–40% sucrose in phosphate buffer, pH 7.3 $\frac{T}{2} = 0.05$ [16]. Protein assays on the gradient fractions were carried out according to the Folin procedure, while C6 assays were based upon restoration of hemolytic activity in C6 deficient serum [11].

Results

Density gradient analysis of rabbit $C(5,6,7)_a$. Figure 1 shows the typical distribution of chemotactic activity in a density gradient to which was added a preparation of rabbit chemotactic factor. The area of chemotactic activity corresponds roughly with the lower half of the zone occupied by C6 (more rapidly sedimenting fractions 7 and 8). It is known that the distribution of C6 is ascribable to C6 existing in a free or noncomplexed form as well as in the form of a complex with C5 and C7 [11]. The finding of chemotactic factor in the lower zone of the C6 profile in figure 1 is in accord with the localization of the trimolecular complex, $C(5,6,7)_a$. In this particular preparation of chemotactic factor the activity is confined to a single zone in the

---

[2] The Principles of Laboratory Animal Care as promulgated by the National Society for Medical Research were observed in these studies.

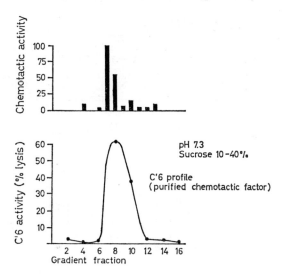

Fig. 1. Analysis by density gradient ultracentrifugation of rabbit preparation of C(5,6,7)ₐ. Activity is confined to a single, relatively fast sedimenting zone.

gradient. In other studies it has been estimated that this chemotactic factor has an approximate sedimentation rate of 12 S (personal observations).

Multiple zones of chemotactic activity by density gradient analysis. In approximately half the analyses by sucrose density gradient ultracentrifugation of rabbit or human preparations rich in C(5,6,7)ₐ, there has appeared a second zone of chemotactic activity. A typical example of this is seen in figure 2 where a preparation of human complement components has been analyzed. The starting material, rich in C5, C6 and C7, was activated by interaction with sensitized erythrocyte stromata containing the first 4 reacting components of complement. The position of C(5,6,7)ₐ is represented by fractions 6–8 that contain C6 and are rich in chemotactic activity. In addition, a second zone of activity is present in the upper portions of the gradient where slowly sedimenting material is found (fig. 2, fractions 12–16). This chemotactic activity falls in the same area as the protein marker cytochrome c, suggesting a material with a molecular weight $< 15,000$. The biphasic distribution of chemotactic activity in this gradient clearly indicates the presence of more than one chemotactic factor in the complement preparation.

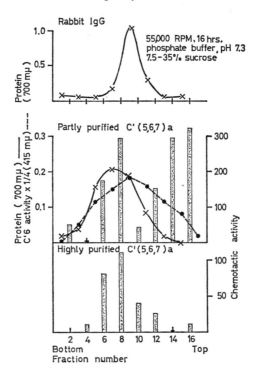

Fig. 2. Density gradient analysis of two preparations of human complement for chemo tactic activity. In upper frame relatively large amounts of C5, C6 and C7 were used, resulting in a biphasic distribution of chemotactic activity. Only a single zone of activity resulted when limited amounts of complement components were used (lower frame).

For the purposes of comparison, highly purified human $C(5,6,7)_a$, kindly supplied by Dr. HANS J. MÜLLER-EBERHARD (La Jolla, Calif.), was also analyzed in a sucrose density gradient. This preparation contained *only* one zone of chemotactic activity which sedimented relatively rapidly in the position characteristic for $C(5,6,7)_a$ (fig. 2, fractions 6–8). It should be noted that this material was generated by the addition of highly purified human C5, C6 and C7 in limiting amounts to sensitized erythrocytes containing the first four components of human complement. Under such conditions of limiting amounts of C5, C6, and C7, the generation of the more slowly sedimenting chemotactic factor does not appear to be favored [17].

Heterogeneity of chemotactic activity in activated rabbit serum. Serum was rendered chemotactically active by incubation with an immune precipitate (see above). In order to determine if the chemotactic activity was completely related in some manner to the presence of C6, antibody to C6 was added in increasing amounts. In one serum (fig. 3, A), complete suppression of chemotactic activity was obtained when 80 μl anti C6 was added to 0.1 ml of serum. The depressing effect on chemotactic activity was directly related to the amount of anti C6 added. On the other hand, a second serum activated similarly showed at best only a 40% reduction in chemotactic activity after addition of anti C6 (fig. 3, B). These data suggest that in some sera all chemotactic activity is related in some way or another to C6 [e.g., as C(5,6,7$_a$)] whereas in other sera only part of the activity is related to C6. The differences in the susceptibility of chemotactic activity in serum to the blocking activity by anti C6 again suggests a heterogeneity of chemotactic factors.

Chemotactic activity in trypsin-treated C5. Elsewhere it is reported that a fragmentation product of C5 is chemotactically active [15]. In table I a typical experiment confirming that finding is presented. Purified human C3

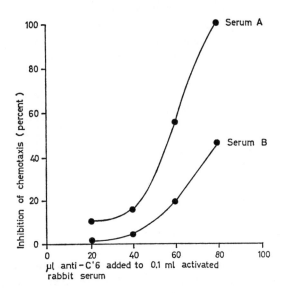

Fig. 3. Differences in ability of antibody to C6 to inhibit chemotactic activity in two activated rabbit sera.

Table I. Relative ability to generate chemotactic activity from human C3 and C5 with trypsin

Material tested	Chemotactic activity[2]
75 µg C3 + 10 µg trypsin[1]	10
150 µg C3 + 10 µg trypsin	20
75 µg C5 + 10 µg trypsin	135
150 µg C5 + 10 µg trypsin	195
150 µg C5 + 20 µg trypsin inhibitor + 10 µg trypsin	25
Blank (medium 199)	

[1] Five minutes at 32°C, then 20 µg soybean trypsin inhibitor was added.

[2] Number of migrated neutrophils in 5 microscopic fields, according to WARD *et al.* [16].

and C5 were each treated with trypsin for 5 min at 32°C, the reaction stopped by the addition of trypsin inhibitor and the solution assayed for chemotactic activity. Considerable activity was found in the trypsin-treated C5 preparation, and the degree of activity was a reflection of the amount of C5 treated with trypsin. On the other hand, C3 proved to be a poor substrate in this regard. This is in line with a prior report where C3 was a considerably less effective substrate than C5 [15]. In the present experiment significant alteration in the immuno-electrophoretic pattern of C5 was not observed after treatment with trypsin, in spite of the fact that substantial chemotactic activity was generated. Gel filtration studies have revealed that the chemotactic factor in trypsin-treated C5 is a fragmentation product with an approximate molecular weight of 8,500 [15].

Discussion

Although it recently seemed that the bioactive products of the complement system could be neatly characterized in terms of one product-one activity, this has not proven to be the case. In the case of anaphylatoxin which has the properties of causing smooth muscle contraction, histamine release from mast cells and increased vascular permeability, it was found that a cleavage product of C3 possessed these activities [3]. Subsequent experiments showed that a cleavage product of C5 also had identical properties [4, 2, 8]. It is now clear that the term 'anaphylatoxin' can refer to bioactive cleavage products of either C3 or C5. To complicate matters, three different substances can cause cleavage of the anaphylatoxin fragment from C3: (a) trypsin [2, 8]; (b) cobra venom factor acting in association with a β-globulin cofactor in serum [9]; and (c) interaction of C3 with intermediate complement complexes consisting of the first three complement components [3]. While each method is productive of material with anaphylatoxin activity, it is not clear if the fragmentation products are, in fact, identical.

Just as the multiorigin of anaphylatoxin has complicated the story, it is now clear that chemotactic activity does not derive from a single complement source. Table II summarizes our current knowledge of complement-associated chemotactic factors. The first described factor, $C(5,6,7)_a$, is the only product with a relatively high molecular weight and, so far as is known, can only be generated by interaction of C5, C6, and C7 with the earlier reacting components of the complement sequence [16, 17]. This factor, like the rest of the chemotactic factors to be described, does not become affixed to the surface of the cell (or surface of an immune precipitate) where it is generated but appears in the fluid phase, even though generation may have occurred at a site on the cell surface. There is no available information concerning the chemical events leading up to the activation of the C(5,6,7) complex, except that more than one component has to be altered for the acquisition of chemotactic activity in the complex [16].

C3 appears to be a suitable substrate for the generation of a chemotactic factor by plasmin, with the resulting cleavage of an acidic fragment of C3 of approximate molecular weight 6,000 [13, 14]. In our hands trypsin has not proven to be an especially effective agent for the cleavage from C3 of a product with chemotactic activity (table I). In studies with DIAS DA SILVA

Table II. Summary of complement-associated chemotactic factors

Complement component	Method of generation of chemotactic activity	Approximate molecular weight
$C(5,6,7)_a$	interaction of C1–C7	> 200,000
C3	trypsin[1]	?
C3	plasmin	6,000
C5	trypsin	8,500
C5	C1–C4	not known

[1] Only limited activity is generated.

and LEPOW, we have not found chemotactic activity in C3 preparations treated with purified C1, C4, and C2 to produce an anaphylatoxin product. Furthermore, human anaphylatoxin from human C3 purified by gel filtration was very active in contracting smooth muscle but was totally devoid of chemotactic activity. These reports are in contrast to those of COCHRANE and MÜLLER-EBERHARD (personal communication) who find chemotactic activity in C3 preparations that are rich in anaphylatoxin activity. It is evident that highly purified cleavage products of complement components will have to be isolated and well characterized biochemically and biologically before definitive conclusions can be drawn about the nature of the various fragments.

C5 also acts as a suitable substrate for the production of a chemotactic factor. The only direct evidence for this conclusion involves the action of trypsin on C5 (table I and reference 15), where a cleavage product of C5 has been characterized. Under the proper conditions, the interaction of C5 with earlier-acting complement components also results in a chemotactic factor of low molecular weight. The only evidence favoring the hypothesis that the chemotactic factor produced by interaction of the first five complement components is also a cleavage product of C5 is the relationship of chemotactic activity to the amount of C5 added, and the analogy with the anaphylatoxin story where a bioactive fragmentation product of C5 can be produced either by the action of trypsin or by interaction with earlier-reacting complement components. It seems possible that the slowly sedimenting chemotactic factor in figure 2 is a fragmentation product of C5, but no direct evidence for this conclusion exists.

There have been recent reports of discrepancies between our earlier findings and those of KELLER and SORKIN [7]. Specifically, it is reported that chemotactic activity can be generated in rabbit serum genetically deficient in C6. Moreover, the ineffectiveness of N-CBZ-a-glutamyl-L-tyrosine to alter chemotactic activity in serum is reported, in contrast to our report where this amino acid derivative abolished chemotactic activity in serum, coincident with dissociation of C(5,6,7)$_a$ [17]. It is not known if, in fact, the chemotactic factor(s) reported by KELLER and SORKIN [5] has any relationship to the complement system, their earlier interpretations being to the contrary. With the multiplicity of chemotactic factors generated from the complement system, and the possibility that other chemotactic factors in serum can be generated without the participation of the complement system, it seems likely that discrepancies between various laboratories will eventually be resolved as the factors are purified and characterized. If this turns out to be the case, it will be very much like the recent history of the anaphylatoxin story where light led to confusion which led to light.

Summary

Heterogeneity of complement-associated factors chemotactic for neutrophils has been demonstrated. Analysis of chemotactically active complement preparations by density gradient ultracentrifugation reveals the presence of the activated trimolecular complex, $C(5,6,7)_a$, alone or, in approximately half the cases, in association with a chemotactic factor that sediments slowly. This latter factor may be a fragmentation product of C5. When antibody to C6 is added to rabbit serum that is chemotactically active, complete suppression of chemotactic activity is attained in some sera but only about 40% suppression in others. This suggests that in some sera chemotactic activity is wholly dependent on C6, whereas in others only part of the activity is related to the presence of C6.

When human C5 is treated with trypsin, chemotactic activity is generated. This factor appears to be a cleavage product of C5 with an estimated molecular weight of 8,500. Similar treatment of C3 results in considerably less chemotactic activity. In contrast to previous studies, interaction of the first four complement components with C5 results in the appearance of a chemotactic factor of relatively low molecular weight. The generation of this C5 dependent factor occurs only if sufficient amounts of C5 are used.

It is now evident that at least three chemotactic factors can be generated from the complement system: $C(5,6,7)_a$, plasmin-split fragment of C3, and a trypsin-split fragment of C5. In addition, there is evidence that C5 may be cleaved into a chemotactically active fragment upon interaction with the first four complement components. These data indicate that several different chemotactic factors can be generated from the complement system. Conditions that favor a particular product are not clearly defined.

References

1. BOYDEN, S.: The chemotactic effect of mixtures of antibody and antigen on polymorphonuclear leukocytes. J. exp. Med. *115:* 453 (1962).
2. COCHRANE, C. G. and MÜLLER-EBERHARD, H. J.: The derivation of two distinct anaphylatoxin activities from the third and fifth components of human complement. J. exp. Med. *127:* 371 (1968).
3. DIAS DA SILVA, W. and LEPOW, I. H.: Complement as a mediator of inflammation. II. Biological properties of anaphylatoxin prepared with purified components of human complement. J. exp. Med. *125:* 921 (1967).
4. JENSEN, J.: Anaphylatoxin and its relation to the complement system. Science *155:* 1122 (1967).
5. KELLER, H. U. and SORKIN, E.: Studies on chemotaxis. I. On the chemotactic and complement fixing activity of γ-globulins. Immunology *9:* 241 (1965).
6. KELLER, H. U. and SORKIN, E.: Studies on chemotaxis. V. On the chemotactic effect of bacteria. Int. Arch. Allergy *31:* 505–517 (1967).
7. KELLER, H. U. and SORKIN, E.: Chemotaxis of leukocytes. Experienta *24:* 641 (1968).
8. LEPOW, I. H.; DIAS DA SILVA, W. and EISELE, J. W.: Nature and biological properties of human anaphylatoxin; in 'Biochemistry of the Acute Allergic Reaction', K. F. AUSTEN and E. L. BECKER, eds., p. 265 (Blackwell Scientific Publications, Oxford 1968).

9. MÜLLER-Eberhard, H. J.: Mechanism of inactivation of the third component of human complement (C'3) by cobra venom. Fed. Proc. *26:* 744 (1967).
10. MÜLLER-EBERHARD, H. J.: Chemistry and reaction mechanisms of complement; in Advances in Immunology, Vol. 8, F. J. DIXON and H. G. KUNKEL, eds., p. 1 (Academic Press, N.Y. 1968).
11. NILSSON, U. R. and MÜLLER-EBERHARD, H. J.: Isolation of β1F-globulin from human serum and its characterization as the fifth component of complement. J. exp. Med. *122:* 277 (1965).
12. SNYDERMAN, R.; GEWURZ, H. and MERGENHAGEN, S. E.: Interactions of the complement system with endotoxic lipopolysaccharide. Generation of a factor chemotactic for polymorphonuclear leukocytes. J. exp. Med. *128:* 259 (1968).
13. TAYLOR, F. B., Jr., and WARD, P. A.: Generation of chemotactic activity in rabbit serum by plasminogen-streptokinase mixtures. J. exp. Med. *126:* 149 (1967).
14. WARD, P. A.: A plasmin-split fragment of C'3 as a new chemotactic factor. J. exp. Med. *126:* 189 (1967).
15. WARD, P. A.: Complement factors involved in chemotaxis of human eosinophils and a new chemotactic factor for neutrophils from C'5. J. Immunol. *101:* 818 (1968). (Abstract.).
16. WARD, P. A.; COCHRANE, C. G. and MÜLLER-EBERHARD, H. J.: The role of serum complement in chemotaxis of PMN's. J. exp. Med. *122:* 327 (1965).
17. WARD, P. A.; COCHRANE, C. G. and MÜLLER-EBERHARD, H. J.: Further studies in the chemotactic factor of complement and its formation *in vivo*. Immunology *11:* 141 (1966).
18. WARD, P. A.; LEPOW, I. H. and NEWMAN, L. J.: Bacterial factors chemotactic for polymorphonuclear leukocytes. Amer. J. Path. *52:* 725 (1968).

Author's address: PETER A. WARD, M. D., Immunology Branch, Armed Forces Institute of Pathology, *Washington, D.C.* (USA).